Breast MRI

Guest Editors

LINDA MOY, MD
CECILIA L. MERCADO, MD

MAGNETIC RESONANCE IMAGING CLINICS OF NORTH AMERICA

www.mri.theclinics.com

Consulting Editors
VIVIAN S. LEE, MD, PhD, MBA
LYNNE STEINBACH, MD
SURESH MUKHERJI, MD

May 2010 • Volume 18 • Number 2

SAUNDERS an imprint of ELSEVIER, Inc.

W.B. SAUNDERS COMPANY
A Division of Elsevier Inc.

1600 John F. Kennedy Boulevard • Suite 1800 • Philadelphia, Pennsylvania 19103-2899

http://www.theclinics.com

MRI CLINICS OF NORTH AMERICA Volume 18, Number 2
May 2010 ISSN 1064-9689, ISBN 13: 978-1-4377-1833-1

Editor: Joanne Husovski

Magnetic Resonance Imaging Clinics of North America (ISSN 1064-9689) is published quarterly by Elsevier Inc., 360 Park Avenue South, New York, NY 10010-1710. Months of issue are February, May, August, and November. Application to mail at periodicals postage rates is pending at New York, NY and at additional mailing offices. Subscription prices are $309.00 per year (domestic individuals), $455.00 per year (domestic institutions), $150.00 per year (domestic students/residents), $345.00 per year (Canadian individuals), $571.00 per year (Canadian institutions), $448.00 per year (international individuals), $571.00 per year (international institutions), and $217.00 per year (international and Canadian students/residents). International air speed delivery is included in all *Clinics* subscription prices. All prices are subject to change without notice. **POSTMASTER:** Send address changes to *Magnetic Resonance Imaging Clinics*, Elsevier Health Sciences Division, Subscription Customer Service, 3251 Riverport Lane, Maryland Heights, MO 63043. Customer Service (orders, claims, online, change of address): Elsevier Health Sciences Division, Subscription Customer Service, 3251 Riverport Lane, Maryland Heights, MO 63043. Tel:1-800-654-2452 (U.S. and Canada); 314-447-8871 (outside U.S. and Canada). Fax: 314-447-8029. E-mail: journalscustomerservice-usa@elsevier.com (for print support); journalsonlinesupport-usa@elsevier.com (for online support).

Reprints. For copies of 100 or more of articles in this publication, please contact the Commercial Reprints Department, Elsevier Inc., 360 Park Avenue South, New York, NY 10010-1710. Tel.: 212-633-3812; Fax: 212-462-1935; E-mail: reprints@elsevier.com.

Magnetic Resonance Imaging Clinics of North America is covered in the *RSNA Index of Imaging Literature, MEDLINE/PubMed (Index Medicus),* and *EMBASE/Excerpta Medica.*

Printed and bound by CPI Group (UK) Ltd, Croydon, CR0 4YY

Transferred to Digital Print 2011

GOAL STATEMENT

The goal of *Magnetic Resonance Imaging Clinics of North America* is to keep practicing physicians up to date with current clinical practice by providing timely articles reviewing the state of the art in patient care.

ACCREDITATION

The *Magnetic Resonance Imaging Clinics of North America* is planned and implemented in accordance with the Essential Areas and Policies of the Accreditation Council for Continuing Medical Education (ACCME) through the joint sponsorship of the University of Virginia School of Medicine and Elsevier. The University of Virginia School of Medicine is accredited by the ACCME to provide continuing medical education for physicians.

The University of Virginia School of Medicine designates this educational activity for a maximum of 15 *AMA PRA Category 1 Credits*™ for each issue, 60 credits per year. Physicians should only claim credit commensurate with the extent of their participation in the activity.

The American Medical Association has determined that physicians not licensed in the US who participate in this CME activity are eligible for a maximum of 15 *AMA PRA Category 1 Credits*™ for each issue, 60 credits per year.

Credit can be earned by reading the text material, taking the CME examination online at http://www.theclinics.com/home/cme, and completing the evaluation. After taking the test, you will be required to review any and all incorrect answers. Following completion of the test and evaluation, your credit will be awarded and you may print your certificate.

FACULTY DISCLOSURE/CONFLICT OF INTEREST

The University of Virginia School of Medicine, as an ACCME accredited provider, endorses and strives to comply with the Accreditation Council for Continuing Medical Education (ACCME) Standards of Commercial Support, Commonwealth of Virginia statutes, University of Virginia policies and procedures, and associated federal and private regulations and guidelines on the need for disclosure and monitoring of proprietary and financial interests that may affect the scientific integrity and balance of content delivered in continuing medical education activities under our auspices.

The University of Virginia School of Medicine requires that all CME activities accredited through this institution be developed independently and be scientifically rigorous, balanced and objective in the presentation/discussion of its content, theories and practices.

All authors/editors participating in an accredited CME activity are expected to disclose to the readers relevant financial relationships with commercial entities occurring within the past 12 months (such as grants or research support, employee, consultant, stock holder, member of speakers bureau, etc.). The University of Virginia School of Medicine will employ appropriate mechanisms to resolve potential conflicts of interest to maintain the standards of fair and balanced education to the reader. Questions about specific strategies can be directed to the Office of Continuing Medical Education, University of Virginia School of Medicine, Charlottesville, Virginia.

The faculty and staff of the University of Virginia Office of Continuing Medical Education have no financial affiliations to disclose.

The authors/editors listed below have identified no professional or financial affiliations for themselves or their spouse/partner:

Sara Bloom, MD; C. Boetes, MD, PhD; Manjil Chatterji, MD; Eduard de Lange, MD (Test Author); Wendy B. DeMartini, MD; Sara C. Gavenonis, MD; Robert L. Gutierrez, MD; Joanne Husovski (Acquisitions Editor); Nola Hylton, PhD; Vivian S. Lee, MD, PhD, MBA (Consulting Editor); H. Carisa Le-Petross, MD, FRCPC; Jessica W.T. Leung, MD; Ritse M. Mann, MD; Cecilia L. Mercado, MD (Guest Editor); Monica Morrow, MD; Linda Moy, MD (Guest Editor); Liane E. Philpotts, MD; Sughra Raza, MD; Susan Orel Roth, MD; Lynne Steinbach, MD (Consulting Editor); Eren D. Yeh, MD

The authors/editors listed below identified the following professional or financial affiliations for themselves or their spouse/partner:

Peter R. Eby, MD is an industry funded research/investigator for GE Healthcare, Ethicon Endo-Surgery, Inc., and Philips Medical.
Constance D. Lehman, MD, PhD is on the Speakers' Bureau and the Advisory Committee/Board for General Electric.
Mary C. Mahoney, MD is on the Speakers' Bureau for Ethicon Endo-Surgery and SenoRx, and is on the Advisory Committee/Board of Hologic.
Virginia Molleran, MD is on the Speakers Bureau for SenoRx.
Suresh Mukherji, MD (Consulting Editor) is a consultant for Philips.
Gillian M. Newstead, MD is an industry funded research/investigator for Philips Health Care, serves on the Advisory Board for Naviscan, and his spouse is a minor stockholder in Hologic.

Disclosure of Discussion of non-FDA approved uses for pharmaceutical products and/or medical devices:
The University of Virginia School of Medicine, as an ACCME provider, requires that all faculty presenters identify and disclose any "off label" uses for pharmaceutical and medical device products. The University of Virginia School of Medicine recommends that each physician fully review all the available data on new products or procedures prior to instituting them with patients.

TO ENROLL

To enroll in the Magnetic Resonance Imaging Clinics of North America Continuing Medical Education program, call customer service at 1-800-654-2452 or visit us online at www.theclinics.com/home/cme. The CME program is available to subscribers for an additional fee of $99.95.

Contributors

GUEST EDITORS

LINDA MOY, MD
Assistant Professor, Department of Radiology,
New York University School of Medicine,
New York, New York

CECILIA L. MERCADO, MD
Assistant Professor of Radiology, Department
of Radiology, New York University Langone
Medical Center, New York, New York

AUTHORS

SARA BLOOM, MD
Surgical Fellow, Breast Service, Department
of Surgery, Memorial Sloan-Kettering Cancer
Center, Evelyn H. Lauder Breast Center,
New York, New York

C. BOETES, MD, PhD
Professor, Department of Radiology,
Maastricht University Medical Center,
Maastricht, The Netherlands

MANJIL CHATTERJI, MD
Clinical Instructor in Radiology,
Department of Radiology, New York
University Langone Medical Center,
New York, New York

WENDY B. DEMARTINI, MD
Assistant Professor of Radiology,
Department of Radiology, University of
Washington School of Medicine; Seattle
Cancer Care Alliance, Seattle, Washington

PETER R. EBY, MD
Assistant Professor of Radiology, Department
of Radiology, University of Washington
School of Medicine; Seattle Cancer Care
Alliance, Seattle, Washington

SARA C. GAVENONIS, MD
Assistant Professor of Radiology, University of
Pennsylvania School of Medicine; Department
of Radiology, Hospital of the University of
Pennsylvania, Philadelphia, Pennsylvania

ROBERT L. GUTIERREZ, MD
Assistant Professor of Radiology, Department
of Radiology, University of Washington School
of Medicine; Seattle Cancer Care Alliance,
Seattle, Washington

NOLA HYLTON, PhD
Professor of Radiology; Director of Breast MRI
Research Program; and Professor of Imaging
Physics, Department of Radiology and
Biomedical Imaging, University of California
San Francisco, San Francisco, California

CONSTANCE D. LEHMAN, MD, PhD
Professor and Vice Chair of Radiology, Director
of Breast Imaging, Department of Radiology,
University of Washington School of Medicine;
Seattle Cancer Care Alliance, Seattle,
Washington

H. CARISA LE-PETROSS, MD, FRCPC
Associate Professor of Radiology, The
University of Texas M.D. Anderson Cancer
Center, Houston, Texas

JESSICA W.T. LEUNG, MD
Medical Director, Breast Health Center,
California Pacific Medical Center, San
Francisco, California

MARY C. MAHONEY, MD
Professor of Radiology, Director of Breast
Imaging, Department of Radiology, Division of
Breast Imaging, University of Cincinnati
Medical Center, Cincinnati, Ohio

RITSE M. MANN, MD
Department of Radiology, Radboud University
Nijmegen Medical Centre, Nijmegen,
The Netherlands

CECILIA L. MERCADO, MD
Assistant Professor of Radiology, Department
of Radiology, New York University Langone
Medical Center, New York,
New York

VIRGINIA MOLLERAN, MD
Assistant Professor of Radiology, Department
of Radiology, Division of Breast Imaging,
University of Cincinnati Medical Center,
Cincinnati, Ohio

MONICA MORROW, MD
Chief Breast Service, Department of Surgery,
Anne Burnett Windfohr Chair of Clinical
Oncology, Memorial Sloan-Kettering
Cancer Center, Evelyn H. Lauder Breast
Center; Professor of Surgery, Weill Medical
College of Cornell University, New York,
New York

LINDA MOY, MD
Assistant Professor of Radiology, Department
of Radiology, New York University Langone
Medical Center, New York,
New York

GILLIAN M. NEWSTEAD, MD
Professor of Radiology, Section Chief Breast
Imaging, Department of Radiology, University
of Chicago, Chicago, Illinois

LIANE E. PHILPOTTS, MD
Chief of Breast Imaging, Co-Director Yale
Breast Center, Associate Professor,
Department of Diagnostic Radiology, Yale
University School of Medicine, New Haven,
Connecticut

SUGHRA RAZA, MD
Associate Director Breast Imaging; Director
Clinical Breast MRI; Director Women's
Imaging Program, Department of Radiology,
Brigham & Women's Hospital; Assistant
Professor, Harvard Medical School, Boston,
Massachusetts

SUSAN OREL ROTH, MD
Professor of Radiology, University of
Pennsylvania School of Medicine; Department
of Radiology, Hospital of the University of
Pennsylvania, Philadelphia, Pennsylvania

EREN D. YEH, MD
Assistant Professor of Radiology, Division
of Breast Imaging, Department of Radiology,
Brigham and Women's Hospital, Dana-Farber
Cancer Institute, Harvard Medical School,
Boston, Massachusetts

CONSULTING EDITORS

VIVIAN S. LEE, MD, PhD, MBA
Professor of Radiology, Physiology, and
Neurosciences; Vice-Dean for Science; and
Senior Vice-President and Chief Scientific
Officer at New York University Langone
Medical Center, New York, New York

LYNNE STEINBACH, MD
Professor of Clinical Radiology and
Orthopaedic Surgery at the University of
California San Francisco, San Francisco,
California

SURESH MUKHERJI, MD
Professor and Chief of Neuroradiology
and Head and Neck Radiology; Professor
of Radiology, Otolaryngology Head Neck
Surgery, Radiation Oncology, Oral Medicine,
and Periodontics at the University of Michigan
Health System, Ann Arbor, Michigan

Contents

Breast Magnetic Resonance Imaging: Current Clinical Indications   155

Eren D. Yeh

> Breast magnetic resonance (MR) is highly sensitive in the detection of invasive breast malignancies. As technology improves, as interpretations and reporting by radiologists become standardized through the development of guidelines by expert consortiums, and as scientific investigation continues, the indications and uses of breast MR as an adjunct to mammography continue to evolve. This article discusses the current clinical indications for breast MR including screening for breast cancer, diagnostic indications for breast MR, and MR guidance for interventional procedures.

The BI-RADS Breast Magnetic Resonance Imaging Lexicon   171

Virginia Molleran and Mary C. Mahoney

> The Breast Magnetic Resonance Imaging Lexicon was designed to standardize interpretation and reporting of breast magnetic resonance (MR) imaging findings, ultimately improving communication between radiologists and clinicians and facilitating patient care. The lexicon includes 3 lesion types: mass, focus, and non-masslike enhancement. The mass category is analogous to the mass category in the mammography lexicon. Non-masslike enhancement is comparable with calcifications in the mammography lexicon. Unique to the MR lexicon is description of lesion enhancement. In addition, description of background enhancement allows assessment and communication of the sensitivity of the study. The Breast MR Imaging Lexicon is reviewed and images provided to illustrate these descriptor terminologies.

Implementing a Breast MR Imaging Program: All Things Considered   187

Sughra Raza

> The role of magnetic resonance (MR) imaging in breast imaging and evaluation has increased rapidly. MR imaging now encompasses diagnostic evaluation as well as screening for breast cancer in high-risk groups, monitoring the extent of disease and the response to chemotherapy. It is expected that the utility of breast MR imaging will continue to increase, requiring additional facilities and expertise. Establishing a breast MR imaging program requires familiarity with several unique issues pertaining to the nature of this imaging modality. This article attempts to address some of these issues, including selection of a magnet based on needs of the particular practice and magnet field strength, selection of a dedicated breast coil, magnet location and siting, advantages and challenges of higher strength magnets such as 3 Tesla, establishing a referral base, scheduling of breast MR examinations, patient safety concerns, and examination interpretation and reporting.

Role of Magnetic Resonance Imaging in Evaluating the Extent of Disease   199

Sara C. Gavenonis and Susan Orel Roth

> Preoperative breast imaging evaluation can contribute useful clinical information to the management of the patient with known breast cancer. Breast magnetic resonance

imaging (MRI) has been used as part of this imaging evaluation, and the ability of breast MRI to detect otherwise occult multifocal and multicentric disease has been demonstrated in multiple studies. The use of MRI for breast cancer staging remains under debate, however. This article reviews some of the current discussion regarding the use of breast MRI in this patient population. It is important to note that this discussion occurs in an evolving context of surgical and breast conservation therapies.

The technical requirements for magnetic resonance imaging (MRI) of the breasts are challenging because high temporal and high spatial resolution are necessary. This article describes the necessary equipment and pulse sequences for performing a high-quality study. Although imaging at 3-Tesla (T) has a higher signal-to-noise ratio, the protocol needs to be modified from the 1.5-T system to provide optimal imaging. The article presents the requirements for performing breast MRI and discusses techniques to ensure high-quality examinations on 1.5-T and 3-T systems.

Ductal carcinoma in situ (DCIS) now accounts for well over 20% of cancers diagnosed in mammography screening programs. This article reviews the biology of DCIS and the unique kinetic and morphologic features of DCIS at MR imaging that allow reliable diagnosis of DCIS lesions, including noninvasive disease that is mammographically occult. Increased detection of DCIS lesions at MR imaging has important implications for high-risk screening programs and for staging of patients with newly diagnosed breast cancer. Future research may provide prognostic information extracted from the MR phenotype of in situ cancer.

Breast cancer is the most common cancer in women. One in 8 women develops breast cancer and approximately 30% of all affected women die of the disease. By performing a nationwide screening program in the Netherlands, a mortality reduction of 1.2% annually was achieved. The screening program is for women between the ages of 50 and 75 years; however, women with an increased risk for developing breast cancer are mostly younger. The role of MRI in this particular group of women has been described in different studies. MRI of the breast in this group of women has a higher sensitivity than mammography, but the highest sensitivity is reached by the combination of these two imaging modalities.

Neoadjuvant chemotherapy is now widely used in the management of locally advanced breast cancer (LABC). Early initiation of systemic therapy can improve overall and disease-free survival for patients with LABC or inflammatory cancer. MR imaging with intravenous contrast and advanced MR imaging techniques provide new opportunities for assessing tumor morphologic changes, tumor vascularity, tumor cellularity, and tumor metabolic features. MR imaging is more reliable than the conventional methods in the assessment of tumor size and vascularity changes during and after chemotherapy. The addition of advanced imaging techniques to further characterize tumor cellularity and metabolic features appears promising. However, there is still no consensus on the role of MR imaging for assessing response to neoadjuvant chemotherapy or on a standardized MR imaging examination in patients receiving neoadjuvant chemotherapy.

The Effectiveness of MR Imaging in the Assessment of Invasive Lobular Carcinoma of the Breast 259

Ritse M. Mann

Invasive lobular carcinoma (ILC) of the breast is, due to its diffuse infiltrative growth pattern, a diagnostic challenge. Even in retrospect, only up to 80% are visible at mammography. Moreover, both mammography and ultrasound tend to structurally underestimate the size of ILC. Breast magnetic resonance (MR) imaging is usually performed after initial cancer detection. In this setting, the sensitivity is approximately 96%. However, multiple cases have been reported in which ILC has been initially detected with MR imaging, thus implying a potential advantage of MR imaging over mammography in screening. The size of an ILC as reported on MR imaging correlates well with size at pathology ($r = 0.89$). Additional tumor foci are detected by MR imaging in approximately one-third of patients, and these foci are subsequently pathologically confirmed in 88%. Hence, preoperative MR imaging of ILC changes management in 28% of patients, often appropriately. Nevertheless, it is still essential to obtain histology prior to large changes in the therapeutic regime based on MR imaging findings, either by second-look ultrasound or by MR imaging–guided biopsy. Using this approach, it has been shown that preoperative MR imaging reduces the rate of reexcisions after breast-conserving surgery from 27% to 9%, without increasing the rate of mastectomies and without extending total therapy time. Finally, the early detection of contralateral carcinomas only visible at MR imaging in approximately 7% of patients with ILC implies that preoperative MR imaging in these patients improves survival, although the magnitude of this effect is unknown.

A Clinical Oncologic Perspective on Breast Magnetic Resonance Imaging 277

Sara Bloom and Monica Morrow

Magnetic resonance (MR) imaging identifies cancer not found by clinical examination or other breast imaging studies, but its effect on patient outcomes is controversial. To date, its use has not been shown to increase the likelihood of obtaining negative surgical margins, decrease the rate of conversion from lumpectomy to mastectomy, or decrease local recurrence. The rate of tumor identification with MR imaging is 2 to 3 times higher than the incidence of local recurrence, resulting in mastectomies that may not be beneficial to the patient. This is also a concern with the use of MR imaging for contralateral cancer detection. The use of MR imaging for early detection of local recurrence does not take into account what is known about the biology of local recurrence because a short interval to local recurrence is associated with poor prognosis. In problem areas, such as evaluation of response to neoadjuvant therapy and detection of cancer presenting as axillary adenopathy, MR imaging provides information that is useful for clinical management.

MR Imaging in the Evaluation of Equivocal Clinical and Imaging Findings of the Breast 295

Jessica W.T. Leung

Because of its high negative predictive value in excluding breast cancer, magnetic resonance (MR) imaging plays a role in the evaluation of selected clinical and imaging findings of the breast, especially when biopsy is not technically feasible. Case selection is very important in ensuring the efficacy of this use of MR imaging because of potential false-positive and (albeit less likely) false-negative results. This article examines the clinical scenarios and imaging findings in which MR imaging is contributory to patient management after conventional workup with equivocal results.

The MR imaging BI-RADS atlas includes a category for probably benign findings, and many radiologists recommend short-term interval follow-up for breast MR imaging lesions. However, the characteristics of those MR imaging findings that could appropriately be considered probably benign are not well defined. This article reviews the published retrospective and prospective data regarding the use and cancer yield of the BI-RADS 3 assessment category as well as the morphology and kinetics of lesions that may be considered suitable for short-term follow-up. Consideration is also given to how the costs, clinical indication for the examination, experience of the reader, and availability of comparisons may affect the use of the BI-RADS 3 category. Based on the evidence that is available, an algorithm is offered with imaging examples as a guide for determining if lesions are appropriate for short-term follow-up. Additional research is needed to fully clarify the distinct morphologic and kinetic characteristics that allow patients to safely avoid biopsy without changing prognosis if malignancy is present.

Although breast magnetic resonance (MR) imaging was initially hindered by the limited availability of coils, protocols, and particularly breast biopsy devices, standardized imaging and specialized equipment necessary to perform high-quality MR imaging of the breast is now readily available. Those performing breast MR imaging should also be capable of performing biopsies, or at least have a close association with a facility that does. Optimal management of patients requires a good understanding of the indications and technique of breast MR imaging biopsies. In this article the indications for breast MR interventional procedures along with the techniques used are described. In addition, the histologic process encountered and recommended strategies for patient management are discussed.

Magnetic Resonance Imaging Clinics of North America

THE CLINICS ARE NOW AVAILABLE ONLINE!

Access your subscription at:
www.theclinics.com

Preface

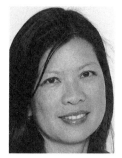 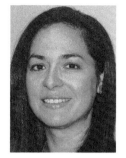

Linda Moy, MD   Cecilia L. Mercado, MD
Guest Editors

In recent years, great advancements have occurred in breast imaging that can be attributed to the marked technological improvements in magnetic resonance (MR) imaging of the breast and to an increase in its usefulness in the evaluation and management of breast disease.

The first part of this publication focuses on the clinical indications and usefulness of breast MR imaging. One of the first articles reviews the BI-RADS Breast MRI lexicon and illustrates various MR imaging descriptors. The content also provides an update on screening of high-risk patients with breast MR and offers valuable information on the management of probably benign lesions identified on breast MR imaging. In addition, the role of MR imaging in the evaluation of specific pathologic entities, such as invasive lobular carcinoma and ductal carcinoma in situ, is discussed. The role of breast MR imaging in the management of patients with breast cancer when evaluating extent of disease and in the management of patients undergoing neoadjuvant chemotherapy is discussed in other articles in this series. The use of breast MR imaging as a problem-solving tool when evaluating selected equivocal clinical and imaging findings is also discussed.

The publication provides valuable information and useful guidelines for the implementation of a breast MR imaging program. Clinical indications and the technique of MR interventional procedures and optimization of MR imaging at the 1.5 Tesla and 3.0 Tesla magnets are also discussed. The content concludes with an interesting article on the current uses of MR imaging of the breast from a breast surgeon's perspective, warning of its potential for over use.

We would like to thank the contributors to this issue who were asked to share their known expertise on MR imaging of the breast. It is hoped that these articles provide a balanced understanding of how to better use MR imaging for the evaluation and management of patients with breast carcinoma or patients at high risk for the disease.

Linda Moy, MD
Department of Radiology
New York University School of Medicine
160 East 34th Street
New York, NY 10016, USA

Cecilia L. Mercado, MD
Department of Radiology
New York University School of Medicine
160 East 34th Street
New York, NY 10016, USA

E-mail addresses:
linda.moy@nyumc.org (L. Moy)
cecilia.mercado@nyumc.org (C.L. Mercado)

Magn Reson Imaging Clin N Am 18 (2010) xiii
doi:10.1016/j.mric.2010.02.014

Breast Magnetic Resonance Imaging: Current Clinical Indications

Eren D. Yeh, MD

KEYWORDS
- Breast • Magnetic resonance • Indications • Breast cancer

Breast cancer is the most common cancer among women. In 2009, approximately 192,370 new cases of invasive breast cancer, and an additional 62,280 in situ breast cancers, will be diagnosed. An estimated 40,170 women are expected to die from breast cancer in 2009. Because of early detection of breast cancers from widespread screening mammography and improvements in treatment, the mortality from breast cancer has decreased almost 30% since 1990.[1]

Mammography is the mainstay of breast imaging. Other imaging technologies such as ultrasound and magnetic resonance (MR) have been found to be useful adjuncts to mammography. Breast MR is highly sensitive in the detection of invasive malignancies, with reported rates of 89% to 100%, although it is somewhat limited with variable specificity, reported at 37% to 97%.[2] As technology improves, as interpretations and reporting by radiologists become standardized through the development of guidelines by expert consortiums, and as scientific investigation continues, the indications and uses of breast MR as an adjunct to mammography continue to evolve.

The specificity of breast MR has gradually improved, likely because of improved technology and increased reader experience. To standardize interpretation among radiologists and to facilitate outcome monitoring, the American College of Radiology (ACR) has developed guidelines for interpretation: the ACR BI-RADS (Breast Imaging Reporting and Data System) MR Imaging Lexicon, the first edition of the MR Imaging Lexicon, in 2003.[3] The BI-RADS MR Imaging Lexicon provides common terminology for describing findings and allows radiologists to communicate findings to referring physicians and with each other in a standardized fashion. It also facilitates comparison of findings across scientific investigations.

One of the current challenges that breast MR faces is that technical parameters are not standardized, varying with equipment and across practice sites, including magnet strength, pulse sequences, spatial resolution, and timing of postcontrast sequences. To address this issue, the ACR has also developed practice guidelines and technical standards for breast MR, the most recent update in 2008.[4] The ACR is also in the process of developing a breast MR accreditation program that will be part of the breast imaging accreditation program and will include technical requirements for optimal breast imaging and the requirement for an MR biopsy program. The current guidelines by the ACR are the foundation for this article on the current clinical indications for breast MR.

The ACR guidelines are designed to assist practitioners in providing appropriate radiologic care for patients.[4] They are not inflexible rules, and the ultimate judgment in determining the appropriateness of specific imaging or a specific procedure must take all circumstances into consideration. MR findings should be correlated with clinical history, physical examination, and results of mammography and other prior breast imaging.

Division of Breast Imaging, Department of Radiology, Brigham and Women's Hospital, Dana-Farber Cancer Institute, Harvard Medical School, 75 Francis Street, RA Building-014, Boston, MA 02115, USA
E-mail address: eyeh@partners.org

Magn Reson Imaging Clin N Am 18 (2010) 155–169
doi:10.1016/j.mric.2010.02.009

The current guidelines published by the ACR recommend breast MR in the following circumstances[4]:

- Screening for the high-risk patient
- Screening the contralateral breast in a patient with a recently diagnosed breast malignancy
- Screening in patients with breast augmentation, for example in patients with postoperative reconstruction and previous free injections.

The diagnostic indications for breast MR are as follows:

- For extent of disease in patients with invasive carcinoma or ductal carcinoma in situ (DCIS)
- In assessing invasion deep to the fascia
- Postlumpectomy with positive margins
- Following patients with neoadjuvant chemotherapy.

In the additional evaluation of clinical or imaging findings, evaluation for recurrence of breast cancer in metastatic cancer of unknown primary or axillary adenopathy, in which a breast origin is suspected, and in lesion characterization, breast MR may be indicated when other imaging modalities, such as mammography and ultrasound, are inconclusive for the presence of breast cancer and biopsy cannot be performed. Breast MR may also be helpful for the additional evaluation of clinical or imaging findings in postoperative tissue reconstruction. Breast MR is also used for guidance for interventional procedures, such as MR core biopsy and MR-guided wire localization (**Table 1**).

SCREENING FOR THE HIGH-RISK PATIENT

In 2007, the American Cancer Society published guidelines for screening for breast cancer with MR as an adjunct to mammography.[5] The guidelines were based on several major clinical trials, the first of which was published by Kuhl and colleagues[6] in 2000, in which 192 asymptomatic women with proven or suspected BRCA mutations were enrolled in a prospective trial comparing MR with conventional imaging. Nine breast cancers were identified, 4 by mammography and ultrasound (44% sensitivity) and all 9 by MR (100% sensitivity).

Since then, there have been several studies worldwide showing benefit to screening subsets of women at high risk for breast cancer with MR.[7] In a review of 8 major clinical trials for MR screening of known or suspected BRCA 1 and BRCA 2 carriers in 4271 patients, 144 breast cancers were found with a 3% cancer yield.[8] Overall, there was a high sensitivity of MR for screening in high-risk populations, with a sensitivity of 71% to 100%, compared with 16% to 40% sensitivity with mammography. The specificity was variable. The call-back rate ranged from 8% to 17% (average 10%), with a benign biopsy rate of 3% to 15% (average 5%). **Figs. 1** and **2** show malignancies detected by screening MR in high-risk patients.

The patients at highest risk for breast cancer are those with a mutation of a breast cancer susceptibility gene. They constitute only 5% to 10% of women with breast cancers, but a familial genetic mutation confers a cumulative lifetime risk of breast cancer between 50% and 85% (19% risk by age 40 years, 50% risk by age 50 years, and 85% risk by age 70 years).[9] The most common of these are the BRCA 1 or 2 mutations, which account for approximately 40% to 50% of familial breast cancer; the others are caused by other familial genes that cannot be tested for at the present time.[7]

Table 1 Indications for performing breast MR imaging	
Breast cancer screening	Screening for the high-risk patient Contralateral breast Breast augmentation
Diagnostic indications	Extent of disease in patient with known breast cancer Following patients with neoadjuvant chemotherapy Breast cancer recurrence Metastatic cancer of unknown primary or axillary adenopathy Lesion characterization when mammography and ultrasound are inconclusive Postoperative tissue reconstruction
Procedure guidance	MR core biopsy MR-guided wire localization

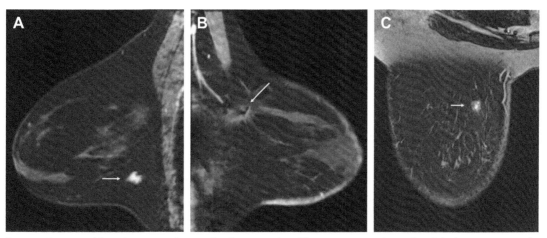

Fig. 1. A 27-year-old, BRCA 1 mutation carrier, just completed lumpectomy and XRT for right breast cancer who presented for a screening MRI. Left breast sagittal post contrast image (A) shows a new 0.8-cm mass with irregular margins, homogeneous enhancement and wash out kinetics. Solid mass identified on correlative ultrasound; ultrasound guided core biopsy yielded invasive ductal carcinoma. Sagittal post contrast image of the right breast (B) shows post treatment changes (arrow). Patient elected bilateral mastectomies. (C) A 55-year-old woman with BRCA 2 mutation who presented for a screening MR. Axial image post-contrast demonstrate a right posterior upper inner breast 1.3-cm non-mass like enhancement (arrow) with heterogeneous enhancement and persistent kinetics. There was no mammographic or sonographic correlate. MR core needle biopsy yielded invasive ductal carcinoma.

The American Cancer Society in 2007 recommended annual MR screening for breast cancer as an adjunct to mammography, based on evidence, for patients with a known BRCA mutation, patients who are a first-degree relative of a BRCA carrier, but untested, or patients with a 20% or greater lifetime risk, as defined by BRCAPRO or other models that are largely dependent on family history.[5] They recommended annual MR screening, based on expert consensus opinion, for patients with radiation to chest between the ages of 10 and 30 years, patients with Li-Fraumeni, Cowden, and Bannayan-Riley-Ruvalcaba syndromes, and first-degree relatives. They reported that there is insufficient evidence to recommend for or against MR screening in patients with a 15% to 20% lifetime risk. They also concluded that there is insufficient evidence for or against MR screening in patients with any one of these risk factors: history of lobular carcinoma in situ, atypical lobular hyperplasia, atypical ductal hyperplasia, heterogeneously or extremely dense breast tissues on mammography, and women with a personal history of breast cancer, including DCIS. They recommended against MR screening, based on expert consensus opinion, in patients with a less than 15% lifetime risk of breast cancer.

Most patients who have had radiation to the chest at a young age, between 10 and 30 years, are Hodgkin lymphoma survivors. Breast cancer is the most common second malignancy among female survivors of treated Hodgkin lymphoma, with a higher risk in those treated for Hodgkin lymphoma before age 30 years, with greater than 40 Gray dose of radiation, and with mantle field radiation compared with mediastinal radiation alone.[10,11] The risk of breast cancer approaches 29% in a woman aged 55 years who is treated for Hodgkin lymphoma at age 25 years.[10] The increased risk of secondary breast cancer emerges after a latency period of 8 to 10 years after treatment. The mammographic and sonographic appearances are similar to sporadic breast cancer; however, the malignancies tend to have unfavorable pathologic characteristics and are invasive cancers more often than DCIS. Dense breast tissues may also limit the sensitivity of screening mammography in young premenopausal women such as Hodgkin survivors. Mammography may be effective at detecting DCIS, but may be inadequate for detection of invasive breast cancer in this high-risk population. Based on expert consensus opinion, the American Cancer Society recently recommended MR imaging as an adjunct to mammography in this high-risk population.

At the Dana-Farber Cancer Institute, the authors recommend annual mammography beginning age 25 and supplement screening with MR in patients with known or suspected BRCA or familial

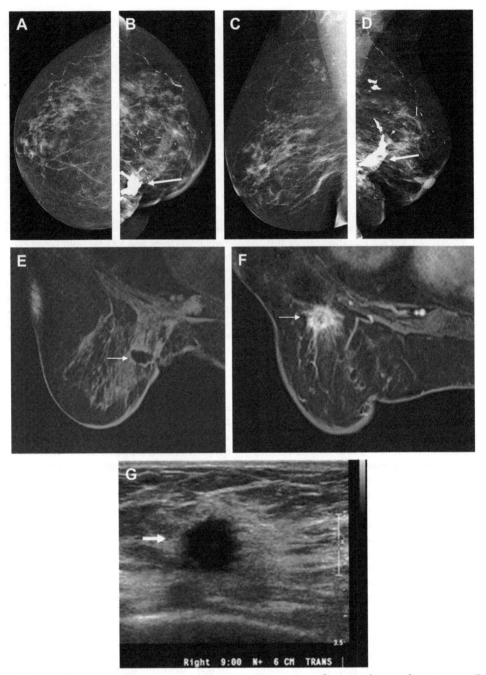

Fig. 2. A 74-year-old woman s/p right lumpectomy and XRT 31 years ago for an early stage breast cancer. Routine mammogram showed right breast post treatment changes on the cranial-caudal (CC) (*B*) and mediolateral oblique (MLO) (*D*) views, with architectural distortion and benign fat necrosis (*arrows*); the left side (*A*, CC; *C*, MLO) was negative. On MR, post treatment changes with large calcifications are present medially (*arrow*, *E*) with no enhancement at the surgical bed. A rim enhancing spiculated mass is present laterally on the post-contrast axial image (*arrow*, *F*) with rapid washout kinetics, highly suspicious for malignancy. Directed ultrasound was performed, demonstrating an 11-mm irregular solid mass in the right breast at 9:00 o'clock, which correlates with the MR finding. The mass was not seen mammographically, in retrospect, due to the far posterior location. Ultrasound core biopsy yielded invasive ductal carcinoma. The patient had a mastectomy.

mutations. In patients with Hodgkins lymphoma treated with mantle radiation, the authors screen beginning 8 years following treatment in patients age 25 or over and supplement screening with MR. If the patient does not live a great distance away and travel is not an impediment, the screening mammogram and MR are offset by 6 months so that the patient receives 1 screening study every 6 months, in the hope that the more frequent screening will detect a developing malignancy earlier.

Further investigation needs to be done in the subset of patients at 15% to 20% increased lifetime risk of breast cancer to determine which of these women benefit from screening MR. This group includes women with a personal history of breast cancer, including DCIS, lobular carcinoma in situ, atypical lobular hyperplasia, atypical ductal hyperplasia, and heterogeneously or extremely dense breast tissues on mammography.

SCREENING FOR THE CONTRALATERAL BREAST

Several single-institution studies have been performed in patients with a newly diagnosed invasive breast cancer with a 3% to 5% detection rate by MR of synchronous cancers in the contralateral breast (range 3%–24%), otherwise occult on clinical breast examination and mammography.[12] In a recent prospective multi-institutional trial of women with a newly diagnosed breast cancer, the American College of Radiology Imaging Network (ACRIN 6667) MRI Evaluation of the Contralateral Breast in Women Recently Diagnosed with Breast Cancer, MR detected 30 contralateral cancers among 969 women with a negative mammogram, at a rate of 3.1%.[13] The sensitivity of MR was 91%, specificity was 88%, and the negative predictive value was 99%. The biopsy rate was 12.5% (121/969), finding 30 cancers, of which 18 were invasive. The mean size of the cancers was 10.9 mm. All were small cancers with a favorable prognosis. No patients had distant metastases, and of the patients with node status known (27/30), none had positive lymph nodes. This result suggests that occult contralateral malignancies are detected by MR at an early stage that is treatable. **Fig. 3** shows a patient in whom MR detected more extensive malignancy than was originally suspected, and an occult contralateral cancer.

If a contralateral suspicious lesion is detected at MR, it is essential that biopsy diagnosis be established before surgical planning, as not all suspicious lesions are malignant.

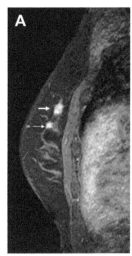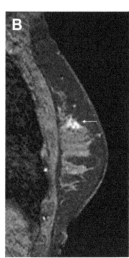

Fig. 3. A 49-year-old woman with new left breast focal asymmetry on mammography; outside ultrasound was negative. MR for problem solving demonstrates two masses in the left breast and non-mass like enhancement on the right. Sagittal post contrast image of the left breast (*A*) shows an oval 1 cm mass with irregular margins superiorly (*thick arrow*) and a second slightly inferior 0.6-cm round mass with irregular margins (*thin arrow*). MR-guided wire-localized surgical biopsies were performed: the superior mass was invasive cancer with ductal and lobular features, and the inferior mass was invasive ductal carcinoma. Sagittal image of the contralateral breast (*B*) demonstrates a mammographically occult 1.4-cm segmental non-mass like enhancement with clumped enhancement (*arrow*). MR-guided wire-localized surgical biopsy showed invasive ductal carcinoma. The patient was treated with bilateral lumpectomies and XRT. (*From* Raza S, Birdwell RL, Ritner JA, et al. Specialty imaging: breast MR: a comprehensive imaging guide. Salt Lake City, UT: Amirsys; 2010. p. 98; with permission.)

IMPLANTS AND BREAST AUGMENTATION

Screening MR may be helpful in patients with augmentation or cosmetic injections. MR has been shown to better visualize tissue around a silicone implant.[14] Detection of malignancy may be challenging with mammography in patients with free injection of materials such as silicone, paraffin, or polyacrylamide gel; MR in these cases may detect malignancy to better advantage. MR may also detect malignancies that occur posterior to an implant, which would not be visualized mammographically because of the posterior location.

MR imaging has been shown to have the highest sensitivity and specificity for the diagnosis of silicone implant rupture without the use ionizing radiation. Sensitivity ranges from 28% to 59% for mammography, and 78% to 81% for MR.[15,16] To optimize detection of implant rupture, no contrast is given to the patient- and silicone-selective sequences, and water-suppression techniques are used. If the clinical indication is to evaluate for possible implant rupture, the technique is not designed to evaluate for breast cancer, as no contrast is given to the patient and the sequences are not optimized for breast cancer detection.

When an implant is surgically placed, the body forms a fibrous capsule of scar tissue around the implant. In patients with a saline implant, a rupture will be clinically evident, with a decrease in the size and contour of the breast, and no imaging will be necessary. In patients with a silicone implant, the implant may be intact, or there may be an intracapsular or an extracapsular rupture. Most silicone implants more than 10 years old have a rupture, most commonly intracapsular. An intracapsular rupture occurs when the envelope breaks, but the silicone remains contained by the fibrous capsule. This may be seen as a linguine sign on MR imaging. Signs of an incomplete envelope collapse on MR are the subcapsular line sign, teardrop sign, and keyhole sign.[17]

An extracapsular rupture represents extrusion of silicone outside the fibrous capsule. On breast MR, silicone may be seen within the breast tissues outside the implant or in the axillary lymph nodes. The signal intensities on the MR sequences obtained will follow silicone.

EXTENT OF DISEASE

MR has been shown in several studies to be more sensitive than physical examination and conventional imaging, including mammography and ultrasound, in determining the extent of disease in patients newly diagnosed with breast cancer. It has been found to be more accurate than mammography, ultrasound, and clinical examination in assessing primary tumor size. MR depicts otherwise unsuspected sites of cancer in 16% (range 6%–34%).[12] **Figs. 3** and **4** show patients in whom MR detected more extensive disease than was originally suspected by conventional imaging.

A recent meta-analysis, including 19 published studies of 2610 women with newly diagnosed breast cancer undergoing preoperative MR, detected multifocal or multicentric cancer occult to conventional imaging in 16% of the patients.[18] MR had a high specificity in this analysis, with 66% of suspicious MR lesions pathologically proven to be malignant. In patients who are possible lumpectomy candidates, determining the extent of disease is important in surgical planning, as the goal is to completely excise the tumor with clean margins with as few surgical procedures as possible. MR has been beneficial in improving surgical planning when assessing for extent of disease.

Patient treatment has been reported to have changed after preoperative MR in 11% to 28% of patients, usually conversion from planned breast conservation to mastectomy.[19,20] In the meta-analysis by Houssami and colleagues,[18] a subset of 13 studies assessed the effect of MR staging on surgical treatment. They found that 11.3% of women were converted from lumpectomy to more extensive surgery, wider or additional excision, or mastectomy, and 8.1% of the women were converted from lumpectomy to mastectomy because of additional sites of malignancy detected with MR.

In posterior breast cancers, assessment of pectoralis muscle invasion is important for surgical planning. MR is the most accurate imaging method for assessing the chest wall and for pectoralis muscle involvement, with a 71% to 100% positive predictive value for pectoralis muscle involvement.[21,22] In patients with posterior breast tumors, signs suggestive of pectoralis muscle invasion are obliteration of the fat plane between the tumor and muscle, and abnormal enhancement of the pectoralis muscle. **Fig. 4**B shows a patient with pectoralis muscle invasion.

MR has been found to be helpful in assessing the extent of disease in cases of invasive lobular carcinoma, in patients with dense breast tissues, and in patients with extensive intraductal component (EIC). Invasive lobular carcinoma histologically has tumor cells infiltrating the stroma in a single-file fashion, and can often be occult to physical examination, mammography, ultrasound, and MR because of its insidious pattern of infiltration.[23,24] MR has been found to be significantly more accurate than mammography (85% compared with 32%) in assessing size and extent of tumor in invasive lobular carcinoma.[25] A recently published study reviewed the current literature on invasive lobular carcinoma to assess the usefulness of MR in the workup of invasive lobular carcinoma, performing a meta-analysis when possible.[26] They found additional ipsilateral lesions detected in 32% of patients and 7% contralateral lesions occult to other modalities, with a sensitivity of 93% and a correlation with pathology ranging from 0.81 to 0.97. The MR findings changed surgical management in 28% of the cases. MR therefore may be helpful in preoperative planning of invasive lobular carcinoma, particularly when breast conservation is being considered.

Young patients and patients with dense breast tissues mammographically and a newly diagnosed

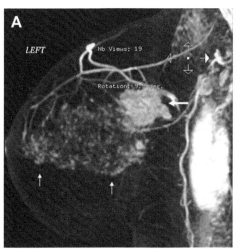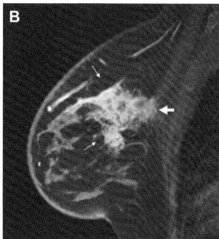

Fig. 4. Two different patients demonstrating extent of disease on MR. (A) A 33-year-old woman who presented with a lump and 3.3-cm mass by mammogram and ultrasound. MR shows the known mass (*large arrow*) with adjacent extensive regional clumped non-mass like enhancement extending to the nipple (*small arrow*), best seen on the MIP image (A). Ultrasound core biopsy yielded invasive ductal carcinoma. The patient was treated with neoadjuvant chemotherapy. (B) A 46-year-old woman with a lump. On the sagittal post contrast image, there is a large enhancing mass with spiculated margins and wash out kinetics (*thin arrows*). There is tenting and enhancement of the adjacent pectoralis muscle, suggesting invasion of the muscle (*thick arrow*). Ultrasound guided core biopsy yielded invasive ductal carcinoma. The patient underwent a mastectomy and invasion of pectoralis muscle with tumor was found.

cancer may benefit from preoperative MR. MR has been found to be more accurate than mammography in assessing tumor extent in patients with dense breast tissues. In one study of patients with multifocal or multicentric carcinoma and dense breast tissues, mammography detected the additional sites of malignancy in 35% and MR 100%.[27]

Invasive breast carcinomas with EIC are associated with DCIS-involved surgical margins and have an increased recurrence rate. The EIC component is nonpalpable, and the size is frequently underestimated on mammography. MR has been found to be more accurate in assessing extent of disease in invasive breast cancers with EIC.[28–30]

Preoperative breast MR to assess extent of disease is particularly important in those patients in whom breast conservation with partial breast irradiation is a treatment consideration. In an effort to decrease the side effects of conventional whole-breast irradiation in lumpectomy patients, investigations are currently ongoing with partial breast irradiation. In a study of 79 patients with breast cancer who were potential candidates for lumpectomy and accelerated partial breast irradiation, additional sites of cancer were observed in 30 patients (38%) on preoperative MR, occult to physical examination and mammography.[31] Of these, 8 (10%) had a malignancy in a different quadrant than the index tumor. The additional sites of occult malignancy would have been outside the treatment area covered by the partial breast irradiation.

To date, there have not been any randomized prospective trials published in the literature assessing the effect of breast MR on mastectomy rates or long-term outcomes such as recurrence rates or mortality. Several studies have shown that additional sites of disease can be found with preoperative MR. However, at this time, it is not certain in which subsets of patients the addition of preoperative MR imaging will result in improved overall survival.

There have been 2 retrospective studies assessing the effect of preoperative breast MR on long-term outcomes. In a study comparing 346 patients, 121 patients of whom had a preoperative MR and 225 patients who did not have a preoperative MR, the in-breast tumor recurrence rate was significantly lower; 1.2% in the patients with the preoperative MR compared with 6.8% in patients without the preoperative MR.[32] The investigators concluded that preoperative MR of the breast is recommended in patients with histopathologically verified breast cancer for local staging. A limitation of the study was that the data were not adjusted for tumor size, nodal status, or use of systemic therapy between groups.

In a more recently published work, 756 women with early-stage invasive breast carcinoma or DCIS who underwent breast-conserving therapy with definitive breast irradiation were studied.[33] Of these, 215 had preoperative breast MR, and 541 women did not. No difference was found in the 8-year local failure rate (3% vs 4%), no difference in overall survival (86% vs 87%), and no difference in freedom from metastases (89% vs 92%). Their conclusion was that preoperative breast MR was not associated with an improvement in outcome after breast conservation with radiation. Limitations of the study were that it was nonrandomized and retrospective. In addition, patients with extensive disease on MR imaging who underwent mastectomy were excluded from the study, which may underestimate the value of MR.

When additional findings are identified at MR, it is important to have a biopsy diagnosis before surgical planning. False-positive enhancing lesions may be the result of benign lesions such as fibroadenomas, sclerosing adenosis, fat necrosis, fibrocystic changes, and normal breast tissue. Multidisciplinary discussions including the surgeon, medical oncologist, radiation oncologist, radiologist, and pathologist are important in the optimal care of patients, and in decisions regarding additional MR imaging findings before changing management, to avoid unnecessary wider excisions or mastectomy.

FOLLOWING NEOADJUVANT CHEMOTHERAPY

Several studies have shown that MR is more accurate than physical examination, mammography, and ultrasound in monitoring response to neoadjuvant chemotherapy in patients with large breast cancers. Survival has been shown to be equivalent in patients with palpable breast cancers undergoing conventional chemotherapy after treatment and those undergoing chemotherapy before surgery, also known as neoadjuvant chemotherapy, followed by surgery and radiation.[34,35]

Potential advantages to having chemotherapy before surgery are reduction of tumor volume permitting breast conservation surgery, earlier treatment of micrometastatic disease, and assessment of tumor response in vivo to specific chemotherapeutic regimens, which may permit the oncologist to tailor preoperative or postoperative chemotherapy more effectively. If the tumor responds early to treatment, then it can be continued, whereas if the tumor does not respond, then the toxic therapy can be changed earlier in the course of treatment. It also allows for the study of biologic markers that may predict response.

MR is helpful when diagnosing a new malignancy before treatment. It can determine size and location of primary tumor, extent of disease, possible nodal involvement, chest wall invasion, and evaluate the contralateral breast for occult disease.

MR during or at the conclusion of chemotherapeutic treatment before surgery is helpful when performed to assess response. MR can distinguish responders from nonresponders. Decrease in tumor size and decrease in tumor vascularity suggest response.

If the tumor is not responding to specific chemotherapeutic agents, changes can be made earlier in the course of treatment so the patient does not continue to receive toxic therapy that is ineffective in reducing the tumor burden. After treatment, the breast MR tumor size correlation with pathology at surgery has been shown to be r = 0.75 to 0.93; more accurate than physical examination, mammography, and ultrasound.[36–39] Accurate prediction of residual tumor size following neoadjuvant chemotherapy is helpful in surgical planning. Among other things, the surgeons need to determine whether the patient is a candidate for lumpectomy and radiation therapy versus mastectomy, and to determine the amount of tissue that needs to be excised during surgery to attain clean margins. **Fig. 5** shows a patient who received neoadjuvant chemotherapy.

MR is not perfect and can overestimate or underestimate residual disease.[36] In cases in which MR overestimates residual disease, the residual enhancement may be caused by reactive inflammation and tumor response and healing. Chemotherapy-induced fibrosis can be difficult to differentiate from residual disease.[40] In cases in which MR underestimates residual disease, decreased enhancement may be the result of small foci of invasive cancer, nests of tumor, or subtypes such as lobular carcinoma, which have been shown to have variable enhancement on MR.[23,41,42] Gadolinium uptake is related to tumor angiogenesis and neovascularity, and lack of these in DCIS may explain the variable uptake seen in residual DCIS.

Certain chemotherapeutic agents may affect the tumor physiology by changing tumor vascularization and vascular permeability, thereby changing MR imaging characteristics. One study has suggested that residual disease on MR is frequently underestimated in tumors treated with taxane-containing regimens.[43] Tumor physiology can potentially be used to optimize the sequence of neoadjuvant chemotherapy in breast cancer. It

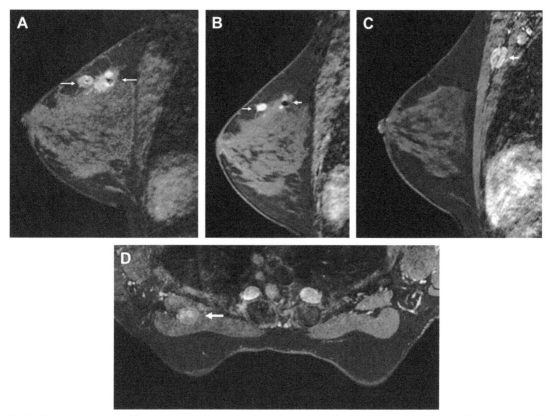

Fig. 5. Pre- and postneoadjuvant chemotherapy, with subsequent development of Rotter's node. A 31-year-old woman presented with a lump. Ultrasound guided core biopsy of two adjacent masses demonstrated invasive ductal carcinoma, poorly differentiated. Sagittal post contrast MR image (*A*) performed prior to neoadjuvant chemotherapy demonstrated the known malignancy, measuring 3.8-cm by MR with artifact from two clips from prior ultrasound guided core biopsies. Following neoadjuvant chemotherapy, a 1-cm residual enhancing mass is present anteriorly on the post contrast sagittal MR (*B, thin arrow*) with artifact from clip posteriorly and minimal posterior enhancement (*B, thick arrow*). The patient was treated with lumpectomy and XRT. She was asymptomatic for two years. On follow up MR a new 2 cm Rotter's node, between the pectoralis major and minor muscles (*C*, sagittal post contrast image; *D*, axial delayed post contrast image) was seen. She subsequently had a left axillary lymph node dissection with 1/14 lymph nodes positives (the Rotter's node was positive).

has been hypothesized that tumors with high interstitial fluid pressure or hypoxia respond poorly to chemotherapy because of poor drug delivery. Paclitaxel significantly reduced the interstitial fluid pressure and improved the oxygenation of tumors, whereas doxorubicin did not cause any significant change.[44]

Clip placement within the tumor mass is crucial before treatment with neoadjuvant chemotherapy, as the tumor may have a complete radiologic and pathologic response. Surgical excision is performed unless the patient has known metastatic cancer, to assess pathologically the extent of residual tumor and to remove all known malignancy. If the tumor is not visible by imaging following neoadjuvant chemotherapy, the clip is used to guide wire-localized surgical excision. The pathologist also uses the clip as a guide in locating the original tumor bed to assess

response. Tumor response to chemotherapy is a predictor of outcome and complete pathologic responders have a significantly better long-term outcome.

EVALUATION FOR RECURRENCE OF BREAST CANCER

Several studies have shown benefits of MR in differentiating scar versus recurrence at the lumpectomy site in patients in whom mammography is indeterminate. Scar older than 6 months postoperatively tends not to enhance with gadolinium, as opposed to malignancy which does enhance.[14,45,46] MR may also be helpful when recurrence is suspected in the setting of postoperative tissue reconstruction with an autologous flap or a silicone implant reconstruction. **Fig. 6** shows

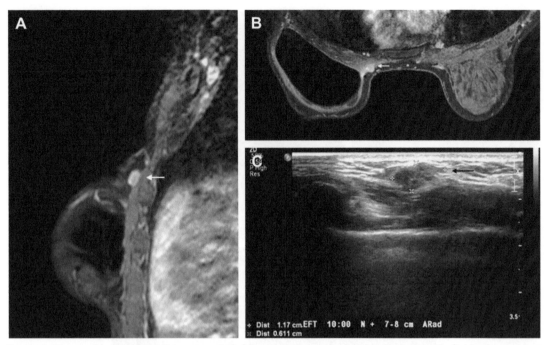

Fig. 6. A 44-year-old asymptomatic woman s/p left mastectomy and saline implant, recently finished treatment. Postcontrast MR shows the mastectomy with saline implant and 1-cm oval enhancing mass in the left superior medial breast (A, sagittal; B, axial). Focal ultrasound of the MR finding showed a 1-cm solid mass with irregular margins (C). Fine-needle aspiration (FNA) was performed with cytology positive for malignancy, consistent with a recurrence.

a patient *status/post* (s/p) mastectomy and implant reconstruction with a recurrence detected by MR.

METASTATIC CANCER OF UNKNOWN PRIMARY AND AXILLARY ADENOPATHY

The incidence of axillary metastases from an occult primary breast cancer is low; less than 1% of breast cancers.[47] In the past, mastectomy with axillary node dissection or, less commonly, whole breast radiation were the most common treatments in patients with axillary nodal metastases from an adenocarcinoma with an unknown primary site. However, in approximately one-third of cases, no tumor is found at pathologic evaluation of the mastectomy specimen.[48–50]

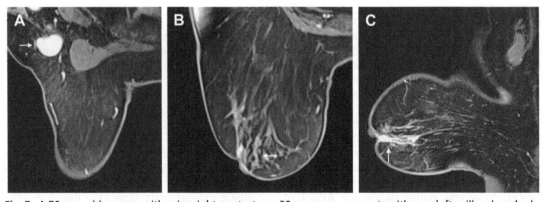

Fig. 7. A 76-year-old woman with prior right mastectomy 20 years ago, presents with new left axillary lymphadenopathy. Ultrasound core biopsy of the lymph node yielded metastatic lobular carcinoma, consistent with spread from a breast carcinoma. MR was performed to assess for breast primary, occult to physical examination and mammogram. MR showed enlarged left axillary lymph node (A) with retroareolar 1.0-cm linear enhancement, on the post contrast axial (B) and sagittal (C) images with persistent delayed kinetics. MR core biopsy yielded invasive lobular carcinoma. Patient had a left modified radical mastectomy with axillary dissection. Pathology was invasive lobular carcinoma, 1.6-cm and 1/14 lymph nodes positive.

Breast MR has been shown to identify a primary breast tumor in 70% to 86% of clinically, mammographically, and ultrasound occult primary breast tumors in patients presenting with metastatic adenopathy of unknown primary.[51–53] The tumor size tends to be small, less than 2 cm. Clinical treatment decisions can be altered by results from the breast MR. If a breast primary malignancy is found, breast conservation may be a treatment option.[54] If the breast MR is negative, mastectomy may not be necessary as a negative breast MR is predictive of a low tumor yield at mastectomy.[50]

Chemotherapeutic regimens would also be tailored to breast cancer if a primary breast malignancy is identified. Moreover, these are often less toxic than chemotherapeutic regimens for an

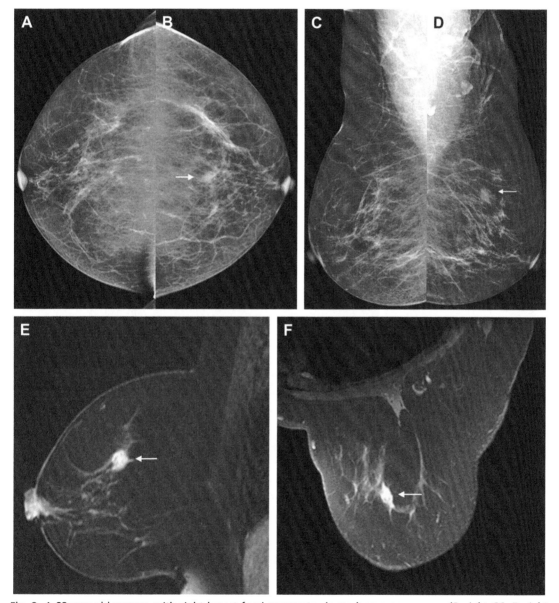

Fig. 8. A 83-year-old woman with right breast focal asymmetry (*arrow*) on mammogram (*B*, right CC; *D*, right MLO, arrows. Left CC (*A*); and MLO (*C*) views are normal) for which MR imaging was recommended. Ultrasound was negative. On MR, a mass with spiculated margins and internal enhancing septations was noted on the sagittal postcontrast. (*E*) and axial delayed postcontrast (*F*) images, wash-out kinetics. Stereotactic core biopsy was performed on the mammographic finding, with pathology of invasive lobular carcinoma. The patient elected mastectomy.

adenocarcinoma of unknown primary. Patients with breast cancer tend to have a more favorable prognosis than other adenocarcinomas; prognostic information is helpful to clinicians in counseling patients.

MR is therefore helpful in determining the presence of an occult primary breast cancer when there are malignant adenocarcinoma axillary metastases and negative physical examination and mammogram. **Fig. 7** shows a patient with malignant axillary adenopathy and occult primary malignancy detected by MR.

PROBLEM SOLVING

MR has been shown to be helpful as a problem-solving tool in cases in which the mammographic and sonographic findings are inconclusive despite a thorough diagnostic workup.[55,56] For example, MR may be performed for problem solving if an asymmetry is seen on 1 view only and cannot be three-dimensionally localized for a mammographic- or sonographic-guided biopsy. In a recent retrospective review of MR examinations with the indication of problem solving for inconclusive findings on mammography, the equivocal findings most frequently leading to MR were asymmetry and architectural distortion.[57] No suspicious MR correlate was found in 100 of 115 cases (87%). In cases in which the breast MR is negative, a final reported recommendation to the referring clinician must be made for the patient's imaging studies.

In the study discussed earlier, MR identified 15 enhancing masses (13%) that correlated with the mammographic abnormality; of these,

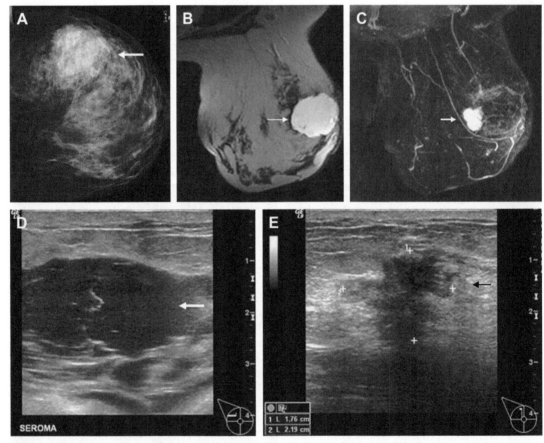

Fig. 9. A 58-year-old woman with recently diagnosed right breast cancer s/p right breast surgical excision at outside hospital with normal breast tissue at pathology, who presented for imaging evaluation to assess for residual tumor. CC view on mammogram (*A*) shows dense breast tissues with a mass laterally (*arrow*). Ultrasound (not shown) showed a seroma. Axial T2-weighted MR image with fat suppression shows a seroma laterally (*B*, *arrow*). Postcontrast axial MIP image shows an enhancing mass at the medial aspect of the seroma cavity. Focal ultrasound was subsequently performed, showing the seroma (*D*) with 2.2-cm irregular hypoechoic mass at the medial aspect of the cavity (*E*). Ultrasound-guided wire-localized surgical excision was performed with confirmation of removal of the malignancy at pathology.

6 were malignant.[57] Eighteen (15.7%) incidental lesions were found, all of which were benign. The investigators concluded that breast MR is a useful adjunct when conventional imaging is equivocal, but caution that strict patient selection criteria are necessary because of the high frequency of false positives. **Fig. 8** shows a patient in whom MR was helpful in problem solving.

MR may also be helpful postoperatively, when additional tumor is suspected to be present within the breast, such as in cases of positive margins or normal breast tissue at pathology. MR is helpful for surgical planning when additional surgery is expected. **Fig. 9** shows a patient in whom malignancy was suspected and an MR was helpful for surgical planning before re-excision.

MR PROCEDURE GUIDANCE

When lesions are identified on breast MR that are occult on mammography and ultrasound, MR is indicated for guidance of interventional procedures such as MR-guided percutaneous core biopsy and MR-guided preoperative wire localization for surgical excision. MR procedures may also be performed in cases in which the MR finding is more confidently seen on MR than on other imaging modalities. It is important to have MR biopsy capability for lesions detected only on MR; this will be a requirement in the new ACR breast MR accreditation program.

SUMMARY

Indications for breast MR continue to evolve as technology improves, interpretations become more standardized, and scientific investigation continues. MR should not be used in place of a full mammographic and sonographic workup. MR is useful as an adjunct to mammography in high-risk screening patients with a lifetime risk greater than 20% to 25%, including BRCA 1 and 2 patients, Hodgkin survivors treated with mantle radiation, patients with unknown primary and axillary metastases, problem solving, and in following response to treatment in patients receiving neoadjuvant chemotherapy. It is currently unclear in which subset of patients with a previous personal history of breast cancer screening is beneficial, or whether patients with intermediate risk factors, such as a previous biopsy diagnosis of atypical lobular hyperplasia or lobular carcinoma in situ, should be screened.

Not all patients with newly diagnosed breast cancer should undergo MR. The potential false positives must be considered and discussed with the patient before recommending MR. The Comparative Effectiveness of MRI in Breast Cancer (COMICE) trial in the United Kingdom is a randomized trial of 1850 patients in progress to evaluate the effect of MR on selection of patients for breast-conserving therapy and the adequacy of breast-conservation surgery.[19]

Further randomized, prospective clinical trials need to be performed to address questions and further delineate indications for breast MR. As the National Comprehensive Cancer Network (NCCN) practice guidelines stress, it is important to have proper equipment, imaging technique, and provider training to achieve high-quality breast MR.[58]

REFERENCES

1. American Cancer Society. Available at: http://www.cancer.org; 2009. Accessed 2009.
2. Kuhl C. The current status of breast MR imaging. Part I. Choice of technique, image interpretation, diagnostic accuracy, and transfer to clinical practice. Radiology 2007;244(2):356–78.
3. American College of Radiology. ACR Breast Imaging Reporting and Data System (BIRADS): breast imaging atlas. 4th edition. Reston (VA): American College of Radiology; 2003.
4. American College of Radiology. Available at: http://www.acr.org. Accessed 2009.
5. Saslow D, Boetes C, Burke W, et al. American Cancer Society guidelines for breast screening with MRI as an adjunct to mammography. CA Cancer J Clin 2007;57(2):75–89.
6. Kuhl CK, Schmutzler RK, Leutner CC, et al. Breast MR imaging screening in 192 women proved or suspected to be carriers of a breast cancer susceptibility gene: preliminary results. Radiology 2000; 215(1):267–79.
7. Kuhl CK. Current status of breast MR imaging. Part 2. Clinical applications. Radiology 2007;244(3): 672–91.
8. Lehman CD. Role of MRI in screening women at high risk for breast cancer. J Magn Reson Imaging 2006;24(5):964–70.
9. Liberman L. Breast cancer screening with MRI–what are the data for patients at high risk? N Engl J Med 2004;351(5):497–500.
10. Lee L, Pintilie M, Hodgson DC, et al. Screening mammography for young women treated with supradiaphragmatic radiation for Hodgkin's lymphoma. Ann Oncol 2008;19(1):62–7.
11. De Bruin ML, Sparidans J, van't Veer MB, et al. Breast cancer risk in female survivors of Hodgkin's

lymphoma: lower risk after smaller radiation volumes. J Clin Oncol 2009;27(26):4239–46.

12. Liberman L. Breast MR imaging in assessing extent of disease. Magn Reson Imaging Clin N Am 2006; 14(3):339–49, vi.

13. Lehman CD, Gatsonis C, Kuhl CK, et al. MRI evaluation of the contralateral breast in women with recently diagnosed breast cancer. N Engl J Med 2007;356(13):1295–303.

14. Heywang SH, Hilbertz T, Beck R, et al. Gd-DTPA enhanced MR imaging of the breast in patients with postoperative scarring and silicon implants. J Comput Assist Tomogr 1990;14(3):348–56.

15. Goodman CM, Cohen V, Thornby J, et al. The life span of silicone gel breast implants and a comparison of mammography, ultrasonography, and magnetic resonance imaging in detecting implant rupture: a meta-analysis. Ann Plast Surg 1998; 41(6):577–85 [discussion: 585–576].

16. Ikeda DM, Borofsky HB, Herfkens RJ, et al. Silicone breast implant rupture: pitfalls of magnetic resonance imaging and relative efficacies of magnetic resonance, mammography, and ultrasound. Plast Reconstr Surg 1999;104(7):2054–62.

17. Soo MS, Kornguth PJ, Walsh R, et al. Intracapsular implant rupture: MR findings of incomplete shell collapse. J Magn Reson Imaging 1997;7(4):724–30.

18. Houssami N, Ciatto S, Macaskill P, et al. Accuracy and surgical impact of magnetic resonance imaging in breast cancer staging: systematic review and meta-analysis in detection of multifocal and multicentric cancer. J Clin Oncol 2008;26(19):3248–58.

19. Orel S. Who should have breast magnetic resonance imaging evaluation? J Clin Oncol 2008; 26(5):703–11.

20. Braun M, Polcher M, Schrading S, et al. Influence of preoperative MRI on the surgical management of patients with operable breast cancer. Breast Cancer Res Treat 2008;111(1):179–87.

21. Morris EA, Schwartz LH, Drotman MB, et al. Evaluation of pectoralis major muscle in patients with posterior breast tumors on breast MR images: early experience. Radiology 2000;214(1):67–72.

22. Kazama T, Nakamura S, Doi O, et al. Prospective evaluation of pectoralis muscle invasion of breast cancer by MR imaging. Breast Cancer 2005;12(4):312–6.

23. Yeh ED, Slanetz PJ, Edmister WB, et al. Invasive lobular carcinoma: spectrum of enhancement and morphology on magnetic resonance imaging. Breast J 2003;9(1):13–8.

24. Kumar V, Abbas AK, Fausto N, et al. Robbins and Cotran pathologic basis of disease. 7th edition. Philadelphia: Elsevier Saunders; 2005.

25. Rodenko GN, Harms SE, Pruneda JM, et al. MR imaging in the management before surgery of lobular carcinoma of the breast: correlation with pathology. AJR Am J Roentgenol 1996;167(6):1415–9.

26. Mann RM, Hoogeveen YL, Blickman JG, et al. MRI compared to conventional diagnostic work-up in the detection and evaluation of invasive lobular carcinoma of the breast: a review of existing literature. Breast Cancer Res Treat 2008; 107(1):1–14.

27. Van Goethem M, Schelfout K, Dijckmans L, et al. MR mammography in the pre-operative staging of breast cancer in patients with dense breast tissue: comparison with mammography and ultrasound. Eur Radiol 2004;14(5):809–16.

28. Ikeda O, Nishimura R, Miyayama H, et al. Magnetic resonance evaluation of the presence of an extensive intraductal component in breast cancer. Acta Radiol 2004;45(7):721–5.

29. Van Goethem M, Schelfout K, Kersschot E, et al. MR mammography is useful in the preoperative locoregional staging of breast carcinomas with extensive intraductal component. Eur J Radiol 2007;62(2):273–82.

30. Schouten van der Velden AP, Boetes C, Bult P, et al. Magnetic resonance imaging in size assessment of invasive breast carcinoma with an extensive intraductal component. BMC Med Imaging 2009;9:5.

31. Godinez J, Gombos EC, Chikarmane SA, et al. Breast MRI in the evaluation of eligibility for accelerated partial breast irradiation. AJR Am J Roentgenol 2008;191(1):272–7.

32. Fischer U, Zachariae O, Baum F, et al. The influence of preoperative MRI of the breasts on recurrence rate in patients with breast cancer. Eur Radiol 2004;14(10):1725–31.

33. Solin LJ, Orel SG, Hwang WT, et al. Relationship of breast magnetic resonance imaging to outcome after breast-conservation treatment with radiation for women with early-stage invasive breast carcinoma or ductal carcinoma in situ. J Clin Oncol 2008;26(3):386–91.

34. Fisher B, Bryant J, Wolmark N, et al. Effect of preoperative chemotherapy on the outcome of women with operable breast cancer. J Clin Oncol 1998; 16(8):2672–85.

35. Bonadonna G, Valagussa P. Primary chemotherapy in operable breast cancer. Semin Oncol 1996; 23(4):464–74.

36. Yeh E, Slanetz P, Kopans DB, et al. Prospective comparison of mammography, sonography, and MRI in patients undergoing neoadjuvant chemotherapy for palpable breast cancer. AJR Am J Roentgenol 2005;184(3):868–77.

37. Segara D, Krop IE, Garber JE, et al. Does MRI predict pathologic tumor response in women with

breast cancer undergoing preoperative chemotherapy? J Surg Oncol 2007;96(6):474–80.

38. Rosen EL, Blackwell KL, Baker JA, et al. Accuracy of MRI in the detection of residual breast cancer after neoadjuvant chemotherapy. AJR Am J Roentgenol 2003;181(5):1275–82.

39. Partridge SC, Gibbs JE, Lu Y, et al. Accuracy of MR imaging for revealing residual breast cancer in patients who have undergone neoadjuvant chemotherapy. AJR Am J Roentgenol 2002;179(5):1193–9.

40. Helvie MA, Joynt LK, Cody RL, et al. Locally advanced breast carcinoma: accuracy of mammography versus clinical examination in the prediction of residual disease after chemotherapy. Radiology 1996;198(2):327–32.

41. Qayyum A, Birdwell RL, Daniel BL, et al. MR imaging features of infiltrating lobular carcinoma of the breast: histopathologic correlation. AJR Am J Roentgenol 2002;178(5):1227–32.

42. Weinstein SP, Orel SG, Heller R, et al. MR imaging of the breast in patients with invasive lobular carcinoma. AJR Am J Roentgenol 2001;176(2):399–406.

43. Denis F, Desbiez-Bourcier AV, Chapiron C, et al. Contrast enhanced magnetic resonance imaging underestimates residual disease following neoadjuvant docetaxel based chemotherapy for breast cancer. Eur J Surg Oncol 2004;30(10):1069–76.

44. Taghian AG, Abi-Raad R, Assaad SI, et al. Paclitaxel decreases the interstitial fluid pressure and improves oxygenation in breast cancers in patients treated with neoadjuvant chemotherapy: clinical implications. J Clin Oncol 2005;23(9):1951–61.

45. Gilles R, Guinebretiere JM, Shapeero LG, et al. Assessment of breast cancer recurrence with contrast-enhanced subtraction MR imaging: preliminary results in 26 patients. Radiology 1993;188(2):473–8.

46. Dao TH, Rahmouni A, Campana F, et al. Tumor recurrence versus fibrosis in the irradiated breast: differentiation with dynamic gadolinium-enhanced MR imaging. Radiology 1993;187(3):751–5.

47. Harris JR. Diseases of the breast. 3rd edition. Philadelphia: Lippincott Williams & Wilkins; 2004.

48. Jackson B, Scott-Conner C, Moulder J. Axillary metastasis from occult breast carcinoma: diagnosis and management. Am Surg 1995;61(5):431–4.

49. Fortunato L, Sorrento JJ, Golub RA, et al. Occult breast cancer. A case report and review of the literature. N Y State J Med 1992;92(12):555–7.

50. Olson JA Jr, Morris EA, Van Zee KJ, et al. Magnetic resonance imaging facilitates breast conservation for occult breast cancer. Ann Surg Oncol 2000;7(6):411–5.

51. Morris EA, Schwartz LH, Dershaw DD, et al. MR imaging of the breast in patients with occult primary breast carcinoma. Radiology 1997;205(2):437–40.

52. Orel SG, Weinstein SP, Schnall MD, et al. Breast MR imaging in patients with axillary node metastases and unknown primary malignancy. Radiology 1999;212(2):543–9.

53. Ko EY, Han BK, Shin JH, et al. Breast MRI for evaluating patients with metastatic axillary lymph node and initially negative mammography and sonography. Korean J Radiol 2007;8(5):382–9.

54. Varadarajan R, Edge SB, Yu J, et al. Prognosis of occult breast carcinoma presenting as isolated axillary nodal metastasis. Oncology 2006;71(5–6):456–9.

55. Sardanelli F, Melani E, Ottonello C, et al. Magnetic resonance imaging of the breast in characterizing positive or uncertain mammographic findings. Cancer Detect Prev 1998;22(1):39–42.

56. Lee CH, Smith RC, Levine JA, et al. Clinical usefulness of MR imaging of the breast in the evaluation of the problematic mammogram. AJR Am J Roentgenol 1999;173(5):1323–9.

57. Moy L, Elias K, Patel V, et al. Is breast MRI helpful in the evaluation of inconclusive mammographic findings? AJR Am J Roentgenol 2009;193(4):986–93.

58. Lehman CD, DeMartini W, Anderson BO, et al. Indications for breast MRI in the patient with newly diagnosed breast cancer. J Natl Compr Canc Netw 2009;7(2):193–201.

The BI-RADS Breast Magnetic Resonance Imaging Lexicon

Virginia Molleran, MD*, Mary C. Mahoney, MD

KEYWORDS

- Breast • MRI • Lexicon • Mass • Focus
- Non-masslike enhancement

Contrast-enhanced magnetic resonance (CE-MR) imaging of the breast has become an important imaging tool in patients with known or suspected breast cancer. Breast MR images are influenced by a variety of technical factors. The wide range of imaging protocols currently in use throughout the world results in variability in appearances of the imaging findings. The need for standardization of MR breast imaging has been recognized, and consensus has been reached regarding many of the most important technical factors such as minimum field strength, the use of dedicated breast coils, and the need for fat suppression and contrast-enhanced images.

Standardization of breast MR imaging has also included development of the breast MR imaging lexicon. The American College of Radiology developed the Breast Imaging Reporting and Data System (BI-RADS) mammography lexicon in 1996 to standardize and improve mammography interpretation and reporting. BI-RADS provided standard descriptors for mammography findings and improved the communication between radiologists and referring clinicians. Similarly, the lexicon for breast MR imaging was developed to clarify reporting of breast MR imaging findings and to establish definitions of the terminology and the implications of these findings for patient care. The lexicon for breast MR imaging was initially published in 2003, and an updated version will be available in 2010.

KINETIC EVALUATION

Early efforts in breast MR imaging developed along 2 pathways: 1 focusing on lesion kinetics and making use of high temporal resolution imaging, and 1 focusing on lesion morphology and using high spatial resolution imaging. This divergence was largely the result of the technical limitations of MR imaging at the time. To perform rapid imaging necessary for kinetic evaluation, spatial resolution had to be sacrificed. To achieve high spatial resolution necessary for detailed morphologic evaluation, longer acquisition times were required, precluding kinetic evaluation. More recently, the importance of using both features in lesion evaluation has been recognized, and current MR imaging technology enables the use of imaging protocols adequate for kinetic and morphologic analysis.

Once tumors reach a size of 2 to 3 mm, they must stimulate growth of new vessels to continue to grow.[1] This process is known as tumor angiogenesis. These new tumor-associated vessels tend to be large and leaky.[2] It is therefore expected that malignant lesions with a greater degree of tumor angiogenesis would show rapid and intense tumor enhancement on contrast-enhanced imaging. Benign lesions, on the other hand, would be expected to have slower and less intense enhancement. This principle is the foundation of kinetic analysis in CE-MR imaging and holds true in many cases. In actuality, lesion enhancement on MR imaging is a more complex

Department of Radiology, Division of Breast Imaging, University of Cincinnati Medical Center, 234 Goodman Street, Cincinnati, OH 45219, USA
* Corresponding author.
E-mail address: mollervm@healthall.com

Magn Reson Imaging Clin N Am 18 (2010) 171–185
doi:10.1016/j.mric.2010.02.001

process, and is affected by many different factors including not only vessel density and vessel permeability but also diffusion rate of contrast material, characteristics of the interstitium, and T1 relaxation time.[3] Observed lesion kinetics are also affected by imaging parameters such as field strength, contrast type, and acquisition time. For adequate kinetic evaluation, dynamic imaging acquisition times should be less than 2 minutes.[4] Invasive malignant lesions tend to reach their peak enhancement within 2 minutes, and longer acquisition times could prevent this peak from being observed.

Kinetics can be quantitatively evaluated in several ways. Parameters such as time to onset of enhancement, rate of enhancement, peak enhancement, and time to peak enhancement have all been studied.[3,5] Some of these measurements require high temporal resolution imaging protocols, which are not in widespread use. Current practice largely makes use of a semi-quantitative type of analysis in which percent change in signal intensity from the baseline pre-contrast value is plotted versus time. The resulting kinetic curve is then divided into 2 phases: early and delayed.

The early phase constitutes the first 2 minutes after contrast, when contrast is generally washing into the lesion. The curve during this period demonstrates the rate of uptake of contrast by the lesion, which is described in the lexicon as slow, medium, or rapid. The specific threshold values used for slow, medium, or rapid uptake vary with imaging protocols.[3] Most invasive malignant lesions show rapid, intense uptake of contrast and will have reached their peak enhancement by the end of this phase.

The remainder of the curve is considered the delayed phase. This part of the curve is evaluated in more of a quantitative manner based on the shape of the curve, which can be described in 3 ways according to the lexicon: persistent, plateau, and washout. A persistent curve shows continuously increasing enhancement throughout the dynamic series. A plateau curve then levels off and maintains a relatively constant value throughout the delayed phase. A washout curve reaches a peak at the end of the initial phase, and then enhancement declines throughout the delayed phase.

Early in the development of breast MR imaging, the focus of kinetic analysis was on the uptake rate and degree of enhancement in the early phase. Although malignant tumors did tend to demonstrate more rapid and intense enhancement than benign lesions, a significant overlap in enhancement rates between benign and malignant lesions was observed,[6,7] resulting in a low specificity. Kuhl

and colleagues[7] showed that including evaluation of the shape of the time-signal intensity curve in the delayed phase could increase specificity. In her study, 83% of benign lesions exhibited a persistent curve and 57% of malignant lesions exhibited a washout curve. There was still overlap, with 5% of benign lesions exhibiting a washout curve and 9% of malignant lesions exhibiting a persistent curve. Analysis of curve shape improved specificity from 37% to 83%. In a later study by Schnall and colleagues[8] 45% of lesions with persistent curves were seen in association with cancer, accounting for 26% of cancers evaluated with kinetics. Thus, the presence of persistent kinetics within a lesion does not exclude cancer, and one should not rely on kinetics alone to determine whether or not a lesion is suspicious. Plateau curves may also be suspicious for malignancy with a sensitivity and specificity for malignancy of 42.6% and 75%, respectively.[9]

When evaluating lesion enhancement, care should be taken to place the region of interest on the most rapidly and intensely enhancing portion of the lesion. This problem is obviated at least to some extent with MR imaging computer-aided diagnosis (CAD) systems, which display kinetic features using color-coded overlays. This allows quick visual assessment of curve types throughout the lesion. Assessment should be based on the most suspicious enhancement type demonstrated in the lesion. In a study by Wang and colleagues[5] using CAD, there was a greater difference in kinetic patterns between benign and malignant lesions when the most suspicious curve, rather than the predominant curve type, was analyzed. Kinetic curves are also affected by motion artifact, which can frequently result in artifactual washout curves. This potential pitfall should be kept in mind particularly when evaluating kinetic overlays generated by MR imaging CAD programs.

BACKGROUND ENHANCEMENT

Background breast parenchymal enhancement on CE-MR imaging is analogous to fibroglandular tissue density on mammography. Prominent background enhancement can obscure lesions and thus lower the sensitivity of the study. As such, an assessment of background enhancement should be included in the breast MR imaging report. Background enhancement is described as none/minimal, mild, moderate, or marked (Fig. 1).

The amount of background enhancement does not necessarily correlate with the amount of parenchymal tissue. Mammographically dense breasts may have no or minimal background enhancement,

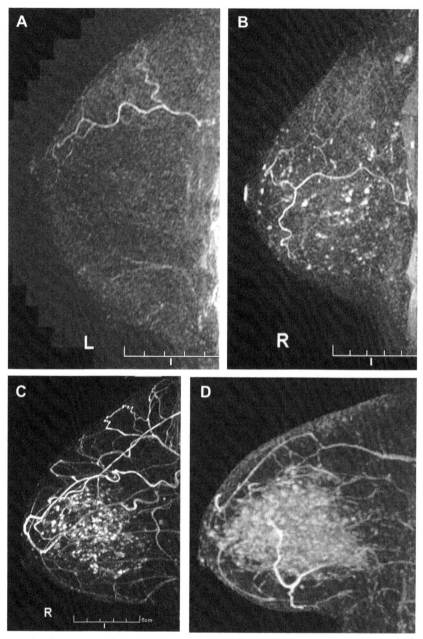

Fig. 1. Background enhancement. (*A*) None/minimal. (*B*) Mild background enhancement consisting of multiple scattered foci. (*C*) Moderate background enhancement with a diffusely stippled pattern. (*D*) Marked background enhancement that could potentially obscure a lesion.

whereas the parenchymal tissues in breasts with scattered fibroglandular densities can have striking enhancement.[10] In addition, there can be significant variations in degree of background enhancement throughout the menstrual cycle. Estrogen causes hyperemia, vasodilatation, and capillary leakiness.[11] This results in increased enhancement of the breast tissue during the first and last weeks of the menstrual cycle, when estrogen is at its peak. Hormonally related parenchymal enhancement can be diffuse, patchy, or focal and nodular, and can sometimes mimic a mass.[11,12] Benign parenchymal enhancement usually shows persistent or plateau curves, but sometimes washout curves can also be seen. To minimize limitations caused by excessive background enhancement, breast

MR imaging should be performed during the second and third weeks of the menstrual cycle when possible.

Background enhancement would also be expected to be increased by other hormonal influences such as hormone replacement therapy and lactation.[13-15] Tamoxifen therapy would be expected to decrease enhancement.[16] Radiation treatment has been shown to cause parenchyma edema and increased enhancement for at least 3 months following completion of radiation.[17]

MORPHOLOGIC EVALUATION

Lesions are assigned to 1 of 3 categories: mass, foci, or non-masslike enhancement.

Masses

The mass category in the MR imaging lexicon is generally the most easily understood, being similar to the mass category in the mammography lexicon. Masses are space-occupying lesions. They have definable shape and definable margins. As such, they may distort or displace the normal breast parenchyma. They may also have different precontrast T1 signal, and therefore may be visible on noncontrast images. Masses always represent pathologic processes, but are not always neoplastic.

Masses are described by shape and margins. Shape may be round, oval, lobular, or irregular (Figs. 2–5). Lobular masses have gently undulating contours. Any mass that cannot be described as round, oval, or lobular is considered irregular. Mass margins may be described as smooth, speculated, or irregular. The term spiculated refers to fine hairlike projections radiating away from the lesion, and is analogous to spiculated margins on mammography. Any margin that cannot be described as smooth or spiculated is described as irregular. A mass with irregular shape and irregular margins would simply be called an irregular mass. In concordance with the mammography lexicon, round or oval masses with smooth margins are more likely to be benign, whereas irregular masses or masses with spiculated margins are more likely to be malignant.

Margins should be evaluated on the first postcontrast series. This is the series on which background parenchymal enhancement should be at its minimum, whereas cancers would be expected to show maximum enhancement. Therefore, the mass margin, which forms the boundary between these 2 tissues, is best defined on this series.

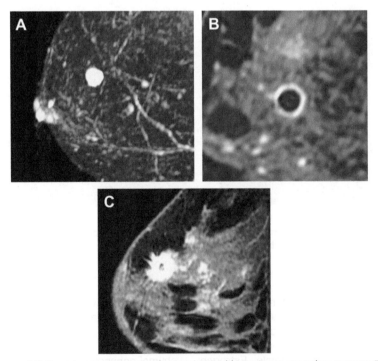

Fig. 2. Round masses. (A) Round mass with smooth margins and homogeneous enhancement. This mass showed persistent kinetics and underwent imaging follow-up with 1-year stability. (B) Cyst with thin uniform rim enhancement. (C) Round mass (invasive ductal carcinoma) with spiculated margins and central necrosis. Associated clumped NMLE suspicious for DCIS.

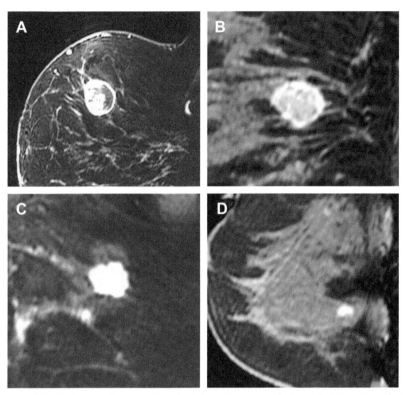

Fig. 3. Oval masses. (A) Triple negative invasive ductal carcinoma with smooth margins and rim and central enhancement. (B) Poorly differentiated invasive ductal carcinoma with irregular margins and rim enhancement. (C) Invasive ductal carcinoma with irregular margins and homogeneous enhancement. (D) Fibroadenoma with smooth margins and homogeneous enhancement.

The resolution of MR imaging is lower than that of mammography. Therefore, some masses that have finely spiculated or indistinct margins on mammography may appear smooth on MR imaging. The negative predictive value of smooth margins is therefore not as high for MR imaging as it is for mammography.

Unique to the MR imaging lexicon is the description of mass internal enhancement. Enhancement may be homogeneous, with smooth uniform enhancement throughout the mass, or heterogeneous, with some areas of the mass enhancing to a greater degree than others, or not at all. Not surprisingly, homogeneous enhancement is more suggestive of a benign lesion, whereas heterogeneous enhancement is more suggestive of a malignant lesion. However, small masses with truly heterogeneous enhancement may appear homogeneous because of resolution limitations. There are also 4 descriptors for more specific enhancement patterns: dark internal septations, enhancing septations, central enhancement, and rim enhancement. Dark internal septations were previously considered virtually pathognomonic of fibroadenomas with a positive predictive value

(PPV) of up to 98%, and were seen in approximately 50% of fibroadenomas (see **Fig. 4**B).[18,19] The septations were felt to correlate with thin collagenous bands within the lesion.[19] However, in a more recent study by Schnall and colleageus[8] 8 of 17 masses with dark internal septations were cancers (see **Fig. 4**C). Dark septations can also be seen in phyllodes tumors and cancers. Rim enhancement is the enhancement descriptor with the highest likelihood of malignancy. However, rim enhancement has a differential diagnosis and can also be seen commonly in fat necrosis. Thin, uniform rim enhancement is a frequent feature of cysts (**Fig. 6**). Breast abscesses can also show rim enhancement. Enhancing internal septations and central enhancement are both features suggestive of malignancy.[20]

In 2002, Liberman and colleagues[21] published a study evaluating the PPV for the lexicon descriptors. They retrospectively assigned lexicon descriptors to 100 lesions, all of which had no known mammographic or sonographic correlates, and all of which were excised. The descriptors with the highest PPVs were spiculated margins, rim enhancement, and irregular shape. When a lesion

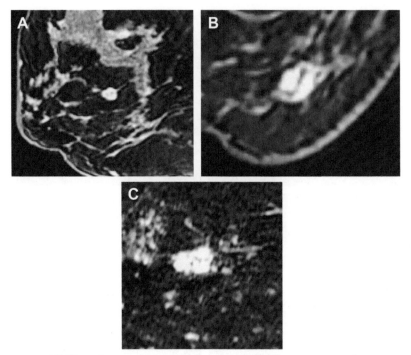

Fig. 4. Lobular masses. (*A*) Fibroadenoma with smooth margins and heterogeneous enhancement. (*B*) Fibroadenoma with smooth margins and dark internal septations. (*C*) Invasive ductal carcinoma with irregular margins and dark septations.

had spiculated margins, 80% of the time it was cancer. When a lesion had rim enhancement, 40% of the time it was cancer. Seventeen percent of lesions with smooth margins were cancers. Although spiculated margins and rim enhancement had a higher PPV for cancer, cancers more frequently had irregular margins and heterogeneous enhancement. This study was limited by relatively low numbers. The same group later published a study evaluating the MR imaging features of mammographically occult invasive cancers.[22] The most common features of invasive cancers presenting as masses were irregular margins (66%) and heterogeneous enhancement (59%). There were equal percentages of washout and plateau kinetics (48%). Among these masses, 10% had smooth margins, 3% had dark septations, and 3% had persistent kinetics.

In a larger study that included 995 biopsied lesions considered suspicious on conventional imaging or clinical examination, Schnall and colleagues[8] evaluated the predictive values of lesion features. They found that for masses, the single feature most predictive of malignancy was margin status. Qualitative evaluation of delayed phase curve shape showed greater predictive value than enhancement rate. Rim enhancement was also highly correlated with malignancy but only present in a small fraction of masses.

In a more recent study, Gutierrez and colleagues[23] performed statistical analysis of 258 lesions identified on MR imaging and determined malignancy risks associated with BI-RADS descriptors. All lesions were considered suspicious from their MR imaging features and underwent biopsy. There were higher odds of malignancy for masses greater than 1 cm, lobular or irregular shape, irregular or spiculated margins, and heterogeneous or rim enhancement. There were lower odds of malignancy for masses less than 1 cm, and masses with smooth margins or homogeneous enhancement. The highest probability of malignancy (68%) was for masses 1 cm or larger in size with irregular margins and heterogeneous enhancement. The lowest probability of malignancy (3%) was for masses 1 cm or less in size with smooth margins and homogeneous enhancement.

When assessing masses with suspicious features, lesion morphology should take precedence over kinetics. A spiculated or irregular mass should be viewed with suspicion regardless of kinetics. When masses have benign features such as oval shape and smooth margins, kinetics plays more of a role. For example, a smooth oval mass with persistent kinetics may be considered probably benign, whereas a smooth oval mass with washout kinetics may deserve biopsy.

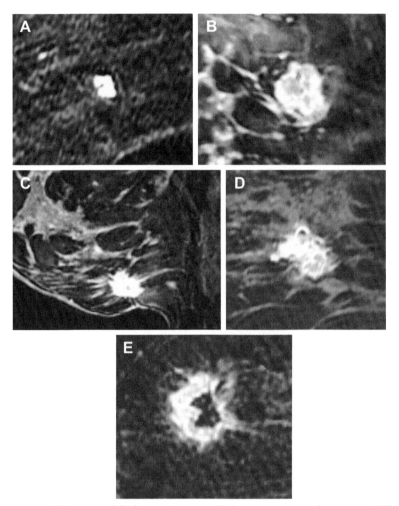

Fig. 5. Irregular masses. (*A*) Invasive lobular carcinoma with homogeneous enhancement. (*B*) Invasive ductal carcinoma with irregular margins and enhancing septations. (*C*) Invasive ductal carcinoma with spiculated margins. (*D*) Invasive ductal carcinoma with irregular margins and enhancing septations as well as central enhancement. (*E*) Invasive ductal carcinoma with irregular and spiculated margins and rim enhancement.

Foci

In contrast to masses, foci are not space-occupying lesions. They have no mass effect or corresponding abnormality on precontrast images. According to the lexicon, foci are small dots of enhancement less than 5 mm in size with no definable shape. They are too small for accurate assessment of margins and internal enhancement features. Foci may be solitary or multiple. When multiple, they should be separated by fat or normal glandular tissue. Foci are not necessarily pathologic and probably frequently represent normal glandular enhancement (**Fig. 7**). In 1 study evaluating the probability of malignancy based on size,[24] only 1 of 37 biopsied lesions (3%) less than 5 mm proved to be cancer. In the more recent study by Gutierrez and colleagues,[23] 6 of 40 (15%)

lesions less than 5 mm in size were cancers on biopsy. However, the investigators indicate that the population of foci from which biopsies were taken in this study likely represented a subset of lesions with suspicious features such as rim enhancement or spiculated margins. Likewise, in the former study, the population of foci evaluated represented lesions considered suspicious enough for biopsy. In a separate study by the same group[25] only 1 cancer occurred among 120 foci that had been assigned a BI-RADS category 3. That focus showed washout delayed-phase kinetics. There were no cancers among 69 foci with purely persistent kinetics. Therefore, the true likelihood of cancer in any given focus remains unclear and probably depends on its morphologic and kinetic features, but is still likely to be very low.

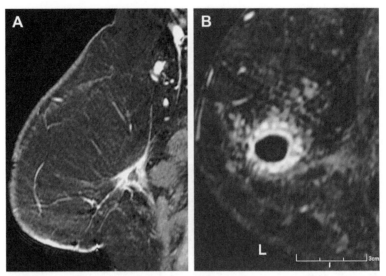

Fig. 6. (*A*) Rim-enhancing fat necrosis in a patient after transverse rectus abdominis muscle flap. (*B*) Inflamed cyst with thick rim enhancement.

The degree of suspicion of a focus also depends heavily on the clinical scenario. Foci that occur in premenopausal patients, particularly when multiple and bilateral, will be much less concerning than solitary foci in postmenopausal patients, particularly when a known cancer is present in the ipsilateral breast. The appearance of a new focus in a postmenopausal patient should also be cause for concern.

Non-masslike Enhancement

The non-masslike enhancement (NMLE) category is analogous to the calcification category in the mammography lexicon. As with calcifications, NMLE is described by morphology (internal enhancement pattern) and distribution. The distribution modifiers can be grouped according to whether they describe patterns reminiscent of ducts and their territories, or patterns more reminiscent of glandular tissue. The duct group consists of ductal, segmental, and linear enhancement (**Figs. 8–10**). Ductal enhancement has shape and positioning similar to a duct. It should be linear, and may or may not branch. It should have an anterior to posterior orientation, pointing toward the nipple anteriorly, and toward the chest wall posteriorly. Segmental enhancement follows the distribution of 1 or more ducts and their branches, usually with a more filled-in appearance, giving it a roughly pyramidal shape with the apex pointing toward the nipple and the base toward the chest wall. The distinction between ductal and segmental enhancement may not always be clear, but differentiating between the 2 is likely not critical, as both features indicate a high suspicion for malignancy. Linear enhancement is enhancement forming a line or sheet, but not necessarily with the orientation of a duct. It may be more transversely or vertically oriented. As such, linear enhancement is not as clearly within a duct as ductal enhancement, and is usually less suspicious.

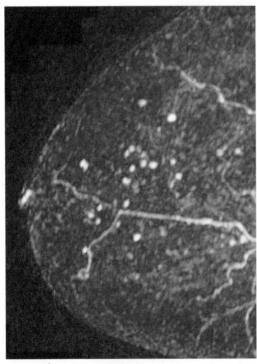

Fig. 7. Multiple scattered foci.

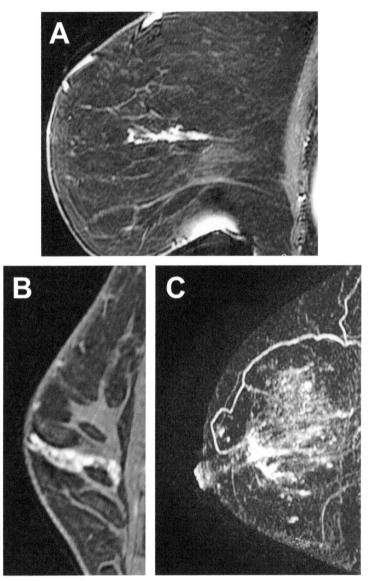

Fig. 8. NMLE with ductal distribution. (*A*) Clumped enhancement in ductal distribution as a result of mucinous carcinoma with low to intermediate-grade DCIS. (*B*) Clumped enhancement in ductal distribution representing DCIS. (*C*) Homogeneous enhancement in ductal distribution with branching. Excisional biopsy demonstrated papillary changes.

The glandular group consists of a focal area of enhancement, regional enhancement, multiple regions of enhancement, and diffuse enhancement. A focal area is the smallest within this group. A focal area of enhancement occupies less than 25% of a quadrant (**Fig. 11**). Regional enhancement covers a larger area, not necessarily corresponding to the distribution of a ductal system (**Fig. 12**). Two or more areas of regional enhancement separated by fat or normal glandular tissue is categorized as multiple regions of enhancement. Diffuse enhancement is enhancement evenly distributed throughout the breast. As with

calcifications, regional and diffuse enhancement are descriptors more commonly associated with benign processes than malignancies. When evaluating NMLE, in particular regional and diffuse enhancement, symmetry is important (**Fig. 13**). Asymmetry should increase the level of concern for malignancy, whereas symmetry can usually confirm the benign nature of an area of NMLE.

Descriptors for internal enhancement are also used for NMLE. As with masses, internal enhancement can be homogeneous or heterogeneous. In addition there are 3 more specific patterns: clumped, stippled/punctuate, and reticular/dendritic. Clumped

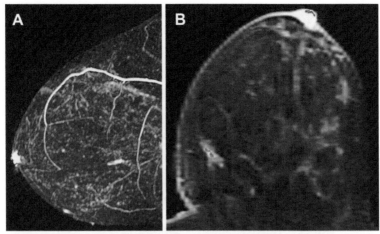

Fig. 9. Linear enhancement. Maximum intensity projection image on core biopsy guided by MR imaging and subsequent excision showed benign breast tissue. The lesion was gone at follow-up.

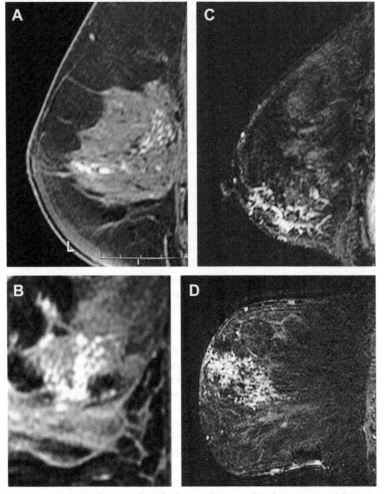

Fig. 10. NMLE with segmental distribution. (A, B) Clumped internal enhancement. (C) Reticular and clumped internal enhancement as a result of high-grade DCIS with invasive ductal carcinoma. (D) Heterogeneous internal enhancement representing intermediate-grade DCIS with atypical ductal hyperplasia.

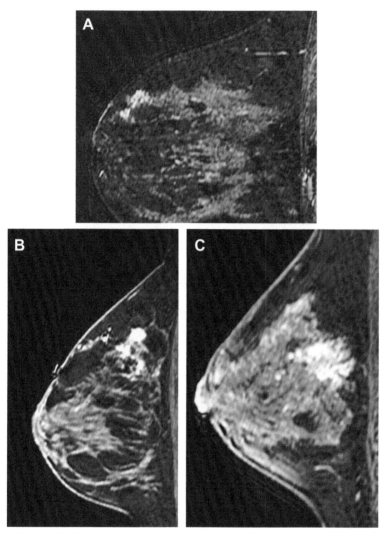

Fig. 11. Focal area NMLE. (*A*) Stippled internal enhancement. (*B*) Clumped internal enhancement representing invasive ductal carcinoma and high-grade DCIS. (*C*) Heterogeneous internal enhancement as a result of invasive ductal carcinoma.

enhancement refers to a close grouping of rounded areas of enhancement, sometimes referred to as a cobblestone pattern (see **Fig. 8**A, B). This pattern is highly suspicious for malignancy. Stippled/punctate enhancement refers to multiple tiny, closely associated dots of enhancement, usually throughout a large area and not conforming to a duct or ducts. This pattern has been increasingly recognized as corresponding to normal glandular tissue or fibrocystic change.[26] The reticular/dendritic pattern is probably the least well understood and least used (see **Fig. 10**C). This is a pattern that one would expect to see in breasts that have undergone involutional changes, with the remaining parenchyma forming thin strands interspersed by fat. In the reticular/dendritic pattern, these strands have become abnormally thickened and distorted, reminiscent

of irregular septal thickening in the lungs at high-resolution chest computed tomography. The reticular dendritic pattern has also been associated with inflammatory carcinoma.[20]

When malignancies present as NMLE, the primary differential diagnosis is between ductal carcinoma in situ (DCIS) and invasive lobular carcinoma.[10] DCIS is by definition not invasive and therefore does not necessarily cause significant tumor angiogenesis. It is not surprising therefore that DCIS has shown variable kinetic patterns and is more likely to show slow or persistent enhancement than invasive ductal carcinoma.[27,28] Similarly, lobular carcinoma generally infiltrates in a single-file pattern without significant desmoplastic reaction and may not cause significant tumor angiogenesis. Thus, these cancers are not

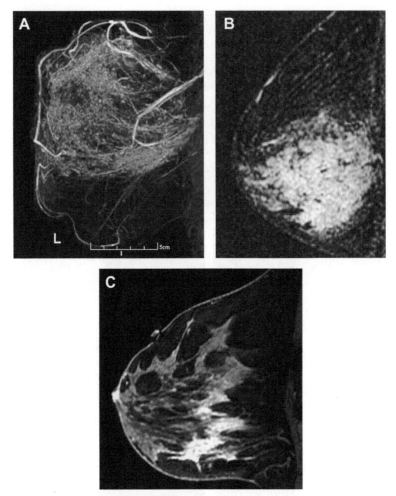

Fig. 12. NMLE with regional distribution. (*A*) Regionally distributed NMLE in a patient with mastitis. This resolved after treatment. (*B*) Regional NMLE with homogeneous internal enhancement in a patient with a large invasive ductal carcinoma. (*C*) Regional benign parenchymal enhancement.

expected to produce rapid enhancement or washout curves[28–30]; therefore, when evaluating NMLE, kinetics may be less important than they are in the setting of masses. NMLE, even with slow enhancement, should be viewed with suspicion in the setting of suspicious distribution and morphologic features.

In the study by Liberman and colleagues[21] the types of non-masslike enhancement with the highest PPV for carcinoma were segmental enhancement (PPV 67%) and clumped linear/ductal enhancement (PPV 31%). Regional enhancement had a PPV of 21%. Schnall and colleagues[8] reported that distribution was the most predictive NMLE feature. Ductal enhancement had a 58.5% likelihood of malignancy, segmental enhancement had a 78% likelihood of malignancy, and regional enhancement

had a 21% likelihood of malignancy. Malignancy rates for internal enhancement patterns were: stippled, 25%; heterogeneous, 53%; clumped, 60%; homogeneous, 67%.

A few studies have looked specifically at ductal and segmental enhancement with somewhat variable PPVs observed. Liberman and colleagues[31] evaluated 88 NMLE lesions classified as ductal and found a PPV of 26%. They found a "trend toward higher frequency of carcinoma" with clumped enhancement, with 35% of lesions with clumped enhancement representing cancer. The likelihood of cancer was not affected by kinetic pattern or lesion size. Morakkabati-Spitz and colleagues[32] reported a PPV of linear or segmental enhancement of 34%. Seventy-one percent of DCIS cases in the study showed linear or

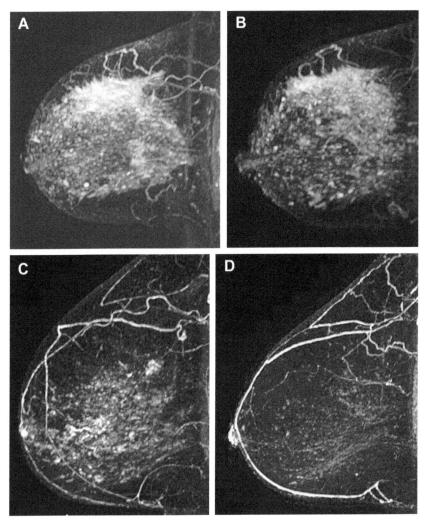

Fig. 13. Importance of symmetry in NMLE. (*A, B*) Bilateral symmetric NMLE in regional distribution, compatible with benign glandular enhancement (*A*, left breast; *B*, right breast). (*C, D*) Asymmetric, heterogeneous regional enhancement in a patient with extensive invasive adenocarcinoma (*C*, left breast; *D*, right breast).

segmental enhancement. All invasive cancers in that study presented as masses rather than NMLE.

Two studies have looked specifically at the lexicon descriptors associated with DCIS. Rosen and colleagues[33] evaluated 64 cases of DCIS. DCIS presented as NMLE much more commonly than invasive cancer (59.4% vs 15.8%). The most common distributions were segmental (42.4%) and focal areas (33.3%). The most common internal enhancement pattern was clumped (51.5%). In a study of 79 pure DCIS lesions, Jansen and colleagues[27] found the most common lesion type was NMLE (81%). Segmental and linear were the most common distributions (33% and 24%, respectively). Clumped was the most common internal enhancement pattern (41%).

PROBABLY BENIGN LESIONS

In most of the studies referred to in this article, the lesions evaluated were all from biopsies and were considered suspicious either from the MR imaging features, or from their features on conventional imaging or clinical examination. Thus, inclusion of those lesions that are considered benign or probably benign at MR interpretation based on their MR features could change the PPVs for the features described earlier. The BI-RADS MR imaging lexicon does not describe specific lesion characteristics that allow assignment of a BI-RADS 3 category. Instead, it states that this should be determined on an "intuitive" basis.[26] Furthermore, criteria for probably benign lesions on mammography cannot necessarily be transferred to MR imaging.[34] This stems, at least in part, from resolution differences between the 2 imaging modalities, as well as the additional information regarding lesion enhancement available with MR imaging.

Several studies have addressed the frequency of malignancy in lesions considered probably benign with somewhat variable cancer rates ranging from 0.6% to 10%.[25] Liberman and colleagues[34] found no statistically significant reliable features that resulted in a less than a 2% chance of malignancy. However, lesions with persistent kinetics and multiple, bilateral round or oval masses had the lowest frequency of subsequent malignancy. Eby and colleagues[25] evaluated lexicon features of 362 lesions considered probably benign, and concluded that foci with 100% persistent enhancement could be considered benign. However, they too give no specific criteria for probably benign lesions. This is an area in which further research is necessary.

ASSOCIATED FINDINGS

Associated findings (**Box 1**) describe secondary signs of cancer that can increase the suspicion of a lesion. These include skin or nipple retraction and skin thickening. They also include findings that can change the staging or surgical management of a cancer: lymphadenopathy, pectoralis or chest wall invasion, nipple invasion, and skin invasion. There are additional descriptors in this category that describe specific benign conditions: hematoma/blood products, precontrast high-duct signal (because of proteinaceous fluid within the

duct), cyst, and abnormal signal void (frequently indicating artifact from a tissue marker).

SUMMARY

The breast MR imaging lexicon has furthered the standardization of breast MR imaging. By providing standard descriptors, the lexicon clarifies reporting of breast MR imaging findings and facilitates lesion management and patient care.

REFERENCES

1. Turkbey B, Kobayashi H, Ogawa M, et al. Imaging of tumor angiogenesis: functional or targeted. AJR Am J Roentgenol 2006;193:304–13.
2. Papetti M, Herman IM. Mechanisms of normal and tumor derived angiogenesis. Am J Physiol Cell Physiol 2002;282:947–70.
3. Kuhl CK. Dynamic breast magnetic resonance imaging. In: Breast MRI: diagnosis and intervention. New York: Liberman and Morris; 2005:7. p. 79–139.
4. Morris EA. Breast MR imaging lexicon updated. Magn Reson Imaging Clin N Am 2006;14(3):293–303.
5. Wang LC, Demartini WB, Partridge SC, et al. MRI-detected suspicious breast lesions: predictive values of kinetic features measured by computer-aided evaluation. AJR Am J Roentgenol 2009;193:826–31.
6. Buadu LD, Murakami J, Murayama A, et al. Breast lesions: correlation of contrast medium enhancement patterns on MR images histopathologic findings and tumor angiogenesis. Radiology 1996;200: 639–49.
7. Kuhl CK, Mielcareck P, Klaschik S, et al. Dynamic breast MR imaging; a signal intensity time course data useful for differential diagnosis of enhancing lesions? Radiology 1999;211:101–10.
8. Schnall MD, Blume J, Bluemke DA, et al. Diagnostic architectural and dynamic features at breast MR imaging: multicenter study. Radiology 2006;238: 42–53.
9. Macure KJ, Ouwerkerk R, Jacobs MA, et al. Patterns of enhancement on breast MR images: interpretation and imaging pitfalls. Radiographics 2006;26:1719–34.
10. Kuhl C. The current status of breast MR imaging Part I. choice of technique, image interpretation, diagnostic accuracy, and transfer to clinical practice. Radiology 2007;244:356–78.
11. Morris EA. The normal breast. In: Breast MRI: diagnosis and intervention. New York: Liberman and Morris; 2005:4. p. 23–44.
12. Kuhl CK, Bieling HB, Gieseke J, et al. Healthy premenopausal breast parenchyma in dynamic contrast-enhanced MR imaging of the breast: normal contrast medium enhancement and cyclical-phase dependency. Radiology 1997;203:137.

Box 1
Associated findings

Nipple retraction or inversion

Precontrast high-duct signal

Skin retraction

Skin thickening

Skin invasion

Edema

Lymphadenopathy

Pectoralis muscle invasion

Chest wall invasion

Hematoma/blood

Abnormal signal void

Cyst

13. Talele AC, Slanetz PJ, Edmister WB, et al. The lactating breast: MRI findings and literature review. Breast J 2003;9(3):237–40.

14. Delille JP, Slanetz JS, Yeh ED, et al. Hormone replacement therapy in postmenopausal women: breast tissue perfusion determined with MR imaging – initial observations. Radiology 2005;235:36–41.

15. Espinosa LA, Daniel BL, Vidarsson L, et al. The lactating breast: contrast-enhanced MR imaging of normal tissue and cancer. Radiology 2005;237:429–36.

16. Heinig A, Lampe D, Kolbi H, et al. Suppression of unspecific enhancement on breast magnetic resonance imaging (MRI) by antiestrogen medication. Tumori 2002;88(3):215–23.

17. Morakkabati N, Leutner CC, Schmiedel A, et al. Breast MR imaging during or soon after radiation therapy. Radiology 2003;229:893–901.

18. Nunes LW, Schnall MD, Orel SG. Update of breast MR interpretation model. Radiology 2001;219:484–94.

19. Hochman MG, Orel SG, Powell CM, et al. Fibroadenomas: MR imaging appearances with radiologic-histopathologic correlation. Radiology 1997;204:123.

20. Erguvan-Dogan B, Whitman GJ, Kushwaha AC, et al. Bi-RADS-MRI: a primer. AJR Am J Roentgenol 2006;187:W152–60.

21. Liberman L, Morris EA, Lee MJ, et al. Breast lesions detected on MR imaging; features and positive predictive value. AJR Am J Roentgenol 2002;179:171–8.

22. Bartella L, Liberman L, Morris EA, et al. Nonpalpable mammographically occult invasive breast cancers detected by MRI. AJR Am J Roentgenol 2006;186:865–70.

23. Gutierrez RL, DeMartini WB, Eby PR, et al. Bi-RADS lesion characteristics predict likelihood of malignancy in breast MRI for masses but not for nonmass-like enhancement. AJR Am J Roentgenol 2009;193:994–1000.

24. Liberman L, Mason G, Morris EA, et al. Does size matter? Positive predictive value of MRI-detected breast lesions as a function of size. AJR Am J Roentgenol 2006;186:426–30.

25. Eby PR, DeMartini WB, Gutierrez RL, et al. Characteristics of probably benign breast MRI lesions. AJR Am J Roentgenol 2009;193:861–7.

26. Ikeda DM, Hylton NM, Kuhl CK. Breast Imaging Reporting and Data System, BiRADS: magnetic resonance imaging. Reston (VA): ACR; 2003.

27. Jansen SA, Newstead GM, Abe H, et al. Pure ductal carcinoma in situ: kinetic and morphologic MR characteristic compared with mammographic appearance and nuclear grade. Radiology 2007;245(3):684–91.

28. Kuhl CK. Concepts for differential diagnosis in breast MR imaging. Magn Reson Imaging Clin N Am 2006;14(3):305–37.

29. Qayyum A, Birdwell RL, Daniel BL, et al. MR imaging features of infiltrating lobular carcinoma of the breast: histopathologic correlation. AJR Am J Roentgenol 2002;178:1227–32.

30. Yeh ED, Slanetz PJ, Edmister WB, et al. Invasive lobular carcinoma: spectrum of enhancement and morphology on magnetic resonance imaging. Breast J 2003;9:13–8.

31. Liberman L, Morris EA, Dershaw DD, et al. Ductal enhancement on MR imaging of the breast. AJR Am J Roentgenol 2003;181:519–25.

32. Morakkabati-Spitz N, Leutner C, Schild H. Diagnostic usefulness of linear and segmental enhancement in dynamic breast MRI. Eur Radiol 2005;14:2010–7.

33. Rosen EL, Smith-Foley SA, DeMartini WB, et al. Bi-RADS MRI enhancement characteristics of ductal carcinoma in situ. Breast J 2007;13(6):545–55.

34. Liberman L, Morris EA, Benton CL, et al. Probably benign lesions at breast magnetic resonance imaging: preliminary experience in high-risk women. Cancer 2003;98(2):377–88.

Implementing a Breast MR Imaging Program: All Things Considered

Sughra Raza, MD[a,b,*]

KEYWORDS

- Breast MR imaging • Magnet selection
- Program development

Contrast-enhanced breast magnetic resonance (MR) imaging has been used as an imaging tool for detection of breast cancer for well over 15 years, with reported sensitivities in the range of 83% to 100% and specificities ranging from 29% to 100%. MR imaging provides not only anatomic and morphologic information but also indirectly reflects functional characteristics by imaging the dynamics of blood flow within lesions. Both features are important in the analysis of enhancing lesions. A 1998 study[1] showed that based on qualitative morphologic analysis alone the sensitivity and specificity of breast MR imaging were 83% and 54%, respectively, whereas quantitative analysis alone showed a sensitivity of 83% and specificity of 66%. Combining morphologic assessment with quantitative analysis improved sensitivity to 93% and specificity to 74%, with considerably higher overall accuracy. Therefore, a major challenge in breast imaging has been to achieve high-resolution anatomic imaging while performing the necessary sequences rapidly enough to document the dynamic enhancement kinetics of masses and nonmass-like lesions.

This has been made possible by technical developments that allow high enough spatial resolution for detailed morphologic assessment and more accurate plotting of the time-intensity curves within the short period of time when breast tumors usually reach peak contrast enhancement and undergo washout. Breast MR imaging is now a well-established and widely accepted imaging modality for breast cancer detection and monitoring, with increasing demand for the examination. A 2008 survey[2] of radiology practices in the United States showed that contrast-enhanced breast MR imaging was offered at 74% of 754 surveyed practices, the majority performing less than 20 examinations per week. Mammography Quality Standards Act–accredited radiologists supervised and interpreted breast MR imaging examinations in most facilities. The majority of practices offered screening breast MR imaging and performed MR-guided interventional procedures, and half reported that interpretation was performed with computer-aided detection. It is highly likely that more and more radiology practices will add breast MR imaging and will offer screening and diagnostic or problem-solving MR imaging.

AMERICAN COLLEGE OF RADIOLOGY BI-RADS LEXICON

Widespread breast MR imaging has been greatly aided by the standardization of imaging protocols, interpretation, and reporting, which has been possible largely because of the American College of Radiology (ACR) Breast Imaging Reporting And Data System (BI-RADS) lexicon, developed specifically for breast MR imaging and published in the fourth edition of the BI-RADS manual in 2003.[3,4] The BI-RADS standards provide guidelines for imaging and interpretation criteria and a common language for clear and concise communication.[5,6]

INDICATIONS FOR BREAST MR IMAGING

Further validation for breast MR imaging was provided in 2007, when the American Cancer

[a] Department of Radiology, Brigham & Women's Hospital, 75 Francis Street, Boston, MA 02115, USA
[b] Harvard Medical School, Boston, MA, USA
* Department of Radiology, Brigham & Women's Hospital, 75 Francis Street, Boston, MA 02115.
E-mail address: sraza1@partners.org

Magn Reson Imaging Clin N Am 18 (2010) 187–198
doi:10.1016/j.mric.2010.02.010
1064-9689/10/$ – see front matter © 2010 Elsevier Inc. All rights reserved.

Society (ACS) published newly expanded guidelines specifying indications for breast MR imaging, including screening for women at high risk (20%–25% lifetime risk), tumor staging, and treatment monitoring.[7] These revised guidelines are based on newer evidence that became available since 2003, which was collected and reviewed by a panel of experts who developed recommendations for women at different defined levels of risk to help identify patients for whom breast MR imaging should be recommended. The ACR supports these guidelines (www.acr.org), and these are detailed elsewhere.

It is likely that the group of women at high risk for breast cancer will benefit from screening with MR imaging, as cancers may be found at an earlier stage, and this will lead to reduction in mortality. Moreover, some experts believe that because of its almost 10 times higher sensitivity, MR imaging will likely replace mammography as the screening modality of choice in high- and intermediate-risk women in the not too distant future.[8]

The role of breast MR imaging for surgical planning in patients with recently diagnosed breast cancer continues to be debated, as the cost/benefit ratio is not entirely clear. Those opposing this role of breast MR imaging believe that because of very high sensitivity, the false-positive rate in breast MR imaging raises the "cost" to an unacceptable level, leading to too many unnecessary mastectomies.[9,10] In a 2007 review Kuhl and colleagues[11] acknowledge that "arguments against the use of breast MR imaging include costs, frequency of false positive diagnoses, lack of availability of minimally invasive biopsy capabilities, lack of evidence by randomized controlled clinical trials, and, last, fear of overtreatment." However, because MR imaging is significantly superior to mammography and ultrasound (US) in detecting intraductal extension of invasive carcinoma, the benefits of preoperative staging MR imaging cannot be ignored. Kuhl and colleagues[11] suggest that rather than letting incidental and "false positive" findings automatically lead to mastectomy, the guidelines for when mastectomy is necessary could be modified as "some small MR imaging detected additional multicentric breast cancer foci will be sufficiently treated by radiation therapy."

Despite controversy and debate, the role of MR imaging in diagnostic and screening breast imaging continues to grow, and there is demand for additional facilities with the best possible equipment, with expert performance and interpretations. Keeping up with fast-changing technical developments while in the process of establishing a new breast MR imaging facility or expanding an existing one can be challenging.

This article attempts to address some of the issues that should be considered in the planning stages of such a facility, and draws attention to some important details of setting up an efficient and organized process for examination performance, interpretation, and reporting.

MAGNET SELECTION

Almost all of the reported literature in breast MR imaging is based on imaging performed on field strength magnets of 1.5 Tesla (T) or greater. More recently, clinical 3-T magnets have become available and are being used at academic institutions as well as in the private practice setting. The specific needs of a particular practice will help determine the optimal magnet. In a multispecialty radiology group, the needs of high-volume users such as neuroradiology, musculoskeletal radiology, and cardiac imaging must be taken into account, and input from colleagues in these specialties should be sought from the beginning. In such a group the advantages and disadvantages of 1.5- versus 3-T magnets in each subspecialty area of imaging would need to be determined.

On the other hand, for an exclusively breast imaging group, a dedicated breast imaging system could be considered. A dedicated system is designed to provide maximal patient comfort in the prone bilateral breast imaging coil, and some systems have an open design to address the not uncommon issue of claustrophobia. There is currently no dedicated breast magnet available at 3 T.

If the magnet is to be used for breast imaging only, financial feasibility to justify such an installation needs to be determined. Factors influencing the cost/benefit ratio of a system used for breast imaging only include the following: is the magnet in an inpatient or outpatient facility; is it to be housed in a newly constructed free-standing facility or in a preexisting space which is to be renovated; is the magnet being added to an existing imaging suite, thereby sharing the operating expenses such as personnel, supplies, utilities, overhead; and will the MR imaging facility be used for diagnostic breast imaging only or also for image-guided interventional procedures. These factors need to be balanced by projected breast imaging volumes. If MR imaging-directed interventional procedures will be performed, not only will the appropriate biopsy-capable breast coils be essential, but the facility will need to be designed to accommodate all other necessary equipment. Whether only diagnostic imaging or interventional procedures also are performed at a free-standing outpatient facility, patient safety mechanisms for emergency situations such as contrast reactions or complications of interventional procedures should be worked out in advance and put in place.

SELECTING MAGNET STRENGTH
Current Status of Breast Imaging at 1.5 T

Breast imaging is inherently challenging because of the need to image both breasts repeatedly over a short time period. As mentioned earlier, high spatial resolution is necessary to assess morphologic features of benign and malignant tumors, whether these are seen as masses or areas of nonmass enhancement. In the case of masses, margins are the most reliable predictors of benign versus malignant pathology,[12,13] and detailed and reproducible margin assessment is best performed on high-resolution images with in-plane spatial resolution less than 1 mm. Because tumor neoangiogenesis is the basis of breast cancer detection on MR imaging, dynamic scanning is essential to evaluate the arterial and venous phases of tumors. To achieve this, it is necessary to image both breasts before contrast administration and then repeatedly and rapidly after contrast is given. In this way images are obtained during the arterial phase to demonstrate the rate of contrast uptake by the tumor, and repeat scans over the next 7 to 8 minutes allow demonstration of the delayed phase or washout characteristics. Most breast cancers have rapid uptake of contrast and, due to the presence of

abnormal tumor vessels, also show rapid washout, which can be reflected by the dynamic sequences.

Fat is seen in MR imaging as very high signal, which can mask enhancement of fibroglandular tissue and of abnormal masses. Historically, this problem has been addressed in the United States by applying fat suppression pulses that render the fat signal null. In Europe, subtraction of the precontrast series from identical postcontrast series has been used to cancel out the signal from fat. Although the latter technique has the advantage that there is no loss of signal, it can be problematic if the patient moves during the dynamic scans causing misregistration, which can lead to the appearance of falsely "enhancing" lesions or nonvisualization of truly enhancing areas. Chemically selective fat suppression is best achieved in a homogeneous magnetic field. At intermediate and low field strength field homogeneity is suboptimal, resulting in uneven fat suppression and image degradation (**Fig. 1**).

At 1.5 T there are well-established and carefully optimized breast imaging protocols using 3-dimensional gradient-echo sequences, with improved signal to noise ratio (SNR), decreased slice thickness (<1 mm), high in-plane resolution of less than 1 mm × 1 mm, shorter acquisition times caused by decreased repetition time (TR)/echo time (TE) (1–2 minutes), and bilateral full coverage, using parallel imaging sequences.[14,15] All these factors ultimately provide breast MR imaging scans with high spatial and temporal resolution, so that detailed morphologic analysis can be performed without sacrificing the ability to characterize enhancement kinetics. Because

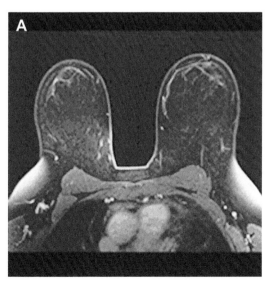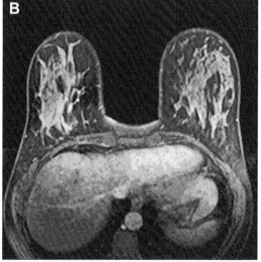

Fig. 1. Homogeneous and adequate fat saturation is necessary to visualize anatomic structures in the axillary regions. Poor fat saturation in the axillae is seen in (*A*) and more optimal fat saturation in (*B*).

there is a linear relationship between magnet strength and SNR, higher field strength such as at 3 T would theoretically provide images of very high spatial resolution. However, in the typical clinical setting the gain in SNR is offset by several technical modifications necessary to obtain quality images in the higher magnetic field. These factors include adjustment of the TR and flip angles, and modification of protocols to keep tissue heating (specific absorption ratio), dielectric effects, and B_1 field inhomogeneities within reasonable limits.

Although there is a paucity of literature comparing diagnostic clarity and accuracy of breast MR imaging using 1.5-T and 3-T magnets, and no definitive evidence has yet been reported that imaging on the higher field strength is more sensitive or accurate, there is increasing evidence that imaging at 3 T is at least as good as at 1.5 T. Specific applications such as MR spectroscopy and diffusion-weighted imaging may prove to be better performed on the higher strength magnet. In 2006 Kuhl and colleagues[16] reported that "differential diagnosis of enhancing lesions is possible with higher diagnostic confidence at 3 T MR imaging." However, the same group then published concerns about limited contrast enhancement at 3 T, saying that "due to spatial B_1 inhomogeneities across the field of view, enhancement of lesions may be reduced to a variable degree."[17] In a response to these concerns, Mountford and colleagues[18] emphasized the importance of protocol design and technique in optimizing the performance of breast MR imaging at 3.0 T, and suggested that the issue of field inhomogeneity can be compensated for by adjusting other parameters in the system.

Advantages at 3 T

The most significant inherent advantage of the higher strength magnet is improved signal strength which, at 3 T is about twice that of a 1.5-T magnet. This higher signal strength provides higher SNR and allows performance of examinations with thinner slices, providing higher in-plane resolution. In addition, chemical shift effect scales in proportion to magnet field strength, doubling from 1.5 to 3 T, and providing improved fat suppression sequences as well as allowing better separation of metabolite peaks for spectroscopy. This finer analysis of the choline peak may provide the ability to distinguish invasive carcinoma from benign lesions and possibly from ductal carcinoma in situ, in vivo.[19,20] With higher signal strength there is also an associated higher susceptibility effect. This effect has clinical applicability in the improved fast spin echo sensitivity

to hemorrhage in certain modified protocols. Higher signal intensity may allow more detailed diffusion-weighted (DW) imaging. The potential role of DW imaging in characterization of breast masses has been studied in recent years. It is currently reported that apparent diffusion coefficient (ADC) values may be a valuable parameter in distinguishing benign from malignant masses. A recently published meta-analysis of 12 published studies evaluating ADC of breast tumors at 1.5 T revealed the pooled sensitivity and specificity to be 89% and 77%, respectively.[21] In contrast, a single-institution report of DW imaging of breast lesions at 3 T showed the sensitivity and specificity to be 95% and 91%, respectively.[22]

Challenges at 3 T

Image quality

The advantages of distinctly better SNR of a 3-T magnet for clinical imaging are balanced by several obstacles, namely higher radiofrequency deposition, increased tissue T1 relaxation times, dielectric resonances, stronger susceptibility effects, and larger chemical shift[23] (**Fig. 2**). To overcome these obstacles, attention to imaging protocol parameters is required. Radiofrequency deposition in tissues scales exponentially with increasing magnet strength, and causes tissue heating. This deposition of energy as heat is quantified as specific absorption ratio (SAR). The International Electrotechnical Commission (IEC) has established SAR limits for clinical examinations at 8 W/kg over 5 minutes or 4 W/kg for the whole body over 15 minutes. Imaging protocols at 3 T

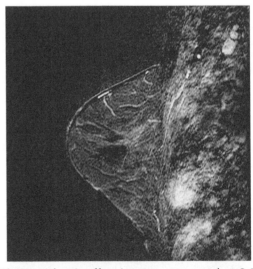

Fig. 2. Dielectric effect is more pronounced at 3 T field strength and is reflected as areas of shading on the image.

can be modified by adjusting the TR and TE to keep the SAR within acceptable limits.

Shading artifact is caused by variations of delivered radiofrequency pulses in a large field of view caused by B_0 inhomogeneity, and surface coil errors can result in B_1 inhomogeneity.

These issues as well as susceptibility artifacts, dielectric effects, and chemical shift artifacts can be addressed by the following modifications:

1. Careful choice of excitation flip angle and TR
2. Using 3-dimensional technique for gradient-echo acquisitions, and small field of view for gradient-echo acquisitions.[18]

Siting issues

Higher field strength magnets are proportionally more sensitive and therefore easily affected by their surroundings. Stationary ferromagnetic objects are less problematic, as their effect on the magnetic field is predictable and stable and therefore can be shielded against. A more difficult problem is caused by moving objects such as elevator banks or ambulance bays, as the effect on the magnetic field is randomly and frequently changing. Thus, placement of a magnet in the vicinity of an ambulance bay or a bank of elevators can have a significant effect on imaging unless minimum distances and/or adequate shielding are provided.

Stability of the ground on which the magnet sits is important. An MR imaging facility located on higher floors within a building may be subject to barely perceptible motion, which can degrade high-resolution imaging with micromotion artifacts, manifesting as image noise or blur. This artifact is more easily visible on images from higher strength magnets, therefore such magnets may be best situated either on the ground floor or a well-reinforced upper floor. Reinforcement for several floors below may be necessary to avoid such micromotion. Because proper siting is critical for optimal imaging results, the potential location for the magnet should be reviewed by engineers from the host institution as well as the manufacturer.

Coil selection

Most vendors manufacture their own breast imaging coils, but the systems are also compatible with coils made by other vendors. There are currently 4-, 7-, and 8-channel coils available on the market. A newer 16-channel bilateral breast surface coil with biopsy capability is also now available. An important consideration when choosing a coil is whether interventional procedures will be performed or not. Some coils are closed and do not allow access for core needle

biopsy or wire localization. At least one of the currently available 16-channel coils allows superior and inferior biopsy access in addition to the lateral and medial approach.

Patient safety and comfort at 3 T

Dizziness anecdotally is not uncommonly experienced by patients when getting up off the scanner and by technologists as they go in and out of the magnetic field, especially during MR-directed interventional procedures; however, scanning at 3 T is generally well tolerated.[24] More important is the issue of patient safety in this magnetic field. A larger number of patients may not safely enter the 3-T field because of the presence of metallic (copper) intrauterine devices (IUDs), certain kinds of stents, certain cochlear or penile implants, many orthopedic devices, and defibrillators. The 2009 Reference Manual for Magnetic Resonance Safety Implants and Devices has exhaustive lists of absolutely contraindicated devices and lists of devices for which caution is recommended.[25] This manual is compiled based on updated guidelines and recommendations from the peer-reviewed literature, including input from multiple national and international organizations.

In summary, breast MR imaging is well established on the 1.5-T magnets. Higher strength magnets should be selected for clinical imaging if there is interest and commitment to the development of newer techniques such as spectroscopy and DW imaging. The decision to install a higher strength magnet should be made with full awareness of the various challenges in siting and installation, protocols and sequences, patient safety issues, and the fact that it would be important to have a backup 1.5-T magnet for patients who cannot safely enter the higher magnetic field. The author's experience suggests that no matter which strength of magnet is selected, one should not expect a "plug and play" system to be delivered. Installation requires detailed calibration and testing.

INSTALLATION AND IMAGING READINESS

Having access to experienced and knowledgeable physicists and MR imaging technologists is absolutely critical in any breast MR imaging facility, but is especially important in the "ramping-up" stage that includes calibration, protocol testing, and establishment of routine protocols.

Once siting issues have been identified and resolved, and the exact location of the magnet installation has been decided, the magnet can be delivered. The arrival and "moving in" of this sizeable piece of equipment is involved and requires detailed preplanning. This scenario may require a street to be closed off during delivery in order for the magnet and crane to be brought in. Direct access to the street may require the creation of an opening in an outer wall (**Fig. 3**). In the author's case, disruption of the main breast imaging reading room occurred for many days. Alternative reading rooms and patient consultation areas had to be planned ahead of time.

Assembly and installation take several days, after which "ramping up" can begin. This procedure usually takes 3 to 5 weeks and includes activating the magnetic field, and ensuring its homogeneity and stability; this is followed by extensive calibrations, quality control steps, and phantom testing as well as sequence testing. The next step is to prepare the magnet for scanning readiness, which consists of protocol testing by a team of technologists, physicists, and engineers working with volunteers. To establish breast imaging protocols, the volunteers must agree to undergo scanning without and with intravenous contrast so that field homogeneity, fat suppression, motion artifacts, and spatial and temporal resolution can all be analyzed and optimized as necessary. The preferred breast surface coils also need to be put through all of the steps of testing. Input from MR physicists with experience in breast imaging and from dedicated breast MR technologists ("supertechs") who have experience and in-depth understanding of the issues specific to breast imaging is important. These people are the key experts in developing the best possible imaging techniques, building protocols, and tailoring sequences, often on an individual patient

basis. Such efforts will help optimize magnet time for each patient, and allow for the most efficient, useful, and diagnostically informative protocols.

REFERRAL BASE

Whether the breast MR imaging facility is a new addition to the practice or supplements previously existing breast MR imaging, it is beneficial to inform the referring doctors of the new service they can expect. This provision is well achieved through a letter succinctly describing the capabilities of the new magnet, the improvements in breast imaging this will provide, a summary of the current ACS/ACR guidelines and accepted indications for breast MR imaging, and the process for requesting such an examination for their patients, including web links and telephone numbers. A consultation hot line is always helpful if personnel and resources are available to offer this service to referring clinicians, being particularly useful for times when questions regarding the appropriateness and safety of an imaging study may arise. If the practice uses an electronic ordering system, it is helpful to include links in the ordering algorithm that will lead requesting physicians to appended sites detailing indications for breast MR imaging, the appropriate scenarios for unilateral versus bilateral examinations, and important patient safety issues and contraindications for MR imaging. Such algorithms should also include a place for the requesting physician to input data from laboratory results of renal function. In cases where renal function is abnormal and administration of MR imaging contrast is contraindicated, the scheduling algorithm can be designed

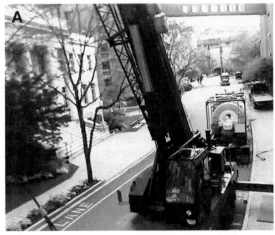
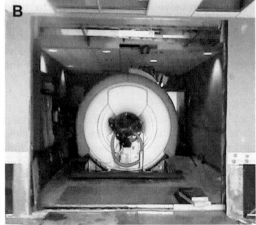

Fig. 3. (*A*) The street with access to the building was closed for the day so a crane could be brought in. (*B*) An outer wall was opened up to move the magnet in.

to block the scheduling of this examination and prompt the requesting doctor to consult a radiologist.

HANDLING BREAST MR IMAGING REQUESTS

If a practice decides to commit a radiologist as a "gatekeeper" to assess all incoming requests for breast MR imaging, each patient can be screened for appropriateness and safety, and the examination can be tailored on an individual case basis. However, this is probably not necessary, as the majority of breast MR imaging examinations can be performed in a standard fashion once the indications and safety issues have been cleared. Referring doctors should be required to provide all pertinent clinical information either in the requisition questionnaire or via electronic medical record, if this is easily accessible to the technologists and radiologists. Patients should be required to bring with them all pertinent breast examinations performed at another facility.

SCHEDULING BREAST MR IMAGING

Many facilities employ central scheduling staff for all examinations being performed in the radiology department. However, because breast MR imaging requirements are especially detailed, the scheduling staff must be trained to screen patients in great detail during a telephone interview. This interview includes history of prior surgery, specifically regarding implanted devices, history of claustrophobia, presence of a copper IUD in premenopausal women, history of previous breast surgery or biopsy, and any history of allergies and allergic reaction to contrast. This detailed questionnaire should be available to the scheduling staff electronically and if the answer to one of the

questions proves to be a contraindication for the examination, the algorithm should ideally block scheduling of the examination and provide a consultation opportunity. For 3-T magnets there are additional questions that must be reliably answered before a patient can be cleared for an examination on this magnet (Fig. 4).

Despite these efforts, it is not rare for a patient to arrive at the breast MR imaging suite and have the examination canceled because of the presence of a forgotten bit of hardware or other contraindication.

EXAMINATION PERFORMANCE

Standard protocols for detection of breast masses and for evaluation of implant integrity should be in place. These protocols may be determined by the breast imaging group or by a departmental MR imaging protocol committee. An excellent guide is available in the form of a 2-part article by Dr Christiane Kuhl.[14,26–29] Experienced and competent breast MR imaging technologists need enough familiarity with breast MR imaging particulars to be able to screen patients carefully, perform the examination, assess quality of each sequence, trouble shoot and repeat any suboptimal sequence, and consult with a radiologist if unable or uncertain about any aspect of the examination. Either the technologists must be trained to start intravenous lines or an intravenous team needs to be routinely available or serve as backup for difficult cases. Guidelines regarding the use of pre-existing central lines for gadolinium administration should be available.

Technologists should review a final screening questionnaire with each patient to ensure safety in the magnet. This questionnaire serves as the final check before the patient enters a high

		FOR ANY PATIENT BEING PERFORMED ON 3T MAGNETS, PLEASE ASK THESE ADDITIONAL QUESTIONS	
❏ YES ❏ NO		Shunt (spinal or intraventricular)	If YES, must be rescheduled to 1.5T system
❏ YES ❏ NO		Neuro Stimulator and/or Spinal Cord Stimulator	If YES, Must be rescheduled to 1.5T system
❏ YES ❏ NO		Magnetically-Activated Implant or Device	If YES, Must be rescheduled to 1.5T system
❏ YES ❏ NO		Do you have an IUD in place.	If YES, Is it copper? If YES, Must be rescheduled to 1.5T system
❏ YES ❏ NO		Heart Valve Prosthesis	If YES, Must have operative notes reviewed *Reviewing technologist initials of approval to perform MRI_____*
❏ YES ❏ NO		Stents (cardiac or vascular), IVC filters	If YES, Must have operative notes reviewed *Reviewing technologist initials of approval to perform MRI_____*
❏ YES ❏ NO		Electronic Implant or Device	If YES, Must have operative notes reviewed *Reviewing technologist initials of approval to perform MRI_____*
❏ YES ❏ NO		Eye Prosthesis or device (i.e. eyelid spring, wire, implant)	If YES, Must have operative notes reviewed *Reviewing technologist initials of approval to perform MRI_____*
❏ YES ❏ NO		Wire Mesh Implant	If YES, Must have operative notes reviewed *Reviewing technologist initials of approval to perform MRI_____*

Fig. 4. Additional questions to clear patients for imaging on a 3-T magnet.

magnetic field, and is sometimes the only time information about a device like a copper IUD may come to light. To address such cases in a practice routinely using a 3-T magnet, a 1.5-T magnet, if available, can serve as backup. Alternatively, there could be an agreement with another facility that could accommodate such patients at short notice.

Most patients feel more comfortable having female technologists position them in the breast coil for imaging. This maneuver requires proper positioning of the breasts to maximize inclusion of all breast tissue for imaging and avoid signal loss that may result from positioning too cephalad or including too much abdominal fat in the coil (**Fig. 5**). Images from each sequence should be reviewed by the technologist as it is completed, to make sure it is of optimal image quality (**Fig. 6**).

BREAST MR IMAGING INTERPRETATION

Radiologists interpreting breast MR imaging should be familiar with all aspects of this examination, such as appropriate indications, proper protocols, expected findings and their significance, as well as potential management options. Familiarity with mammography and breast US allows proper correlation between these imaging modalities. Working closely with breast surgeons, pathologists, and medical and radiation oncologists also allows the radiologist to provide a comprehensive and efficient service addressing common questions and concerns. In light of the above considerations, it is often ideal if breast imagers perform breast MR imaging interpretations.

BACKGROUND PATIENT DATA

Even more than in mammography and breast US, it is important to interpret breast MR imaging in the context of individual patients' pertinent history and risk factors for breast cancer. At the time of breast MR imaging, each patient should complete a history sheet similar to that used in mammography practices. If breast MR imaging examinations from multiple locations in the practice are interpreted at a central location, patient history sheets need to be made available to the interpreting radiologist, either by having them scanned into PACS (picture archiving and communications system) and thus being readily accessible (a difficult task at times) or by faxing them to the central location.

Most PACS allow radiologists to customize hanging protocols by individual preference. These protocols typically include methodical viewing of all image sequences and comparison to any previous breast MR examinations on the patient. A typical bilateral breast MR examination comprises anywhere from 800 to more than 2000 images; therefore, developing a habitual and systematic approach to viewing each sequence is essential. This approach makes reading more efficient and decreases the chance of forgetting to look at a particular sequence. In addition, the use of computer-aided diagnosis has a different role in MR imaging compared with mammography,

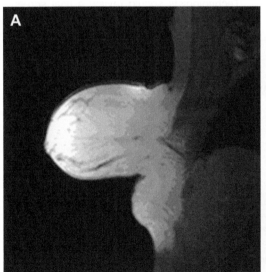
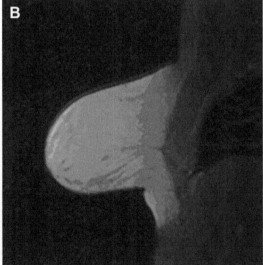

Fig. 5. Sagittal gradient-echo MR 3-plane localizer shows poor positioning of the right breast (*A*) which is too cephalad within the coil, resulting in signal loss superiorly and inclusion of abdominal fat inferiorly. (*B*) Good positioning results in a homogeneous signal.

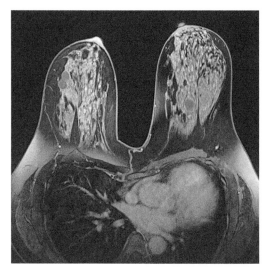

Fig. 6. Suboptimal fat saturation is seen in the axillary regions in an otherwise high-resolution scan. A technologist assessing this scan for quality would repeat with modifications to achieve better visualization.

as it efficiently provides quantitative analysis of enhancement kinetic curves.[30,31] Whereas many breast imaging groups have historically assessed the kinetic curve of a lesion by visual inspection of the dynamic pre- and postcontrast sequences, computer-aided diagnosis may provide more accurate analysis based on signal intensity measurements independent of the relative change in visualization caused by increasing enhancement of surrounding normal parenchyma.

CORRELATIVE BREAST IMAGING

Comparison to and correlation with all pertinent previous breast imaging studies allows the radiologist to make appropriate recommendations for patient management. For example, in the case of mammographic or US findings deemed suspicious enough to recommend biopsy, and a negative MR study, the biopsy recommendation should remain unchanged and the biopsy should be performed with the appropriate image guidance. In such a case, the final BI-RADS assessment of the MR imaging examination should reflect the previous recommendations or make it clear that those recommendations remain, despite the negative MR imaging.

REPORTING

For maximum ease in communication among radiologists and between radiologists, pathologists, and referring doctors, it is best to practice consistent and accurate use of the breast MR imaging

ACR BI-RADS lexicon.[3] The lexicon provides a structure within which interpretation can be facilitated and reported. Breast MR imaging findings are divided into focus/foci, masses, and non-mass-like enhancement. For focus/foci, detailed analysis is by definition not possible. For masses, the lexicon suggests describing shape, margins, internal enhancement, and enhancement over time (kinetics). For nonmass-like enhancement, the detailed analysis should include distribution of the enhancement, internal pattern, and kinetics. For each finding there are prescribed descriptors for morphology and distribution. Enhancement kinetics are described by initial and delayed phases. The initial phase may reflect rapid, medium, or slow contrast uptake within the first 90 seconds after contrast administration. The delayed phase is defined as change in enhancement after peak enhancement has been reached, or after the first 2 minutes. This change may be described as 1 of 3 time-intensity curve types. Type I is a Persistent curve, describing progressively greater than 10% increase in signal intensity over the time of the dynamic sequence, frequently associated with benign pathology. Type II or Plateau curve is one in which there is a leveling off of the signal intensity remaining within 10% of peak enhancement. A type III or Washout curve describes a greater than 10% decrease in signal intensity after the peak. The latter is most highly associated with malignant lesions (87%–92% positive predictive value).[32]

The final assessment categories parallel those for mammography and US,[33] with the addition of a subcategory of BI-RADS 3, which allows for a very short interval follow-up based on the premise that a certain pattern of enhancement may be related to physiologic hormonal effects of the menstrual cycle and thus may appear different when scanned at a different point in the cycle. The use of BI-RADS 3 in breast MR imaging may not necessarily follow the established paradigm based on mammography.[34,35] Recent research is beginning to identify appropriate lesion types and situations where 6-month follow-up may be appropriate. However, conclusions and recommendations are still in the process of being studied. One point reported in the primary literature is that enhancing foci with type I or persistent enhancement kinetics have an exceedingly low chance of malignancy, and therefore may be interpreted as BI-RADS 2 rather than 3.[36]

REPORT TEMPLATES

Given the need to include technical details of the examination in each report, it is easiest to use

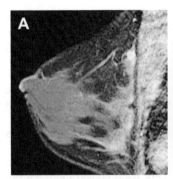
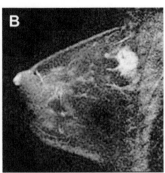

Fig. 7. (A) This 42-year-old BRCA-positive patient was found to have a small rim-enhancing lesion on surveillance MR imaging. Focused US and biopsy with either US or MR guidance was recommended. The clinician was notified but this communication was not recorded in the report. The patient was not notified of correct findings and returned 6 months later with a palpable mass, seen as an enlarged mass on MR imaging (B) a to be a high-grade invasive ductal carcinoma.

standardized templates in the dictation or reporting system. These templates can be developed by radiologists in the group to reflect the group style or by individual radiologists for their own use. The technical parameters such as magnet strength, standard protocols, and amount of contrast given should be included. Any reaction to contrast should be documented in the report and in the electronic medical record. Recommendations for modified future use of contrast should be made as needed.

If the template contains blocks where blanks can be filled in for each case, a great deal of consistency can be maintained between reports. This consistency makes it less likely to inadvertently forget to describe any aspect of interpretation and reporting, and more importantly, makes reports from the group easily, clearly, and more efficiently understood by the referring clinicians.

COMMUNICATION OF RESULTS

The report should include documentation of conveying positive results and recommendations to the referring clinician, preferably with confirmation that results were received. In addition, recommendations for management of positive results such as image-guided biopsy or targeted US should be not only conveyed to the referring doctor, but arrangements for the recommended procedures should be facilitated by providing contact information of the biopsy coordinator or scheduling staff. One way to achieve this is to convey results and recommendations to the referring doctor via e-mail and copy the e-mail to the biopsy coordinator or practice manager, thus minimizing the chance of patients "falling through the cracks" or getting lost to follow-up (**Fig. 7**). Taking

such action is especially important in situations where patients do not routinely receive copies of the actual report and depend on their primary physicians for information about their examination results. By current standards in the United States, it is the responsibility of the interpreting radiologist to contact the referring doctor with any positive or "actionable" examination findings and recommendations for management, so as not to lose track of patients who need diagnosis and treatment.

SUMMARY

Awareness and knowledge of the numerous factors regarding magnet and coil selection, location and siting, patient safety, examination scheduling, performance, interpretation, and reporting will aid in proper planning and establishment of an efficient and high-quality breast MR imaging program.

ACKNOWLEDGMENTS

The author would like to thank the following for their invaluable contributions and comments during the preparation of this manuscript Dr Robyn L. Birdwell, Dr Carolyn Mountford, Dr Peter Stanwell, and Lisa Bussolari.

REFERENCES

1. Liu PF, Debatin JF, Caduff RF, et al. Improved diagnostic accuracy in dynamic contrast enhanced MRI of the breast by combined quantitative analysis. Br J Radiol 1998;71(845):501–9.
2. Bassett LW, Dhaliwal SG, Eradat J, et al. National trends and practices in breast MRI. AJR Am J Roentgenol 2008;191(2):332–9.

3. Ikeda D, Hylton M, Kuhl C, et al. Breast imaging reporting and data system, BI-RADS: magnetic resonance imaging (BI-RADS: MRI). Reston (VA): American College of Radiology; 2003.

4. Ikeda DM, Hylton NM, Kinkel K, et al. Development, standardization, and testing of a lexicon for reporting contrast-enhanced breast magnetic resonance imaging studies. J Magn Reson Imaging 2001;13: 889–95.

5. Gutierrez RL, DeMartini WB, Eby PR, et al. BI-RADS lesion characteristics predict likelihood of malignancy in breast MRI for masses but not for non-masslike enhancement. AJR Am J Roentgenol 2009;193:994–1000.

6. Tardivon AA, Athanasiou A, Thibault F. Breast imaging and reporting data system (BIRADS) magnetic resonance imaging illustrated cases. Eur J Radiol 2007;61(2):216–23.

7. Saslow D, Boetes C, Burke W, et al. American Cancer Society guidelines for breast screening with MRI as an adjunct to mammography. CA Cancer J Clin 2007;57(2):75–89.

8. Hall F. The rise and impending decline of screening mammography. Radiology 2008;247:597–601.

9. Morrow M, Harris JR. More mastectomies: is this what patients really want? J Clin Oncol 2009; 27(25):4038–40.

10. Morrow M. Should routine breast cancer staging include MRI? J Clin Oncol 2008;26(3):352–3.

11. Kuhl C, Kuhn W, Braun M, et al. Pre-operative staging of breast cancer with breast MRI: one step forward, two steps back? Breast 2007; 16(2):34–44.

12. Tozaki M, Igarashi T, Fukuda K, et al. Positive and negative predictive values of BI-RADS-MRI descriptors for focal breast masses. Magn Reson Med Sci 2006;5(1):7–15.

13. Liberman L, Morris EA, Lee MJ, et al. Breast lesions detected on MR imaging: features and positive predictive value. AJR Am J Roentgenol 2002; 179(1):171–8.

14. Rausch D, Hendrick RE. How to optimize clinical breast MR imaging practices and techniques on your 1.5 T system. Radiographics 2006;26: 1469–84.

15. Hendrick RE. Breast MRI: fundamentals and technical aspects. New York (NY): Springer; 2007.

16. Kuhl CK, Jost P, Morakkabati N, et al. Contrast-enhanced MR imaging of the breast at 3.0 and 1.5 T in the same patients: initial experience. Radiology 2006;239(3):666–76.

17. Kuhl CK, Kooijman H, Gieseke J, et al. Effect of B1 inhomogeneity on breast MR imaging at 3.0 T. Radiology 2007;244(3):929–30.

18. Mountford CE, Stanwell P, Ramadan S. Breast MR imaging at 3.0 T. Radiology 2008;248(1): 319–20.

19. Stanwell P, Mountford C. In vivo proton MR spectroscopy of the breast. Radiographics 2007;27(Suppl 1):S253–66.

20. Thomas MA, Lipnick S, Velan SS, et al. Investigation of breast cancer using two-dimensional MRS. NMR Biomed 2009;22(1):77–91.

21. Tsushima Y, Takahashi-Taketomi A, Endo K. Magnetic resonance (MR) differential diagnosis of breast tumors using apparent diffusion coefficient (ADC) on 1.5 T. J Magn Reson Imaging 2009; 30(2):249–55.

22. Lo GG, Ai V, Chan JKF, et al. Diffusion-weighted magnetic resonance imaging of breast lesions: first experience at 3T. J Comput Assist Tomogr 2009; 33(1):63–9.

23. Kuhl CK. Breast MR imaging at 3T. Magn Reson Imaging Clin N Am 2007;15(3):315–20, vi.

24. Szameitat AJ, Shen S, Sterr A. The functional magnetic resonance imaging (fMRI) procedure as experienced by healthy participants and stroke patients—a pilot study. BMC Med Imaging 2009; 9:14.

25. Shellock FG. Reference manual for magnetic resonance safety, implants and devices: 2009 edition. Los Angeles (CA): Biomedical Research Publishing Company; 2009.

26. Kuhl C. The current status of breast MR imaging. Part I. Choice of technique, image interpretation, diagnostic accuracy, and transfer to clinical practice. Radiology 2007;244(2):356–78.

27. Kuhl CK. Current status of breast MR imaging. Part 2. Clinical applications. Radiology 2007;244(3):672–91.

28. Morris E, Liberman L, editors. Breast MRI: diagnosis and intervention. New York (NY): Springer; 2005.

29. Raza S, Birdwell RL, Ritner JA, et al. Breast MRI: a comprehensive imaging guide. Salt Lake City (UT): Amirsys; 2009.

30. Baltzer PA, Renz DM, Kullnig PE. Application of computer-aided diagnosis (CAD) in MR-mammography (MRM): do we really need whole lesion time curve distribution analysis? Acad Radiol 2009; 16(4):435–42.

31. Baltzer PA, Freiberg C, Beger S. Clinical MR-mammography: are computer-assisted methods superior to visual or manual measurements for curve type analysis? A systematic approach. Acad Radiol 2009;16(9):1070–6.

32. Ritner JA. Kinetic curves. In: Raza S, Birdwell RL, Ritner JA, et al, editors. Breast MRI: a comprehensive imaging guide. Salt Lake City (UT): Amirsys; 2009.I.1. p. 36–47.

33. Raza S. MR BI-RADS lexicon. In: Raza S, Birdwell RL, Ritner JA, et al, editors. Breast MRI: a comprehensive imaging guide. Salt Lake City (UT): Amirsys; 2009. I.1. p. 22–35.

34. Birdwell RL, Chikarmane SA, McCarthy N, et al. Use of the mammography-derived BI-RADS 3

assessment for breast MR; is it a good fit? [abstract]. Presented at Radiological Society of North America scientific assembly and annual meeting program. Oak Brook, IL, 2008.

35. Moy L, Levy A, Mercado C, et al. BI-RADS 3 lesions on MRI: classification, outcomes and frequency of malignancy [abstract]. Presented at the annual scientific meeting of the American Roentgen Ray Society. Orlando, FL, 2007.

36. Eby PR, DeMartini WB, Gutierrez RL, et al. Characteristics of probably benign breast MRI lesions. AJR Am J Roentgenol 2009;193:861–7.

Role of Magnetic Resonance Imaging in Evaluating the Extent of Disease

Sara C. Gavenonis, MD, Susan Orel Roth, MD*

KEYWORDS

- Breast magnetic resonance imaging
- Extent of disease • Multifocal/multicentric
- Breast conservation versus mastectomy

The main goal of preoperative breast imaging evaluation in the patient with known cancer is to assess accurately the extent of disease. This information then can be used to guide surgical treatment planning. In cases where the disease appears localized, breast-conserving surgery likely will be successful. In contrast, when the disease appears to be multifocal or multicentric, mastectomy likely will be required. In addition, imaging evaluation of the contralateral breast can result in the detection of clinically unsuspected synchronous cancer, which also may affect surgical management.

Beyond mammography and breast ultrasound, breast magnetic resonance imaging (MRI) has emerged as a tool that can be applied toward the preoperative imaging evaluation of patients with known cancer. The ability of breast MRI to depict the extent of cancer has been well-documented in the literature.[1–13] MRI has been reported to detect multifocal disease in the ipsilateral breast in 10% to 44% of cases.[4,5,11,14–16] The utility of breast MRI in the detection of multicentric disease also has been widely reported, with additional cancer detected in 11% to 54% of cases.[2,5–7,14,15,17–22] In addition, many of these cases were MRI-demonstrated but mammographically and clinically occult (Figs. 1 and 2).[23] Given the potential of MRI to detect unsuspected multifocal or multicentric cancer, it has been suggested that the addition of MRI to the preoperative imaging work-up of patients with newly diagnosed breast cancer can aid in surgical and definitive treatment. This implies that breast MRI has the theoretical potential to reduce the number of surgical procedures to obtain negative margins of resection or to convert patients from planned breast-conservation therapy (BCT) to mastectomy when multifocal or multicentric cancer is found. It also has been postulated that the detection of additional areas of cancer in the ipsilateral breast on MRI may result in a lower rate of in-breast recurrence following BCT.

In addition to evaluating the extent of disease in the ipsilateral breast, it also has been demonstrated that MRI can be used to evaluate the contralateral breast. Historically, the reported incidence of synchronous bilateral breast cancer detected on physical examination or mammography is 3% to 6%.[24–26] With the application of breast MRI, there are now multiple single-institution and multicenter trial reports indicating the ability of MRI to detect synchronous cancers in the contralateral breast that were otherwise mammographically and clinically occult. Rates of approximately 3% to 19% of patients examined have been reported.[24–26] The study by Lehman and colleagues[26] had the largest number of patients (969), and the rate of contralateral disease detected by MRI was 3.1%. Approximately half of

Department of Radiology, Hospital of the University of Pennsylvania, 1 Silverstein, 3400 Spruce Street, Philadelphia, PA 19104, USA
* Corresponding author.
E-mail address: Susan.Roth@uphs.upenn.edu

Magn Reson Imaging Clin N Am 18 (2010) 199–206
doi:10.1016/j.mric.2010.02.002
1064-9689/10/$ – see front matter © 2010 Published by Elsevier Inc.

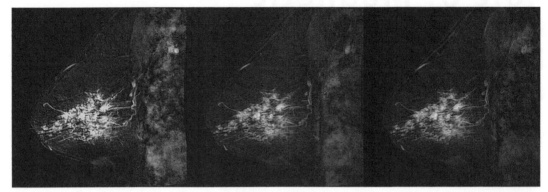

Fig. 1. Breast MRI demonstrates the extent of disease. Sequential subtraction images from dynamic contrast-enhanced breast MRI demonstrate the extent of disease in this patient with biopsy-proven DCIS (dynamic enhanced series were obtained at approximately 90 seconds, 180 seconds, and 270 seconds after injection as per protocol at the authors' institution). Anteroposterior extent of enhancement is from the nipple to the posterior breast, and was only demonstrated on breast MRI. Surgical plan was for mastectomy.

the lesions detected on MRI have been invasive cancers, and the other half have been ductal carcinoma in situ (DCIS).[24–26] Breast MRI can detect synchronous cancers in the contralateral breast, information that can help to optimize clinical therapy for the patient.

PITFALLS OF MRI STAGING OF BREAST CANCER

One of the major limitations of MRI of the breast is false-positive enhancement of benign lesions, including fibroadenomas, fat necrosis, fibrocystic changes, and presumably normal breast tissue.[27] False-positive enhancement is one main pitfall in the application of MRI for breast cancer staging (Fig. 3). False-positive rates in the setting of breast cancer staging have varied among studies, with an average rate of approximately 20%.[19,28,29] In a study of 70 women with percutaneously diagnosed breast cancer who were being considered for BCT, MRI detected additional sites of cancer in the ipsilateral breast in 27% of patients.[19] Biopsy was recommended for MRI-detected additional lesions in the ipsilateral breast in 51% of women. The positive predictive value (PPV) was 52%, with an overall rate of 24% of women with MRI-recommended biopsies for findings that ultimately were found to be benign.[19] The PPV was higher for lesions in the same quadrant as the index lesion as compared with lesions in different

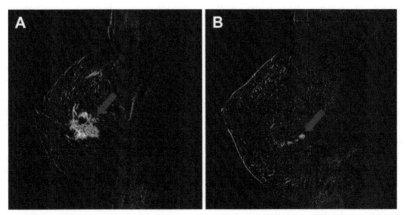

Fig. 2. Breast MRI demonstrates the extent of disease. (A) Index tumor site in the outer right breast (arrow), as demonstrated on a subtraction image from a breast MRI. Prior ultrasound-guided core biopsy and clip placement revealed poorly differentiated invasive mammary carcinoma. (B) Subtraction image from a breast MRI demonstrates enhancing foci in a linear pattern in the posterior central right breast (arrow), separate from the index tumor site and only demonstrated on breast MRI. MRI-guided biopsy of these findings revealed high-grade in situ ductal carcinoma.

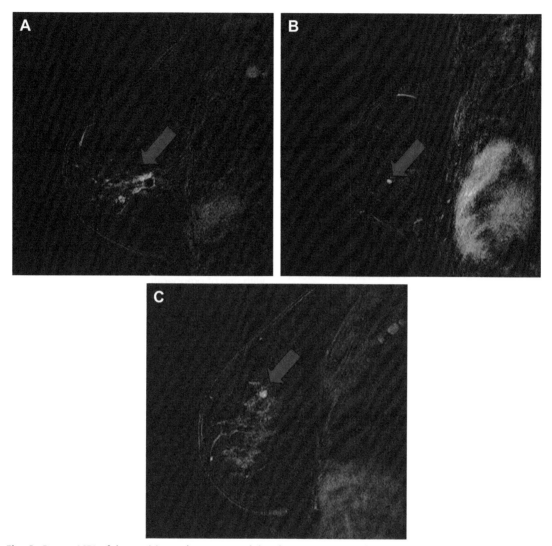

Fig. 3. Breast MRI—false-positive enhancement. (*A*) Subtraction image from a breast MRI demonstrates the patient's known DCIS from prior percutaneous biopsy (*arrow*). (*B*) Subtraction image from a breast MRI demonstrates an enhancing mass (*arrow*) in a different quadrant of the ipsilateral breast. MRI-guided biopsy demonstrated fibroadenoma. (*C*) Subtraction image from a breast MRI demonstrates an enhancing mass in the contralateral breast (*arrow*). MRI-guided biopsy demonstrated fibroadenoma.

quadrants (64% vs 31%). A similar finding was reported by Bedrosian and colleagues,[21,30] where a higher percentage of enhancing lesions in the same quadrant as the index cancer were malignant compared with findings in a different quadrant.

Despite the relatively high PPV for breast MRI that is higher than the reported PPV for mammographically detected suspicious lesions, these reports that demonstrate the performance of breast MRI also indicate that many of these recommended biopsies for MRI-detected suspicious lesions will yield benign results. Thus, there is still

potential theoretical delay in definitive surgical therapy for these patients with additional enhancing findings detected on preoperative breast MRI, especially if the findings are found to be benign. False-positive MRI findings in the setting of breast cancer staging may result in high cost, increased patient anxiety, additional surgical procedures that may compromise the cosmetic results for those patients who do undergo BCT, and potentially an increase in the mastectomy rate. The range of these costs and the quantifiable potential impact on patient management remain to be determined definitively.

IMPACT OF PREOPERATIVE BREAST MRI ON CLINICAL MANAGEMENT

Multiple studies demonstrate that the addition of MRI will result in a change in therapeutic approach, with reported rates of change ranging from 4% to 43%, with most of these rates at about 20%.[4,7,13,19,21,29,31-37] The findings on MRI were reported as true positive in 4% to 32% of cases, and false positive in a lower percentage.[4,7,13,19,21,29,31-37] In cases where the enhancement proved to be benign, this resulted in unnecessary additional surgery, or delay in definitive surgery because of the need for percutaneous biopsy.

Given that there are false positives in breast MRI, a caveat to keep in mind is that before any final surgical treatment decision, tissue diagnosis should be obtained of suspicious findings if the results will affect clinical recommendations relating to BCT versus mastectomy. Balancing the known pitfalls of breast MRI and its false positives with the clinical goal of accurate assessment of extent of disease is also an evolving process, and an area of continued investigation.

PREOPERATIVE STAGING WITH BREAST MRI—CURRENT CONTROVERSIES

The data are clear that MRI permits detection of mammographically, sonographically, and clinically occult multifocal cancer in selected patients with presumed unifocal disease. There is an ongoing debate, however, over the use of MRI for preoperative cancer staging. Much of the controversy appears to center around the clinical impact of the additional sites of disease that are detected only on MRI. In terms of short-term benefit, will the addition of MRI result in improved surgical planning, ultimately resulting in a decrease in number of surgical procedures to obtain negative margins? In terms of long-term benefit, will the addition of MRI result in reduced recurrence rates and improved overall survival?

Investigation into the use of MRI for preoperative breast cancer staging has demonstrated both negative and positive results. In one study that compared patients who underwent surgery with and without a routine preoperative MRI, MRI use was reported to not be associated with improved margin status, but instead was reported to be associated with a treatment delay and an increased mastectomy rate.[38] In addition, a recent meta-analysis of breast MRI accuracy and impact on surgical management reported an 11.3% conversion rate from wide local

excision to more extensive surgery.[39] This analysis also alluded to the false positives that MRI finds, and concludes that additional studies need to be done.

Recently, a multicenter, randomized controlled trial was reported from the United Kingdom.[40] The comparative effectiveness of MRI in breast cancer (COMICE) trial included approximately 1623 women with a breast cancer diagnosis, with 816 patients receiving a preoperative breast MRI, and 807 not receiving one. The group without preoperative MRI underwent conventional breast imaging with mammography and ultrasound. Reoperation rate within 6 months was reported as 19% in the MRI group, and 19% in the group without a preoperative MRI. The conclusions included that no significant benefit in terms of reduction in reoperation rate was achieved with use of preoperative breast MRI.

As counterpoint, however, a report of preoperative MRI associated with more completely excised invasive cancer also has been published.[41] In addition, preoperative MRI again has been reported to be useful in the surgical management of patients eligible for different management choices.[42] Furthermore, a prospective single-institution study also was reported recently by Siegmann and colleagues[43] that assessed that location's experience with the impact of preoperative bilateral breast MRI on the clinical management of patients. They reported that the findings of preoperative breast MRI examinations changed the clinical management in 48 of the 119 study patients (approximately 40%). In 36 of these women, additional sites of malignancy were demonstrated that clarified the surgical management (17 with conversion to mastectomy). In 12 patients, the MRI-detected lesions ultimately were found to be benign. In comparison to the 30.3% of patients where breast MRI clarified the extent of the malignancy by detecting additional sites of malignancy, the false positives in 10.1% of patients was deemed relatively acceptable.

Also important to remember is that the increased use of breast MRI may not be the only factor influencing changes in surgical management and the reports of increased mastectomy rate. In another recently published analysis,[44] the year of surgery and a preoperative breast MRI were reported as independent significant predictors of the type of surgery a breast cancer patient received. Although patients with an MRI were reported to be more likely to undergo mastectomy than those without (54% vs 36%, $P<.0001$), the year of surgery (2004 to 2006) at this institution also was associated with an increased mastectomy rate (29% in 2003 to 41% in 2006, *P*<.0001). In this latter group, the rate of mastectomy increased in patients without *MRI*. Factors such as increased awareness and information about genetic status and family history have been discussed as possible influences on this trend, with potential choices for mastectomy being made even for early stage breast cancer, and even without a breast MRI. Furthermore, increased knowledge about and development of breast reconstruction options also may factor into any trend in increased mastectomy rates. A recent report suggests that women are much more likely to choose mastectomy when informed with breast reconstruction options.[45] Thus, there also may be other variables and influences on the recently reported increase in mastectomy rate for breast cancer patients beyond breast MRI.

There are many potential explanations for these conflicting reports on the impact of preoperative MRI on surgical management. One explanation may be differences in patient populations in each study. It is possible that the selective application of breast MRI in certain populations will help optimize the use of this tool in the preoperative breast imaging evaluation of the patient with known cancer. It is also important to note that no imaging test is universally 100% sensitive and 100% specific. Given the variable histology of breast cancer, individual patient variability, and variation in current clinical application, there is much to influence the false-positive rate of any breast imaging study, including breast MRI. Further investigation needs to be done in the application of breast MRI in patients with known breast cancer.

CONTRALATERAL BREAST CANCER SCREENING—CURRENT DISCUSSION

Although MRI can be used to detect clinically and mammographically unsuspected synchronous bilateral breast cancer, many questions remain. The clinical significance, specifically the survival benefit, of the detection of these occult synchronous cancers, especially the noninvasive cancers, has not been addressed definitively. Furthermore, the detection of these contralateral cancers must be weighed against the added time, expense, and additional costs associated with MRI and MRI-guided biopsy. Also, what is the natural history of these contralateral findings? Would these contralateral cancers have ever manifested clinically, especially if systemic chemotherapy was planned for treatment of the

index cancer? Additional investigation appears to be necessary.

WHAT OF IMPACT ON LOCAL RECURRENCE AND OVERALL SURVIVAL?

The available data on the impact of breast MRI on local recurrence following breast conservation therapy and on overall survival are not definitive. In a retrospective study from Fischer and colleagues,[16] results of a lower in-breast recurrence rate were reported in a group of breast cancer patients who had received preoperative breast MRI (n = 121, recurrence rate 1.2%) versus in a group of patients where no preoperative breast MRI was obtained (n = 225, recurrence rate 6.8%), *P*<.001. It is important to interpret these results with caution, given there were many variables between the two groups that may not have been optimally controlled for, such as tumor size and nodal status. Additional studies need to be done to clarify the effect of preoperative breast MRI on local recurrence rates.

In another retrospective study, Solin and colleagues[46] reported on a single-institution analysis of 756 women who underwent BCT (28% of whom had a staging MRI) and found no significant difference in 8-year rates of relapse-free survival (3% with MRI vs 4% without MRI) and no significant difference in the 8 year rates of overall survival (94% with MRI vs 95% without MRI). It is important to note the limitations of this study when interpreting these results. Although this report appears to indicate no impact of breast MRI on survival, this nonrandomized, retrospective study may have underestimated the theoretical value of breast MRI given that patients with extensive disease detected on MRI were excluded. Given that current methods of breast conservation do have low rates of local failure, the necessary power to detect a small difference may not have been achievable in a single-institution study.

Optimally, a randomized controlled clinical trial would be the ideal method to demonstrate any impact that preoperative staging with MRI would have on recurrence rate following BCT and overall survival. However, it may not be possible to power this study within the practical confines of the current world of breast cancer diagnosis and treatment. The clinical utility of breast MRI is widely known, and it is no longer an early experimental imaging examination. Thus, practical recruitment into both cohorts would be difficult. Extrapolating surrogate markers for improved survival that have been delineated through mammography studies, such as size of tumor detected, percentage of cancers which are in situ, and nodal status, ultimately may be the best compromise between the theoretical and practical considerations in the evolving evaluation of breast MRI as an imaging tool for preoperative staging of breast cancer.

In the context of existing BCT methods (lumpectomy and whole breast irradiation) versus mastectomy, the survival of patients treated with BCT has been reported to be equal to that of those treated with mastectomy.[47,48] This has supported some of the reports that preoperative breast MRI has little impact on patient survival. Existing retrospective studies, however, should be interpreted in this context of existing treatments. It is important to remember that BCT continues to evolve. New advances such as partial breast irradiation may make breast MRI particularly more relevant, as sites of multifocal and multicentric disease that previously may have been treated with postoperative whole breast irradiation may now not fall within the treatment field if partial breast irradiation is used.[49,50]

MRI DETECTION AND STAGING OF BREAST CANCER: WHAT QUESTIONS REMAIN?

Many questions remain unanswered about breast MRI in the context of the patient with known cancer. For example, would certain subgroups of patients (defined by breast density or age) with certain tumor subtypes (eg, lobular) preferentially benefit from a preoperative MRI? Are there subsets of patients who are most at risk for having multifocal or multicentric cancer that would benefit most from MRI? Additional clinical investigation is needed in an attempt to find answers to these questions.

Additional questions include

> Just because MRI can detect additional areas of cancer, what is the true clinical impact?
> What is the natural history of enhancing lesions that are only detected on MRI?
> Does it matter what size the finding is?
> If BCT includes whole breast irradiation, would the findings have been treated without altering the surgical plan?
> And what of findings in the contralateral breast that may not have ever become clinically apparent?
> For patients who undergo subsequent chemotherapy, would these incidental cancers have been treated successfully without altering the surgical management?
> For breast cancer patients who do undergo this examination, what is the risk–benefit ratio?

Clinical investigation continues in an effort to find answers to these questions.

SUMMARY

There is little debate over the ability of breast MRI to detect additional sites of cancer during a preoperative breast cancer imaging evaluation. The current discussion appears to center around the clinical impact this information has, and what quantifiable clinical benefit this imparts to patients. Though MRI is currently the most accurate imaging method for determining extent of disease in the ipsilateral breast, this ability for improved detection of additional foci of breast cancer has not necessarily translated into better patient outcome universally. Perhaps the complementary information breast MRI can provide should be obtained if it is determined clinically that this would affect clinical management, in the context of the known tumor histology, receptor status, and any other mammographic/sonographic findings. The careful application of this powerful breast-imaging tool is paramount, as is the careful integration of the information it provides into the clinical picture of the patient. It should not be universally approved or condemned, nor should the imaging information from breast MRI trump suspicious mammographic, sonographic, or clinical findings. In the appropriate setting, breast MRI can be invaluable in the patient with known breast cancer. Furthermore, issues of technical quality, cost, and availability need to be addressed. Much has been learned from clinical investigation about the capabilities and potential of MRI of the breast. There is much more to learn as the application of this powerful breast-imaging tool is refined.

REFERENCES

1. Harms SE, Flamig DP. MR imaging of the breast: technical approach and clinical experience. Radiographics 1993;13(4):905–12.
2. Harms SE, Flamig DP, Hesley KL, et al. MR imaging of the breast with rotating delivery of excitation off resonance: clinical experience with pathologic correlation. Radiology 1993;187(2):493–501.
3. Morris EA, Schwartz LH, Dershaw DD, et al. MR imaging of the breast in patients with occult primary breast carcinoma. Radiology 1997;205(2):437–40.
4. Orel SG, Schnall MD, Powell CM, et al. Staging of suspected breast cancer: effect of MR imaging and MR-guided biopsy. Radiology 1995;196(1):115–22.
5. Boetes C, Mus RD, Holland R, et al. Breast tumors: comparative accuracy of MR imaging relative to

mammography and US for demonstrating extent. Radiology 1995;197(3):743–7.

6. Esserman L, Hylton N, Yassa L, et al. Utility of magnetic resonance imaging in the management of breast cancer: evidence for improved preoperative staging. J Clin Oncol 1999;17(1):110–9.

7. Fischer U, Kopka L, Grabbe E. Breast carcinoma: effect of preoperative contrast-enhanced MR imaging on the therapeutic approach. Radiology 1999;213(3):881–8.

8. Weinstein SP, Orel SG, Heller R, et al. MR imaging of the breast in patients with invasive lobular carcinoma. AJR Am J Roentgenol 2001;176(2):399–406.

9. Rodenko GN, Harms SE, Pruneda JM, et al. MR imaging in the management before surgery of lobular carcinoma of the breast: correlation with pathology. AJR Am J Roentgenol 1996;167(6):1415–9.

10. Orel SG, Reynolds C, Schnall MD, et al. Breast carcinoma: MR imaging before re-excisional biopsy. Radiology 1997;205(2):429–36.

11. Fischer U, Baum F, Luftner-Nagel S. Preoperative MR imaging in patients with breast cancer: preoperative staging, effects on recurrence rates, and outcome analysis. Magn Reson Imaging Clin N Am 2006;14(3):351–62, vi.

12. Liberman L. Breast MR imaging in assessing extent of disease. Magn Reson Imaging Clin N Am 2006;14(3):339–49, vi.

13. Tillman GF, Orel SG, Schnall MD, et al. Effect of breast magnetic resonance imaging on the clinical management of women with early stage breast carcinoma. J Clin Oncol 2002;20(16):3413–23.

14. Mumtaz H, Hall-Craggs MA, Davidson T, et al. Staging of symptomatic primary breast cancer with MR imaging. AJR Am J Roentgenol 1997;169(2):417–24.

15. Mumtaz H, Davidson T, Hall-Craggs MA, et al. Comparison of magnetic resonance imaging and conventional triple assessment in locally recurrent breast cancer. Br J Surg 1997;84(8):1147–51.

16. Fischer U, Zachariae O, Baum F, et al. The influence of preoperative MRI of the breasts on recurrence rate in patients with breast cancer. Eur Radiol 2004;14(10):1725–31.

17. Harms SE, Flamig DP, Hesley KL, et al. Fat-suppressed three-dimensional MR imaging of the breast. Radiographics 1993;13(2):247–67.

18. Drew PJ, Chatterjee S, Turnbull LW, et al. Dynamic contrast-enhanced magnetic resonance imaging of the breast is superior to triple assessment for the preoperative detection of multifocal breast cancer. Ann Surg Oncol 1999;6(6):599–603.

19. Liberman L, Morris EA, Dershaw DD, et al. MR imaging of the ipsilateral breast in women with percutaneously proven breast cancer. AJR Am J Roentgenol 2003;180(4):901–10.

20. Furman B, Gardner MS, Romilly P, et al. Effect of 0.5 Tesla magnetic resonance imaging on the surgical management of breast cancer patients. Am J Surg 2003;186(4):344–7.

21. Bedrosian I, Mick R, Orel SG, et al. Changes in the surgical management of patients with breast carcinoma based on preoperative magnetic resonance imaging. Cancer 2003;98(3):468–73.

22. Berg WA, Gutierrez L, NessAiver MS, et al. Diagnostic accuracy of mammography, clinical examination, US, and MR imaging in preoperative assessment of breast cancer. Radiology 2004;233(3):830–49.

23. Liberman L, Bracero N, Morris E, et al. MRI-guided 9-gauge vacuum-assisted breast biopsy: initial clinical experience. AJR Am J Roentgenol 2005;185(1):183–93.

24. Lee SG, Orel SG, Woo IJ, et al. MR imaging screening of the contralateral breast in patients with newly diagnosed breast cancer: preliminary results. Radiology 2003;226(3):773–8.

25. Liberman L, Morris EA, Kim CM, et al. MR imaging findings in the contralateral breast of women with recently diagnosed breast cancer. AJR Am J Roentgenol 2003;180(2):333–41.

26. Lehman CD, Gatsonis C, Kuhl CK, et al. MRI evaluation of the contralateral breast in women with recently diagnosed breast cancer. N Engl J Med 2007;356(13):1295–303.

27. Orel SG, Schnall MD. MR imaging of the breast for the detection, diagnosis, and staging of breast cancer. Radiology 2001;220(1):13–30.

28. Teifke A, Hlawatsch A, Beier T, et al. Undetected malignancies of the breast: dynamic contrast-enhanced MR imaging at 1.0 T. Radiology 2002;224(3):881–8.

29. Van Goethem M, Schelfout K, Dijckmans L, et al. MR mammography in the preoperative staging of breast cancer in patients with dense breast tissue: comparison with mammography and ultrasound. Eur Radiol 2004;14(5):809–16.

30. Bedrosian I, Schlencker J, Spitz FR, et al. Magnetic resonance imaging-guided biopsy of mammographically and clinically occult breast lesions. Ann Surg Oncol 2002;9(5):457–61.

31. Tan JE, Orel SG, Schnall MD, et al. Role of magnetic resonance imaging and magnetic resonance imaging–guided surgery in the evaluation of patients with early-stage breast cancer for breast conservation treatment. Am J Clin Oncol 1999;22(4):414–8.

32. Gatzemeier W, Liersch T, Stylianou A, et al. [Preoperative MR mammography in breast carcinoma. Effect on operative treatment from the surgical viewpoint]. Chirurg 1999;70(12):1460–8 [in German].

33. Hlawatsch A, Teifke A, Schmidt M, et al. Preoperative assessment of breast cancer: sonography

versus MR imaging. AJR Am J Roentgenol 2002; 179(6):1493–501.

34. Schelfout K, Van Goethem M, Kersschot E, et al. Preoperative breast MRI in patients with invasive lobular breast cancer. Eur Radiol 2004;14(7):1209–16.

35. Schelfout K, Van Goethem M, Kersschot E, et al. Contrast-enhanced MR imaging of breast lesions and effect on treatment. Eur J Surg Oncol 2004; 30(5):501–7.

36. Lehman CD, Blume JD, Thickman D, et al. Added cancer yield of MRI in screening the contralateral breast of women recently diagnosed with breast cancer: results from the International Breast Magnetic Resonance Consortium (IBMC) trial. J Surg Oncol 2005;92(1):9–15 [discussion: 15–6].

37. Pediconi F, Catalano C, Padula S, et al. Contrast-enhanced magnetic resonance mammography: does it affect surgical decision-making in patients with breast cancer? Breast Cancer Res Treat 2007; 106(1):65–74.

38. Bleicher RJ, Ciocca RM, Egleston BL, et al. Association of routine pretreatment magnetic resonance imaging with time to surgery, mastectomy rate, and margin status. J Am Coll Surg 2009;209(2):180–7 [quiz: 294–5].

39. Houssami N, Ciatto S, Macaskill P, et al. Accuracy and surgical impact of magnetic resonance imaging in breast cancer staging: systematic review and meta-analysis in detection of multifocal and multicentric cancer. J Clin Oncol 2008;26(19):3248–58.

40. Turnbull L, Brown S, Harvey I, et al. Comparative effectiveness of MRI in breast cancer (COMICE) trial: a randomised controlled trial. Lancet 2010; 375(9714):563–71.

41. Pengel KE, Loo CE, Teertstra HJ, et al. The impact of preoperative MRI on breast-conserving surgery of invasive cancer: a comparative cohort study. Breast Cancer Res Treat 2009;116(1):161–9.

42. Braun M, Polcher M, Schrading S, et al. Influence of preoperative MRI on the surgical management of

patients with operable breast cancer. Breast Cancer Res Treat 2008;111(1):179–87.

43. Siegmann KC, Baur A, Vogel U, et al. Risk-benefit analysis of preoperative breast MRI in patients with primary breast cancer. Clin Radiol 2009; 64(4):403–13.

44. Katipamula R, Degnim AC, Hoskin T, et al. Trends in mastectomy rates at the Mayo Clinic Rochester: effect of surgical year and preoperative magnetic resonance imaging. J Clin Oncol 2009;27(25): 4082–8.

45. Alderman AK, Hawley ST, Waljee J, et al. Understanding the impact of breast reconstruction on the surgical decision-making process for breast cancer. Cancer 2008;112(3):489–94.

46. Solin LJ, Orel SG, Hwang WT, et al. Relationship of breast magnetic resonance imaging to outcome after breast-conservation treatment with radiation for women with early stage invasive breast carcinoma or ductal carcinoma in situ. J Clin Oncol 2008;26(3):386–91.

47. Fisher B, Jeong JH, Anderson S, et al. Twenty-five-year follow-up of a randomized trial comparing radical mastectomy, total mastectomy, and total mastectomy followed by irradiation. N Engl J Med 2002;347(8):567–75.

48. Veronesi U, Cascinelli N, Mariani L, et al. Twenty-year follow-up of a randomized study comparing breast-conserving surgery with radical mastectomy for early breast cancer. N Engl J Med 2002; 347(16):1227–32.

49. Al-Hallaq HA, Mell LK, Bradley JA, et al. Magnetic resonance imaging identifies multifocal and multicentric disease in breast cancer patients who are eligible for partial breast irradiation. Cancer 2008; 113(9):2408–14.

50. Tendulkar RD, Chellman-Jeffers M, Rybicki LA, et al. Preoperative breast magnetic resonance imaging in early breast cancer: implications for partial breast irradiation. Cancer 2009;115(8):1621–30.

Optimizing 1.5-Tesla and 3-Tesla Dynamic Contrast-Enhanced Magnetic Resonance Imaging of the Breasts

Manjil Chatterji, MD, Cecilia L. Mercado, MD,
Linda Moy, MD*

KEYWORDS

- Breast • Breast cancer • MR imaging
- Dynamic contrast enhancement • 3Tesla MR imaging

Dynamic contrast-enhanced (DCE) magnetic resonance (MR) imaging of the breast is a highly accurate imaging tool for the detection of primary and recurrent breast cancer, with reported sensitivities in the range of 83% to 100%.[1–3] The American Cancer Society recommends that women with a lifetime risk of breast cancer greater than 20% undergo an annual MR imaging screening examination in addition to screening mammography.[4] A recent American College of Radiology (ACR) Imaging Network trial supports the role of MR imaging in staging women who have biopsy-proven cancer.[5] The demand for contrast-enhanced breast MR imaging in these patient populations continues to increase. A 2008 survey of radiology practices in the United States showed that breast MR imaging was offered at 74% of 754 surveyed practices.[6] Given increased demand, it is predicted that additional radiology practices will offer this examination in a screening and diagnostic setting in the near future.

Increased clinical use of breast MR imaging has also been facilitated by the standardization of interpretation and reporting among radiologists. In 2003 the ACR published the fourth edition of the Breast Imaging Reporting and Data System (BI-RADS) manual, which contained the first edition of the MR Imaging Lexicon.[7,8] The BI-RADS MR Imaging Lexicon provides a common language for describing findings and allows radiologists to communicate findings to referring physicians in a uniform, clear, and concise fashion.

At present, one of the challenges that breast MR faces is the wide range of specificities, ranging from 29% to 100%.[1–3] A reason for this variable specificity is that the technical aspects of performing breast MR imaging have not been standardized. Most of the technical parameters, including equipment (magnet strength and breast coil), spatial and temporal resolution, pulse sequences, and timing of the dynamic contrast sequences, vary widely between practice sites. To address these issues, the ACR and the European Society of Breast Imaging have developed practice guidelines and technical standards for breast MR imaging, updated in 2008.[9,10] The ACR is also developing a breast MR accreditation program, which will include technical requirements for optimizing this examination. Further improvement and standardization of the imaging protocol should lead to improvements in the characterization of lesions detected on breast MR imaging. This article reviews the basic principles of DCE breast MR imaging and discusses the technical parameters necessary for a high-quality examination. The

Department of Radiology, New York University Langone Medical Center, 160 East 34th Street, New York, NY 10016, USA
* Corresponding author.
E-mail address: linda.moy@nyumc.org

Magn Reson Imaging Clin N Am 18 (2010) 207–224
doi:10.1016/j.mric.2010.02.011
1064-9689/10/$ – see front matter © 2010 Elsevier Inc. All rights reserved.

article also discusses the advantages, limitations, and considerations for performing breast MR imaging at 3T.

PATIENT FACTORS

Given the wide overlap of breast cancer presentations on MR imaging, an effective approach to breast MR imaging protocol must include a multisequence assessment of benign and potentially malignant lesions. In premenopausal women, the MR imaging examination should be performed during the second week of the menstrual cycle (days 7–14), because uptake of contrast medium is dependent on the phase of the menstrual cycle. Good positioning of the patient is another essential factor for a high-quality study. It is essential for the patient to be comfortable and to have both breasts symmetrically centered within the coil. Both breasts are placed as deeply in the coil as possible with the nipples pointing downward. More breast coverage may be obtained by placing both arms at the side of the body and not above the patient's head.[10] The authors apply mild compression of breasts in the medial to lateral direction to decrease motion artifact and to decrease the number of slices needed to cover each breast (we scan in the sagittal plane) (Fig. 1).[11] Whenever possible a female technologist positions the patient in the coil for screening and/or diagnostic breast MR imaging examination. A female MR technologist always assists the authors with MR-guided interventional procedures because the breasts may need to be manipulated to visualize the index lesion. Most MR technologists have been trained to position the breast by observing stereotactic biopsies (performed on a prone table device). Once the patient has been positioned, localizer images are obtained. The technologist reviews these scout images to ensure that both breasts have been included in their entirety and are centered within the coil (Fig. 2). During the study, images from each sequence are reviewed by the technologist as they are processed to ensure optimal image quality and to evaluate for additional MR applications (eg, diffusion, spectroscopy). Suboptimal sequences are repeated by the technologist.

EQUIPMENT: MAGNET AND COIL

Conventional breast MR imaging is routinely performed on 1.5T magnets, 3T magnets, and some lower-field dedicated breast magnets. The technical requirements for breast MR imaging at 1.5T are listed in Table 1, which appears at the end of this article, and are reviewed later. Although there are no guidelines for performing the examination at 3T, the authors assume that imaging parameters at 3T should also meet the minimal technical requirements for a breast MR imaging performed on a 1.5T magnet. For an in-depth discussion of the technical aspects of breast MR imaging, see Ref.[12]

Proper dedicated equipment is necessary to optimize a breast MR imaging examination. The use of dedicated bilateral breast coils and high-field magnets are 2 essential components of this study, and are discussed in this section. A high signal-to-noise ratio (SNR) is a highly desirable variable in diagnostic breast MR imaging to maximize lesion characterization. The SNR is directly proportional to magnetic field strength (B_0), which at high strengths also affords higher spatial resolution. A high magnetic field also ensures adequate signal homogeneity and application of chemically selective fat suppression. The field homogeneity may be suboptimal for low-field magnets, resulting

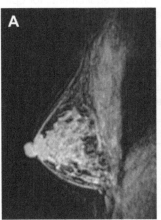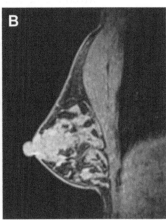

Fig. 1. Motion artifact. (A) Sagittal noncontrast T1-weighted MR image at 3T magnet shows considerable motion artifact when no compression is used. (B) Sagittal noncontrast T1-weighted MR image at 3T shows no motion artifact after mild compression is applied.

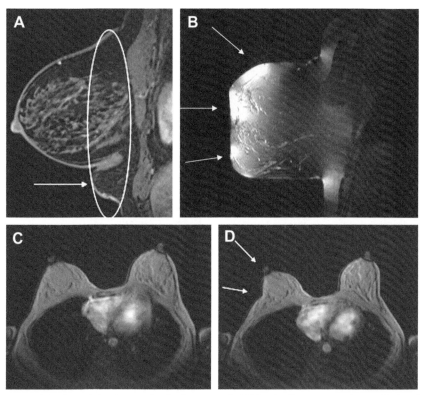

Fig. 2. Improper positioning of the breasts in the breast coil. (*A*) Sagittal contrast-enhanced T1-weighted image with fat saturation MR image at 1.5T magnet shows poor positioning of the breast, which is too cephalad within the coil, resulting in signal loss superiorly, and inclusion of the upper abdomen (*arrow*). The approximate location of coil apertures is circled. (*B*) It is difficult to position a woman with large breasts. Sagittal noncontrast T1-weighted MR image shows signal intensity changes where the breast tissue is in proximity to coil elements (*arrows*). (*C*) Axial localizer image shows the breasts are now correctly positioned. (*D*) Axial localizer image shows the lateral left breast is not pulled down into the coil and the nipple deviated laterally (*arrows*).

in uneven fat suppression and image degradation and it may impair lesion conspicuity.

A dedicated breast coil system that can image both breasts with the patient in the prone position enhances the clinical usefulness of breast MR imaging (**Fig. 3**). Advances in multichannel radio-frequency (RF) coil design have greatly improved signal homogeneity; they also provide a higher SNR (**Fig. 4**). Typically, 4-channel bilateral breast coils are matched to maximize parallel imaging techniques (discussed in the next section), although recent advances have pushed the coil array up to 32 receiver coils. In most clinical departments, a multipurpose body coil can be used as the transmit coil, whereas the dedicated breast coil is used as the receiver coil. Mediolateral

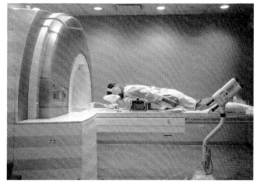

Fig. 3. The patient is lying prone on a breast coil and the arms are placed at the side of the body.

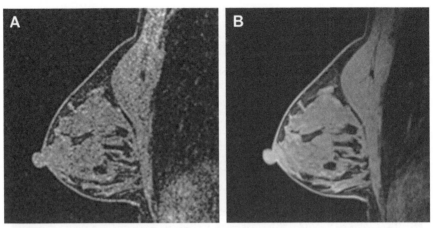

Fig. 4. Increased SNR by using a dedicated breast coil. (*A*) Sagittal noncontrast T1-weighted MR image performed with the body coil as the receiver coil is noisy. (*B*) The sequence is repeated with the breast coil as the receiver coil and shows higher SNR.

coil selection with open design also provides added interventional flexibility, allowing access for MR-guided core needle biopsy or wire localization in complex cases. In addition, given the imaging time required for diagnostic breast MR imaging and the marked degradation of image quality with patient motion, coil comfort with judicious padding and streamline design while providing adequate compression are added considerations in coil selection.

Although unilateral breast coils are available, bilateral coil design is highly desirable for modern imaging, especially in those patients with known carcinoma. Comparison of physiologic fibroglandular enhancement between breasts can often serve as an internal standard, particularly in premenopausal midcycle and postmenopausal women receiving hormonal therapy. In addition, in those patients with known carcinoma, evaluation of the contralateral breast, axilla, and chest wall can aid in preoperative staging. Bilateral breast imaging also reduces wraparound artifacts found in unilateral imaging when the contralateral breast falls out of the field-of-view (FOV). Wraparound artifact occurs when the FOV is too small, and the signal from tissue outside the selected FOV wraps around or aliases into the acquired image (**Fig. 5**).[11] Therefore, the selected FOV should be large enough to include full coverage of both breasts and to maximize spatial resolution.[12–14] In addition, special techniques such as phase oversampling can be used to mitigate wrap artifact, albeit at the expense of the SNR.[14]

PITFALLS AND TECHNICAL ARTIFACTS

As discussed earlier, voluntary patient motion greatly limits diagnostic MR image quality. Respiratory and cardiac motion may degrade image quality. Because motion always propagates in the phase-encoding direction, proper selection of the phase-encoding direction minimizes artifact from cardiac and respiratory motion. For breast MR imaging, the correct choice of the phase-encoding direction is left to right for axial images and superior to inferior for sagittal images. Prone positioning of the breasts decreases wraparound

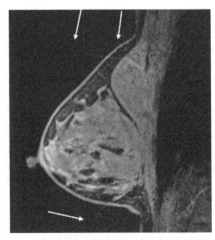

Fig. 5. Incorrectly sized FOV. Sagittal noncontrast T1-weighted MR image shows wraparound artifact (*arrows*) because the selected FOV was too small.

artifacts, and affords dependent positioning of the breasts with minimal cardiac and respiratory interference. In addition, prone positioning separates the breast parenchyma from the chest wall, increasing conspicuity of the fibroglandular tissue and chest wall interface. Coil selection is a balance between SNR, signal uniformity, interventional access, patient comfort, and cost.

Fat has a high signal on MR imaging and may obscure enhancing masses on the postcontrast images (**Fig. 6**). To increase lesion conspicuity most European techniques rely solely on subtraction of the postcontrast from the precontrast images to identify suspicious enhancing lesions. Subtraction is a postprocessing technique that subtracts a precontrast data set from a postcontrast data set on a pixel-by-pixel basis. The subtraction images are created automatically on the scanner. The advantages to using subtraction technique include no loss of signal, independence from magnetic field homogeneity, and no increase in scanning time. However, the SNR is low on the subtracted images, and the images may be plagued by misregistration from patient motion and automated technique error in slice positioning. In the United States, lesion conspicuity is enhanced by a chemically selective fat suppression to make the fat signal null. With both approaches, significant motion artifact during the dynamic phase causes misregistration and leads to the appearance of falsely enhancing lesions or nonvisualization of enhancing lesions (**Fig. 7**). At the authors' institution, we use fat suppression and subtraction in the evaluation of the dynamic postcontrast images.

Chemical shift artifact and magnetic susceptibility may also affect image quality. Chemical shift artifact is misregistration of spatial information caused by difference in the resonant frequency of water and fat. This artifact is seen in the frequency encoding direction, and is a result of incorrect mapping of the signal from lipid relative to that of water.[15] The number of pixels over which the chemical shift occurs is dependent on the bandwidth per pixel of the imaging sequence. It can be corrected by increasing the bandwidth and by using fat suppression techniques.[11–14] Magnetic susceptibility artifact is caused by the presence of an object in the FOV with a higher or lower magnetic susceptibility. It is most noticeable around metallic objects, and the size of the artifact is dependent on the size and composition of the metallic object.[14] This artifact appears more prominently on the gradient echo sequences, commonly used in DCE breast MR imaging. Most breast biopsy clips are now made of titanium, and the presence of a metallic clip may be difficult to identify on MR images.

IMAGING PROTOCOL

Sample DCE breast MR imaging protocols at 1.5T and 3T are presented in **Tables 2** and **3** appearing at the end of this article. The parameters listed are guidelines; clinical practices may need an experienced MR technologist to modify the protocol on a case-by-case basis. At the authors' institution, a precontrast T1-weighted image without fat saturation is first obtained. This sequence is useful to identify regions of fat in benign lymph nodes or fat

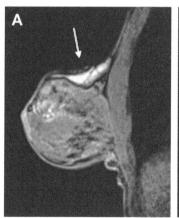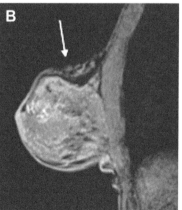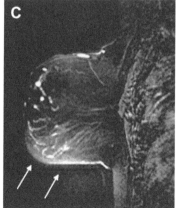

Fig. 6. Problems with fat suppression (*A*) Sagittal contrast-enhanced T1-weighted image with fat saturation MR image shows no fat suppression in the superior breast (*arrow*), leaving fatty tissue bright. (*B*) The center frequency is adjusted by the technologist and fat suppression is achieved (*arrow*). (*C*) Sagittal contrast-enhanced T1-weighted image with fat saturation MR image shows inhomogeneous fat suppression in the inferior breast, most likely as a result of field inhomogeneity.

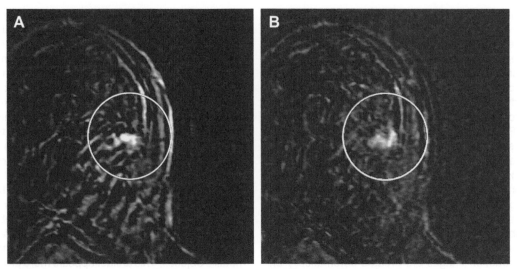

Fig. 7. If a patient moves during the dynamic scans, misregistration of the subtraction images can lead to the appearance of falsely enhancing lesions or nonvisualization of truly enhancing areas. (*A*) Subtraction image of an axial contrast-enhanced T1-weighted image with fat saturation MR image shows non-mass-like enhancement (*circle*) that was interpreted as being secondary to normal physiologic enhancement. Note the significant motion artifact. (*B*) The patient returns 6 months later and now an irregular mass (*circle*) can be appreciated. MR-guided core biopsy yielded DCIS.

necrosis. It also serves to delineate anatomic landmarks in problem cases in conjunction with other sequences. In addition, regions of subtle architectural distortion are often better characterized on this sequence. Moreover, the authors find it easier to identify the metallic clips deployed to demarcate biopsy sites on this sequence compared with the gradient echo sequences. Next, a precontrast fat-saturated T2-weighted sequence is obtained. This fluid-weighted sequence is essential for the diagnosis of simple cysts, but can also reveal internal architecture within a complex cyst. The T2-weighted sequence is often used to confirm the expected high signal seen with certain lesions, such as fibroadenoma or lymph nodes. Next, a precontrast T1-weighted sequence with a fat suppression pulse is performed to serve as the mask for the postcontrast images.

The final and most important sequence depends on the injection of intravenous gadolinium (discussed later). Sequential postcontrast three-dimensional (3D) T1-weighted gradient echo with fat saturation sequences are obtained in a dynamic fashion to assess the enhancement kinetics of suspicious lesions in relation to the expected background fibroglandular enhancement. These postcontrast sequences can then be subtracted from the precontrast T1 sequence to assess underlying contrast enhancement in those lesions with hemorrhage or proteinaceous material.

Subtraction images are also invaluable in postoperative cases in which there may be extensive inherent foci of T1 hyperintensity along the surgical bed, confounding the diagnosis of residual/recurrent disease.

The peak enhancement for most invasive cancers is within the first 2 minutes after the injection of contrast medium. Therefore, short dynamic imaging acquisition times, between 60 and 120 seconds per acquisition, are necessary.[16] Not all cancerous lesions adhere to this rule, and many have mixed or heterogeneous patterns of enhancement. Imaging should continue for 6 to 7 minutes after injection. During multiphase dynamic imaging, the normal background fibroglandular tissue enhances progressively, resulting in decreasing tumor-to-background conspicuity. At present, there is no consensus for the number of dynamic acquisitions that need to be obtained for assessing temporal information. At a minimum, the dynamic T1-weighted sequence should be obtained for at least 3 time points: 1 before and 2 after contrast administration.[10] At the New York University Langone Medical Center, the DCE breast MR imaging protocol consists of 1 precontrast sequence followed by 4 postcontrast sequences. The authors also use short repetition time (TR) and short echo time (TE) to maximize T1 weighting and to minimize acquisition times.

CONTRAST MEDIUM

Injection of intravenous gadolinium is essential to assess the malignant potential of lesions discovered at MR imaging. Although there was hope for noncontrast techniques in breast MR imaging early in development, it has become clear that gadolinium serves a crucial role for lesion detection and characterization. Free elemental gadolinium is toxic when injected, but after chelation to a conjugate base, the unpaired electrons in gadolinium interact with adjacent tissues, causing relaxation of T1 greater than T2 and T2* times. In this way, hypervascular lesions (including cancer) are exposed to the paramagnetic effects of gadolinium as it circulates through the blood, and appear brighter than the surrounding tissues on T1-weighted images. Typical dosing involves injection of 0.1 mmol/kg at 2 mL/s. The gadolinium injection is typically followed by a saline flush (20–30 mL). Gadolinium is cleared by the kidneys through glomerular filtration, and has a half-life of approximately 90 minutes. In patients with renal dysfunction and impaired glomerular filtration rate (GFR), gadolinium can be diffusely deposited in the body, resulting in a multiorgan fibrosis known as nephrogenic systemic fibrosis. The US Food and Drug Administration (FDA) now recommends that at-risk patients should be screened for renal insufficiency (GFR < 30 mL/min/1.73 m^2) before receiving gadolinium (current FDA guidelines can be found at http://www.fda.gov/).

The principles of contrast enhancement, and therefore, breast cancer detection on MR imaging, are based on tumor angiogenesis. These abnormal tumor vessels tend to be large and leaky.[17] Breast cancers typically show rapid uptake of contrast, early, intense peak enhancement, and rapid washout of contrast. Benign lesions and normal tissue have slower and less intense enhancement. The proper timing of postcontrast pulse sequences is critical for the detection of subtle non-masslike lesions. Longer acquisition times may prevent the peak tumor enhancement from being observed. In addition, timing the postcontrast sequences to optimize the center of k-space is essential. K-space is defined by the space covered by the phase and frequency encoded data. The outer rows of k-space contain high-spatial frequencies and provide fine details regarding the margins of a lesion, whereas the inner rows of the matrix contain the low-spatial frequencies, which provide contrast.

As stated earlier, there is continuous imaging of both breasts, with a temporal resolution of 1 to 2 minutes. The breasts are repeatedly and rapidly imaged for 6 to 7 minutes after contrast administration. Then a semiquantitative analysis of the percent change in signal intensity from the precontrast value is plotted over time. This kinetic analysis generates a time-signal intensity curve that is divided into 2 phases: early and delayed. The early phase is defined as the first 2 minutes after contrast administration, and characterizes the initial wash-in of contrast into a lesion. The BI-RADS lexicon describes the initial uptake of contrast as fast, medium, or slow.[7] The specific threshold values used for fast, medium, or slow uptake vary with imaging protocols.[18] Most invasive cancers have reached their peak enhancement by the end of this early phase. The delayed phase is defined as the change in enhancement after the first 2 minutes, or after the curve starts to change. This part of the curve is classified into 3 types based on its shape: persistent, plateau, and washout.

Persistent (type 1) curve is one in which the signal intensity continues to increase with time, throughout the dynamic series.

Plateau (type 2) curve is a curve in which the signal intensity levels off after initial enhancement and does not change with time. Plateau curves have a sensitivity and specificity for malignancy of 42% and 75%, respectively.[18]

Washout (type 3) curve reaches a peak at the end of the initial phase, followed by a decrease in the signal intensity throughout the delayed phase. This curve is most frequently associated with malignant lesions (76%–92% positive predictive value).[18,19]

In 1999, Kuhl and colleagues[18] showed that the additional analysis of the time-signal intensity curve could increase specificity of breast MR imaging from 37% to 83%. In their study, a type 1 curve was associated with a 6% likelihood of malignancy. A type 2 curve is associated with a 64% likelihood of malignancy and a type 3 curve is associated with an 87% likelihood of malignancy. There was still overlap, with 5% of benign lesions exhibiting a washout curve and 9% of malignant lesions exhibiting a persistent curve. In a more recent study by Schnall and colleagues,[19] 45% of lesions with persistent curves were malignant. Those lesions that show washout should be viewed with a high suspicion for malignancy in conjunction with other imaging indices of cancer. The investigators stressed the importance of using the enhancement kinetic curves in conjunction with morphologic analysis of the lesion to avoid false reassurance of an atypical malignant lesion or, conversely, to avoid overcalling benign lesions. This was reemphasized by Liu and colleagues,[20] who found morphology and kinetic curve assessment combined yielded the highest sensitivity and specificity for cancer detection.

SPATIAL VERSUS TEMPORAL RESOLUTION

Despite advances in MR imaging techniques, spatial and temporal resolutions remain competing interests in characterizing breast cancer. With only 1 bolus gadolinium injection, characterization of lesion morphology with thin slices (ie, spatial resolution) must be tempered with the sequence acquisition time (ie, temporal resolution), which provides enhancement kinetic and time-signal intensity curve analysis. Thicker slices (>3 mm) increase partial volume effects. Thin section thickness increases the sensitivity for lesion detection, but may decrease the SNR (**Fig. 8**). Increasing spatial resolution also increases the acquisition time, thereby decreasing temporal resolution.

In 2005, Kuhl and colleagues[21] evaluated the performance of a modified protocol that offered increased spatial resolution, low-temporal resolution (32 cm FOV 400 × 512 matrix, 3 mm slice thickness for 3.0 × 0.8 × 0.6 mm voxel size) every 69 seconds, compared with a standard low-spatial resolution, high temporal resolution imaging technique (32 cm FOV 256 × 256 matrix, 3 mm slice thickness for 3.0 × 1.25 × 1.25 mm voxel size) every 116 seconds. In assessing 54 lesions in 30 patients with this modified dynamic protocol, these investigators found that a higher spatial resolution detected subtle morphologic features (spicules, septations). Also, no diagnostically relevant kinetic information was lost by scanning at the lower temporal resolution because the time-course pattern curve was unchanged. Thirteen of 26 (50%) malignant lesions were correctly upstaged using the modified protocol, whereas no cancer was incorrectly downgraded. The investigators concluded that the increased spatial resolution improved their diagnostic confidence in cancer detection.[21] This study allowed for the reconciliation of the European and United States techniques. There is now a consensus that a significant amount of detail is gained when the in-plane pixel size is decreased from greater than 1 cm to a submillimeter in-plane voxel. This additional detail should be obtained while maintaining an adequate temporal resolution of 1 to 2 minutes. As technology evolves with the advent of faster-acquisition strategies, this compromise between spatial and temporal resolution will be revisited.

A recent advancement in MR imaging has been the development of parallel imaging, which allows simultaneous acquisition of multiple channels of data without loss of spatial resolution. This technique exploits the use of multiple receiver coils to derive spatial localization, reducing the need for repeat phase-encoding steps.[22] Parallel imaging speeds image acquisition by a factor called the acceleration factor. It is recommended for breast MR imaging to keep the acceleration factor between 2 and 3, otherwise there are image artifacts and significant loss of SNR.[12] This approach allows data to be acquired at higher spatial resolution with greater FOV coverage within the same acquisition time or enables higher temporal resolution for kinetic analysis. One disadvantage is a penalty of SNR by 30% when parallel imaging techniques are used if all other parameters are maintained. Most sequences listed in this article use a parallel imaging factor of 2, thereby

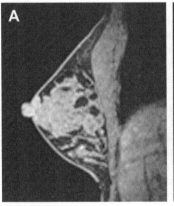
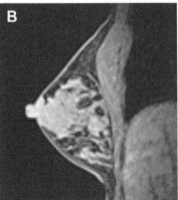
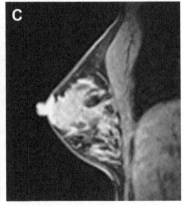

Fig. 8. Effect of section thickness on image quality. Sagittal noncontrast T1-weighted with fat saturation MR images obtained with (*A*) 1-mm, (*B*) 2-mm, and (*C*) 3-mm section thickness shows partial volume averaging increases with section thickness.

decreasing the examination time. Average acquisition time of a breast MR imaging with contrast is typically less than 30 minutes. The authors have used parallel imaging to dramatically shorten scan times for full bilateral coverage, and have been able to obtain simultaneous bilateral sagittal imaging. These techniques also reduce wraparound artifacts and other imaging artifacts at 1.5T and 3T imaging.

What should be sacrificed if your clinical scanner is older or is not equipped with these new technologies? The authors believe that the following scanning parameters should be maintained: 3D gradient echo sequences, full coverage of both breasts, and a submillimeter in-plane resolution. Using the shortest possible TR and TE values keeps the acquisition times less than 2 minutes. One may consider sacrificing an isotropic voxel, foregoing the ability to reformat in other planes without losing spatial resolution, if high spatial resolution may be maintained in the imaging plane.[12] Also, the slice thickness may be increased up to 3 mm if necessary.

IMAGING PLANE

The selection of imaging plane is based on interpreting physicians' preferences and technical capabilities of the MR imaging systems in various clinical practices. The authors acquire images in a sagittal plane, which affords a higher spatial resolution at the expense of SNR. The sagittal plane has a smaller FOV and facilitates homogenous fat saturation. In the authors' experience, acquiring images in the sagittal plane may highlight areas of architectural changes not so well appreciated on axial images. A large drawback is that bilateral sagittal imaging requires at least twice the number of sections required for bilateral axial imaging, increasing the demands on an MR system for rapid imaging. On the other hand, bilateral axial images allow for the assessment of symmetry and the detection of subtle lesions. Also, the physiologic non-masslike areas of enhancement often seen in premenopausal women are easier to assess on axial imaging. There are fewer slices, allowing for less trade-off between spatial or temporal resolution. In any case, if isotropic voxel size is obtained in either orientation, the sequences can be interpreted using multiplanar 3D analysis tools.

WHY MOVE TO BREAST MR IMAGING AT 3T?

The technical requirements for breast MR imaging are challenging because acquisitions of both breasts must be completed within 2 minutes to capture information about the peak arterial enhancement. Continuous dynamic scanning for 6 to 7 minutes allows assessment of the delayed phase of contrast enhancement. With longer acquisition times, the differential enhancement between a cancer and fibroglandular tissue may not be accentuated. At the same time, a slice thickness of 2 mm or less and a submillimeter voxel size ensure the high spatial resolution necessary for characterization of a lesion based on size, shape, margins, and internal enhancement patterns. Although the sensitivity of DCE breast MR imaging on a 1.5T magnet is high, the wide range of specificities emphasizes that further improvement in the MR characterization of the breast lesion is essential.

Recent published reports suggest 3T MR systems are superior to 1.5T MR systems in the brain, musculoskeletal system, and for MR angiography.[23–25] 3T MR imaging systems are becoming increasingly used in the clinical setting. A 2008 survey of trends in breast MR imaging in the United States found 9.5% of clinical practices were using 3T magnets to perform this examination.[6] Because the SNR in MR is proportional to the magnetic field strength (B_o), the additional SNR at 3T should translate into higher spatial resolution and faster imaging times for breast MR imaging. The other advantage is improved fat suppression as a result of the greater spectral separation of fat and water at 3T. However, the gain in SNR is offset by technical modifications, along with physical and safety considerations, that are necessary to obtain high-quality images at 3T. Parameter adjustments are necessary to account for changes in the tissue contrast, B_o field inhomogeneity, B_1 field inhomogeneity, tissue heating, and chemical shift effects.[26,27] Therefore, the SNR at 3T is approximately 1.7 to 1.8 times that at 1.5T.[28] The effects of these issues on the image quality are discussed later and various approaches to overcome these challenges are proposed.

The paradigm for breast MR imaging at 3T is similar to that for a study at 1.5T. The conventional protocols are modified to work more effectively at 3T and mimic the image quality of 1.5T, with some expected improvements in SNR, spatial resolution, and acquisition time.[26] A few published reports conclude that the image quality at 3T is at least as good as at 1.5T. In 2006 Kuhl and colleagues[29] prospectively studied 37 patients with 53 lesions who underwent breast MR imaging twice, once at 1.5T and once at 3T. They found image quality was higher at 3T. These investigators concluded that "at 3T, the differential diagnosis of enhancing lesions was possible with a higher diagnostic confidence."[29] Additional prospective blinded studies comparing both systems are needed. However, it is difficult to make a direct comparison, as the sequence parameters and coils for 1.5T and 3T are different. On a practical level, many institutions may not have 1.5T and 3T magnets readily available.[26]

The same investigators then published concerns about limited contrast enhancement at 3T, stating that "due to spatial B_1 inhomogeneities across the FOV, enhancement of lesions may be reduced to a variable degree."[27,30] This surprisingly lower enhancement of lesions may have contributed to the overall higher specificity. In a response to these concerns, Mountford and colleagues[31] emphasized the "importance of protocol design and technique in optimizing the performance of breast MR imaging at 3T." The adjustment of other parameters in the imaging protocol may compensate for B_1 field inhomogeneity.

Two recent studies performed at 3T have reported a sensitivity of 100%, with specificities of 72.2% to 93.9%.[32,33] These studies have shown incremental benefits of 3T compared with 1.5T with respect to image quality and efficiency. It remains to be seen whether breast MR imaging at 3T will lead to improvement in lesion detection, more accurate diagnosis, or improved patient outcome in clinical practice (**Fig. 9**).

TECHNICAL CONSIDERATIONS FOR OPTIMIZING IMAGE QUALITY AT 3T

There are several challenges to obtaining high image quality at 3T, including increased T1 relaxation times, RF inhomogeneity, and accentuation of certain MR imaging artifacts. Therefore, scanning

parameters must be modified to address these constraints of the 3T systems.

The T1 relaxation times of tissues are longer at 3T and may lead to decreased accentuation of tissue contrast; however, the T1 relaxivity of gadolinium chelates at 3T is relatively constant when compared with 1.5T. Both changes, coupled with the increased SNR at 3T, may lead to greater contrast between enhancing and nonenhancing breast tissue for the same dose of contrast. Adjustments of TR, TE, and flip angle can usually compensate for these effects and maintain image quality.[26] Caution with these parameter modifications is advised because the lengthening of TR increases acquisition times. Higher bandwidths may be required and lead to a loss of some SNR. Similarly, parallel imaging may be used to reduce TR and tissue heating, but again this occurs at the expense of SNR.

In theory, uniform fat saturation may be more difficult to achieve at 3T because it may be more difficult to maintain a uniform magnetic field (B_o). However, separation of the signal peaks for fat and water is greater at 3T, and therefore correct identification of the fat peak is easier with higher field magnets. The authors find the increased spectral separation of fat and water resonance frequencies at 3T leads to more uniform and effective (more nulling of the fat signal) fat saturation.

RF HOMOGENEITY

Newer high sensitivity multichannel phased-array breast coils are needed to harness the increased signal of higher field magnets. At present, 7, 8, 16, and 32 multichannel coils are available for

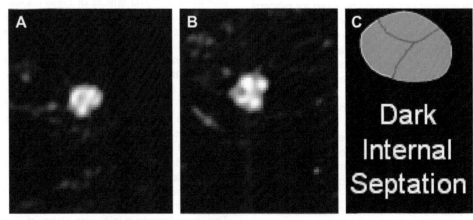

Fig. 9. Increased spatial resolution at 3T. A 45-year-old high-risk woman with a known fibroadenoma. (*A*) Contrast-enhanced T1-weighted MR image with fat saturation MR image at 1.5T magnet shows a lobulated enhancing mass with a suggestion of several dark septations. (*B*) Contrast-enhanced T1-weighted MR image with fat saturation MR image at 3T magnet shows the dark septations more clearly. (*C*) The dark septations that may be seen in a fibroadenoma.

breast MR imaging at 3T. RF (B_1) homogeneity is difficult to achieve and maintain with increasing field strength because the interactions between coils and biologic tissue become significant (rather than being determined by the coil design alone).[26] RF inhomogeneity leads to variation in signal intensity across an image. Reducing RF (B_1) field inhomogeneity requires improvement in coil design, with multiple close elements. Several vendors have developed multichannel breast coils that can be adjusted to accommodate larger and smaller breasts. These newer designs may reduce focal field inhomogeneity and improve SNR and patient comfort.

MR IMAGING ARTIFACTS

There may be greater chemical shift effects, greater susceptibility artifacts, and dielectric effects, all of which may compromise uniform enhancement of both breasts at 3T. With higher signal strength there is also associated higher susceptibility effect. Shorter TE and lower flip angles can help compensate for the stronger susceptibility effects seen at 3T. Dielectric effects appear as nonuniformity of signal or shading in MR images and are seen more commonly with a larger FOV, higher field magnet, and with multichannel coils. A chemical shift artifact is caused by the difference in chemical shift (Larmor frequency) of fat and water. The artifact manifests itself as a misregistration between the fat and water pixels in an image and is accentuated at any fat-water interfaces along the frequency axis. To reduce the chemical shift artifact at 3T, the bandwidth must be increased, but leads to a reduction in SNR.[14,26] Also, frequency selective fat suppression improves as spectral separation increases with higher field strength, and may compensate for chemical shift effects.[34] Overall, optimization of the image protocol at 3T shares similar principles to adjustments made at 1.5T. These modifications include selecting an FOV just large enough to provide full coverage of both breasts, adjustments of the TR/TE, increasing bandwidths, and decreasing flip angles.[31]

The synergistic effect of parallel imaging and 3T imaging has reduced the trade-off between spatial and temporal resolution. In addition to significantly shorter acquisition times, parallel imaging can address some of the challenges of imaging at 3T mentioned earlier. Parallel imaging techniques limit tissue heating by reducing the RF exposure and the scan time.[26,35,36] Improved signal homogeneity may also be achieved with this technique.[26,35,37] Parallel imaging also reduces image artifacts and distortions caused by susceptibility effects.

Although parallel imaging involves a penalty in SNR, new multichannel breast coils and higher field strengths can compensate for this loss in signal and provide high-quality images.[38]

FUTURE MR IMAGING PROTOCOLS AT 3T

The benefit of higher spatial resolution at 3T holds particular promise for improved assessment of small, non-masslike lesions (usually fibroglandular enhancement) and improved detection of ductal carcinoma in situ (DCIS).[39] DCIS often presents as a non-masslike lesion in a linear distribution, with clumped internal enhancement pattern.[40–42] However, DCIS has variable enhancement kinetics, with most lesions enhancing less than invasive cancers.[42] A higher spatial resolution may lead to better assessment of the margins and internal enhancement pattern of these non-masslike lesions (**Figs. 10** and **11**).

Another area of active research is a more refined analysis of the time-signal intensity curve. The higher temporal resolution at 3T imaging suggests that a quantitative analysis of the changes in signal intensity with time may improve lesion characterization and specificity. Various parameters derived from the time-signal intensity curve, including time to onset of enhancement, maximum slope of enhancement, time to peak enhancement, degree or percent change over baseline, peak enhancement, and signal enhancement ratios, may be quantitatively measured with high temporal resolution protocols. Early studies on the uptake rate of contrast and the rate of enhancement found a significant overlap in enhancement rates between benign and malignant lesions.[18,43] Because field strength, T1 relaxation time, and temporal resolution affect lesion kinetics, several investigators have suggested that the higher temporal resolution at 3T may allow for a more detailed evaluation of the initial uptake of the contrast medium. Boetes and colleagues[44] noted improved diagnostic accuracies at high temporal resolution using the greater number of time points. Veltman and colleagues[45] found that imaging with a high temporal resolution (every 4.1 seconds) during the initial phase followed by high spatial resolution analysis with a slower dynamic analysis (86 seconds) improved lesion classification and diagnostic accuracy.

CHALLENGES AT 3T

Although the FDA has concluded that clinical MR magnets 8-T or less pose nonsignificant risk for patients, issues regarding patient safety must be addressed before ultrahigh-field imaging is

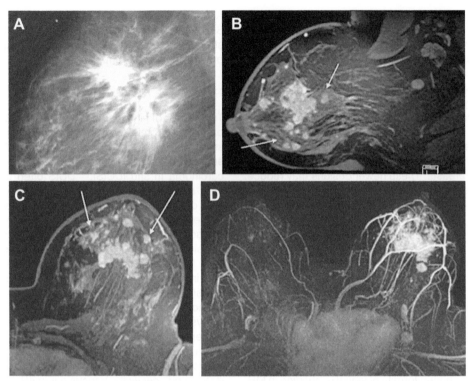

Fig. 10. Breast MR imaging at 3T magnet. A 60-year-old woman presents with a palpable mass in the left breast. (*A*) On mammography, a large spiculated mass is seen, corresponding to the palpable lump. (*B*) Sagittal and (*C*) axial contrast-enhanced T1-weighted MR images with fat saturation show an irregular mass with multiple satellite lesions (*arrows*). Biopsy yielded invasive ductal carcinoma. (*D*) Maximum intensity projection image shows the enhancing masses in the left breast.

routinely performed. These concerns include deposition of RF energy, implanted medical devices, acoustic noise, and patient comfort. They may pose a more practical limit and are discussed in this section.

SPECIFIC ABSORPTION RATE

The deposition of RF energy in tissue grows exponentially with increasing field strength and frequency, and may cause tissue heating and possibly skin burns. This RF absorption of energy

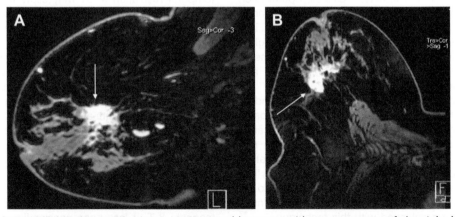

Fig. 11. Breast MR imaging at 3T magnet. A 65-year-old woman with an asymmetry of the right breast on mammography. (*A*) Sagittal and (*B*) axial contrast-enhanced T1-weighted MR images with fat saturation show an irregular enhancing mass (*arrows*). Biopsy yielded invasive lobular carcinoma.

as heat is known as specific absorption rate (SAR). SAR-induced temperature changes of a human body are a significant safety issue of high-field strengths. The energy deposited in a patient's tissues is fourfold higher at 3T than at 1.5T. The International Electrotechnical Commission has established the following limits on SAR[46]:

1. No more than 4 W/kg averaged over the entire body for a duration of 15 or more minutes
2. No more than 8 W/kg in any gram of tissue in the head or torso for a duration of 5 or more minutes.

The authors modified their imaging parameters at 3T to keep within the SAR limits imposed by the FDA. Sequence modifications for RF-intensive pulse sequences such as diffusion-weighted imaging (DWI) become technically challenging at high-field magnets. These adjustments included decreasing slices per TR, decreasing flip angle, lengthening TR, increasing interecho spacing, and prolonging the RF pulse duration. However, these modifications led to reduced anatomic coverage, alteration of tissue contrast, and diminished SNR. The addition of parallel imaging has negated some of these trade-offs, albeit at loss of SNR.

To date, we have not encountered any SAR limit in our practice. In addition, no SAR limit has been reported in the literature. Our patients complain of feeling very warm if they are undergoing a long examination (eg, routine protocol for contrast-enhanced breast MR imaging followed by a protocol to evaluate for implant rupture, approximately 50 minutes in total). This discomfort is more of an annoyance rather than a safety issue. We address this discomfort by turning on fans that are beneath the coil.

MEDICAL DEVICES

Another important safety issue is the effect of a 3T magnet on implanted medical devices. Image artifacts related to implanted devices are likely to increase with increasing field strength. Higher field systems may lead to heating or motion of these devices. Imaging centers should have a backup 1.5T magnet for patients who cannot safely enter the higher magnetic field. Most medical devices considered safe at 1.5T are also considered safe at 3T. However, there is a wide range of medical devices including copper intrauterine devices, certain types of aneurysm clips, cardiac stents, and orthopedic devices that have not been proven to be safe at higher magnetic fields. Our nurses

and technologist use MR imaging safety Web sites and reference manuals to identify the devices have been proven to be safe at 3T.[47] If the type of medical device cannot be identified (eg, by obtaining an intraoperative report), we perform the examination on a 1.5T system.

A common side effect is noise related to the vibration of the gradient coils. Acoustic noise level increases at higher field strength because the forces experienced by changing gradient currents are proportional to field strength.[26] Routine safety measures, such as ear plugs and head phones, are usually sufficient to reduce ambient noise to acceptable levels. The use of parallel imaging techniques reduces k-space sampling and also leads to decreased noise and acquisition times. Additional safety concerns include the side effects of motion through large magnetic fields, usually causing mild transient vertigo and difficulty in balancing after leaving the 3T magnet. These patients are monitored before leaving the imaging facility to ensure their safety.

ADDITIONAL APPLICATIONS OF THE 3T MAGNETS

The benefits of parallel imaging and 3T imaging coupled with the development of new multi-channel coils may permit functional MR techniques (proton MR spectroscopy, DWI, perfusion-weighted imaging) to reach a point of clinical usefulness. These MR techniques give insight into organ function and complement the vascular information provided by DCE breast MR imaging. MR spectroscopy of the breast detects increased levels of choline metabolites, which is a marker for increased cell turnover. A choline resonance peak at 3.2 parts per million is detected primarily in malignant breast lesions.[48,49] MR spectroscopy may improve the characterization of lesions detected on breast MR imaging, even for enhancing non-masslike lesions.[50] Most published studies have been performed at 1.5T magnets and focused on lesions of 2 cm or more. At 3T imaging the wider separation of metabolite peaks may improve the quality of proton MR spectroscopy of the breast, especially in smaller lesions and possibly regions of DCIS. The authors' data show that MR spectroscopy at 3T may detect choline metabolites in lesions approximately 1 cm in size, and may lead to wider adoption of this technology in clinical practice.[51]

Another promising technique in characterization of breast masses is DWI. DWI uses motion-sensitive gradients to measure the diffusion of water in tissue. The MR imaging signal obtained with diffusion weighting is reduced in intensity proportional to the water mobility.[38] Several studies have shown that the apparent diffusion coefficients (ADC) of benign and malignant breast tissues differ. Breast cancers exhibit restricted diffusion (ie, lower ADC values), possibly because of their increased cellularity (**Fig. 12**). Tsushima and colleagues[52] performed a meta-analysis of 12 published studies evaluating ADC of breast tumors at 1.5T, and found a pooled sensitivity and specificity of 89% and 77%, respectively. The higher SNR at 3T may allow more detailed DWI, as suggested by 2 recent reports of DWI of breast lesions at 3T that showed sensitivities and specificities of 95% to 96% and 91% to 94%, respectively.[53,54] Also, breast cancers have high signal on diffusion-weighted images, suggesting the potential for DWI to be incorporated into a noncontrast breast MR imaging screening technique.

The development of high-field MR imaging systems has been driven by the expected improvements in SNR ratio, contrast-to-noise ratio, spatial-temporal resolution trade-off and spectral separation. Specialized multichannel coils have been developed to achieve such potential. The synergistic effect of parallel imaging and 3T imaging has reduced the trade-off between spatial or temporal resolution. The authors have used the increased SNR to obtain a high spatial resolution at comparable imaging times to 1.5T.

Benefits of high-field strength scanning

- More homogenous and effective fat saturation facilitates MR image interpretation
- Improved image quality as a result of a higher spatial resolution

- Higher spatial resolution may aid in the evaluation of small subcentimeter lesions and improved detection of DCIS
- Rapid imaging time may permit enhanced temporal assessment of contrast agent uptake and distribution
- The faster scans reduce image degradation as a result of patient motion; also, a shorter examination time allows imaging of claustrophobic, uncooperative, or anxious patients to tolerate the study.

The drawbacks are

- The maximal theoretic benefits cannot be achieved because competing effects come into play. Higher magnetic field strengths have disadvantages that need to be overcome compared with 1.5T. These disadvantages include stronger susceptibility effects, longer T1 relaxation times, shorter in-phase TEs, and higher RF deposition. Susceptibility effects may distort images acquired with a gradient echo pulse sequence, the type of sequence that is typically used for breast MR imaging.
- An increased SAR can result in excessive heating in the patient. RF energy deposition in tissue increases exponentially with field strength, therefore SAR limitations are reached sooner at 3T.
- Some metal implants and medical devices have not been shown to be safe at 3T. Therefore these patients should be imaged on the 1.5T systems.
- The 3T MR imaging system is more expensive than the 1.5T system, although

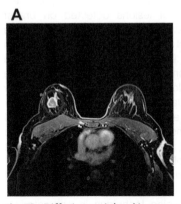
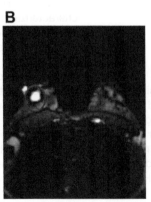
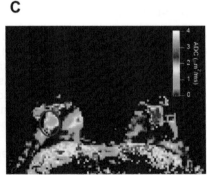

Fig. 12. Diffusion-weighted image at 3T magnet. A 45-year-old woman with a 1.5-cm invasive ductal carcinoma in the right breast. (*A*) Axial contrast-enhanced T1-weighted MR images with fat saturation shows an irregular rim enhancing mass (*circle*). (*B*) On axial DWI, b = 800 s/mm², the lesion appears hyperintense (*arrow*). (*C*) ADC map shows a lower apparent diffusion in the lesion (*circle*).

examinations performed on both magnets have similar reimbursement rates.

SUMMARY

Breast MR imaging has emerged as a useful imaging modality for detection of breast cancer. A high-quality breast MR imaging requires a high-field magnet (1.5T or 3T) and use of a dedicated multichannel breast coil. Modern breast MR protocols are optimized for the simultaneous acquisition of high spatial resolution and high temporal resolution images, which are necessary for accurate assessment of breast lesion morphology and a semiquantitative enhancement kinetic analysis. It remains to be seen if the enhanced resolution of images at 3T, coupled with functional imaging for lesion characterization, will continue to improve lesion detection and characterization. Despite potential challenges in per-

---

Table 1
General guidelines for optimizing DCE breast MR imaging at 1.5T

High magnetic field strength with good magnetic field homogeneity across both breasts
Dedicated bilateral breast coil with prone positioning
Full coverage of both breasts
Homogenous fat suppression over both breasts
Selection of a phase-encoding direction to minimize artifacts
3D contrast-enhanced T1-weighted gradient echo sequences[a]
Short acquisition times of 1–2 minutes. Use the shortest possible TRs and TEs to keep total acquisition time short
Intravenous administration of a gadolinium chelate at a dose of 0.1 mmol/kg at a rate of 1–2 mL/s
Section thickness 1–3 mm[b]
High in-plane resolution (<1 mm × 1 mm)
High SNR per pixel
High temporal resolution (1–2 minutes)
Continuous dynamic imaging for 6–7 minutes
Subtraction or fat suppression

[a] Ideally with parallel imaging sequences, with an acceleration factor ≤2.
[b] With technologic improvements, thin slices ≤1 mm may be achieved.

Table 2
Parameters for breast MR imaging at 1.5T at our institution

	Imaging Sequence	
Parameter	Sagittal T2-weighted	Sagittal T1-weighted Gradient Recalled Echo (GRE)
TR (ms)	6100	4.33
TE (ms)	113	1.32
Fat saturation	Yes	Yes
Flip angle	180	10
FOV (mm)	300	340
Matrix	256 × 256	448 × 448
Slice thickness (mm)	4	.9
No. of sections	66	176
Voxel size (mm)	0.9 × 0.7 × 4	1.1 × 0.8 × 0.9
Bandwidth (Hz/pixel)	150	350
Imaging time (min:s)	2:10	6:31

Table 3
Parameters for breast MR imaging at 3T at our institution

	Imaging Sequence	
Parameter	Sagittal T2-weighted	Sagittal T1-weighted GRE
TR (ms)	7220	4:01
TE (ms)	84.0	1:52
Fat saturation	Yes	Yes
Flip angle	130	12
FOV (mm)	270	270
Matrix	320 × 320	448 × 448
Slice thickness (mm)	3	1 mm
No. of sections	80	224
Voxel size (mm)	1.3 × 0.8 × 3.0	1.1 × 0.9 × 0.9
Bandwidth (Hz/pixel)	252	450
Imaging time (min:s)	5:34	6:19

forming breast MR imaging, high-quality images may be obtained on 1.5T and 3T systems by understanding key issues and by following appropriate techniques.

REFERENCES

1. Davis PL, McCarty KS Jr. Sensitivity of enhanced MRI for detection of breast cancer: new, multicentric, residual, and recurrent. Eur Radiol 1997;7(Suppl 5):289–98.
2. Orel SG, Schnall MD. MR imaging of the breast for the detection, diagnosis, and staging of breast cancer. Radiology 2001;220:13–30.
3. Heywang-Kobrunner SH, Viehweg P, Heinig A, et al. Contrast-enhanced MRI of the breast: accuracy, value, controversies, solutions. Eur J Radiol 1997;24:94–108.
4. Saslow D, Boetes C, Burke W, et al. American Cancer Society guidelines for breast screening with MRI as an adjunct to mammography. CA Cancer J Clin 2007;57(2):75–89.
5. Lehman CD, Gatsonis C, Kuhl CK, et al. MRI evaluation of the contralateral breast in women with recently diagnosed breast cancer. N Engl J Med 2007;356(13):1295–303.
6. Bassett LW, Dhaliwal SG, Eradat J, et al. National trends and practices in breast MRI. AJR Am J Roentgenol 2008;191(2):332–9.
7. American College of Radiology. ACR breast imaging reporting and data system (BIRADS): breast imaging Atlas. 4th edition. Reston (VA): American College of Radiology; 2003.
8. Ikeda D, Hylton M, Kuhl C, et al. Breast imaging reporting and data system, BI-RADS: magnetic resonance imaging (BI-RADS: MRI). Reston (VA): American College of Radiology; 2003.
9. American College of Radiology. Available at: http://www.acr.org/SecondaryMainMenuCategories/quality_safety/guidelines/breast/mri_breast.aspx. Accessed January 30, 2010.
10. Mann RM, Kuhl CK, Kinkel K, et al. Breast MRI: guidelines from the European Society of Breast Imaging. Eur Radiol 2008;18(7):1307–18.
11. Rausch D, Hendrick RE. How to optimize clinical breast MR imaging practices and techniques on Your 1.5T system. Radiographics 2006;26:1469–84.
12. Hendrick RE. Breast MRI: fundamentals and technical aspects. New York (NY): Springer; 2007. ISBN: 978-0-387-73506-1.
13. Harvey JA, Hendrick RE, Coll JM, et al. Breast MR imaging artifacts: how to recognize and fix them. Radiographics 2007;27(Suppl 1):S131–45.
14. Ojeda-Fournier H, Choe KA, Mahoney MC. Recognizing and interpreting artifacts and pitfalls in MR imaging of the breast. Radiographics 2007;27(Suppl 1):S147–64.
15. Hood MN, Ho VB, Smirniotopoulos JG, et al. Chemical shift: the artifact and clinical tool revisited. Radiographics 1999;19(2):357–71.
16. Kuhl CK. Concepts for differential diagnosis in breast MR imaging. Magn Reson Imaging Clin N Am 2006;14(3):305–37.
17. Papetti M, Herman IM. Mechanisms of normal and tumor derived angiogenesis. Am J Physiol Cell Physiol 2002;282:947–70.
18. Kuhl CK, Mielcareck P, Klaschik S, et al. Dynamic breast MR imaging; a signal intensity time course data useful for differential diagnosis of enhancing lesions? Radiology 1999;211:101–10.
19. Schnall MD, Blume J, Bluemke DA, et al. Diagnostic architectural and dynamic features at breast MR imaging: multicenter study. Radiology 2006;238:42–53.

20. Liu PF, Debatin JF, Caduff RF, et al. Improved diagnostic accuracy in dynamic contrast enhanced MRI of the breast by combined quantitative analysis. Br J Radiol 1998;71(845):501–9.

21. Kuhl CK, Schild HH, Morakkabati N. Dynamic bilateral contrast-enhanced MR imaging of the breast: trade-off between spatial and temporal resolution. Radiology 2005;236(3):789–800.

22. Dietrich O, Nikolaou K, Wintersperger BJ, et al. iPAT: application for fast and cardiovascular MR imaging. Electromedica 2002;70:133–45.

23. DeLano MC, Fisher C. 3T MR imaging of the brain. Magn Reson Imaging Clin N Am 2006; 14(1):77–88.

24. Bolbos RI, Zuo J, Banerjee S, et al. Relationship between trabecular bone structure and articular cartilage morphology and relaxation times in early OA of the knee joint using parallel MRI at 3 T. Osteoarthritis Cartilage 2008;16(10):1150–9.

25. Kaufmann TJ, Huston J 3rd, Cloft HJ, et al. A prospective trial of 3T and 1.5T time-of-flight and contrast-enhanced MR angiography in the followup of coiled intracranial aneurysms. AJNR Am J Neuroradiol 2009. [Epub ahead of print].

26. Hecht EM, Lee RF, Taouli B, et al. Perspectives on body MR imaging at ultrahigh field. Magn Reson Imaging Clin N Am 2007;15(3):449–65, viii.

27. Kuhl CK. Breast MR imaging at 3T. Magn Reson Imaging Clin N Am 2007;15(3):315–20, vi.

28. Erturk SM, Alberich-Bayarri A, Herrmann KA, et al. Use of 3.0-T MR imaging for evaluation of the abdomen. Radiographics 2009;29(6):1547–63.

29. Kuhl CK, Jost P, Morakkabati N, et al. Contrast-enhanced MR imaging of the breast at 3.0 and 1.5 T in the same patients: initial experience. Radiology 2006;239(3):666–76.

30. Kuhl CK, Kooijman H, Gieseke J, et al. Effect of B1 inhomogeneity on breast MR imaging at 3.0 T. Radiology 2007;244(3):929–30.

31. Mountford CE, Stanwell P, Ramadan S. Breast MR imaging at 3.0 T. Radiology 2008;248(1):319–20.

32. Pinker K, Grabner G, Bogner W, et al. A combined high temporal and high spatial resolution 3 Tesla MR imaging protocol for the assessment of breast lesions: initial results. Invest Radiol 2009;44(9): 553–8.

33. Elsamaloty H, Elzawawi MS, Mohammad S, et al. Increasing accuracy of detection of breast cancer with 3T MRI. AJR Am J Roentgenol 2009;192(4): 1142–8.

34. Merkle EM, Dale BM, Paulson EK. Abdominal MR imaging at 3T. Magn Reson Imaging Clin N Am 2006;14(1):17–26.

35. Zhu Y. Parallel excitation with an array of transmit coils. Magn Reson Med 2004;51(4):775–84.

36. Zhang C, Yip CY, Grissom W, et al. Reduction of transmitter B1 inhomogeneity with transmit SENSE slice-select pulses. Magn Reson Med 2007;57(5): 842–7.

37. Katscher U, Bornert P, Leussler C, et al. Transmit SENSE. Magn Reson Med 2003;49(1):144–50.

38. Partridge SC. Future applications and innovations of clinical breast magnetic resonance imaging. Top Magn Reson Imaging 2008;19(3):171–6.

39. Gutierrez RL, DeMartini WB, Eby PR, et al. BI-RADS lesion characteristics predict likelihood of malignancy in breast MRI for masses but not for nonmasslike enhancement. AJR Am J Roentgenol 2009;193:994–1000.

40. Raza S, Vallejo M, Chikarmane SA, et al. Pure ductal carcinoma in situ: a range of MRI features. AJR Am J Roentgenol 2008;191(3):689–99.

41. Kuhl CK, Schrading S, Bieling H, et al. MRI for diagnosis of pure ductal carcinoma in-situ; a prospective observational study. Lancet 2007; 370:485–92.

42. Jansen SA, Newstead GM, Abe H, et al. Pure ductal carcinoma in situ: kinetic and morphologic MR characteristics compared with mammographic appearance and nuclear grade. Radiology 2007; 245:684–91.

43. Buadu LD, Murakami J, Murayama A, et al. Breast lesions: correlation of contrast medium enhancement patterns on MR images histopathologic findings and tumor angiogenesis. Radiology 1996;200: 639–49.

44. Boetes C, Barentsz JO, Mus RD, et al. MR characterization of suspicious breast lesions with a gadolinium-enhanced TurboFLASH subtraction technique. Radiology 1994;193:777–81.

45. Veltman J, Stoutjesdijk M, Mann R, et al. Contrast-enhanced magnetic resonance imaging of the breast: the value of pharmacokinetic parameters derived from fast dynamic imaging during initial enhancement in classifying lesions. Eur Radiol 2008;18(6):1123–33.

46. Guidance for Industry and FDA Staff: criteria for significant risk investigation of MR diagnostic devices. Available at: http://www.fda.gov/cdrh/ode/guidance/793.html 2003. Accessed July 14, 2003.

47. Shellock FG. Reference manual for magnetic resonance safety, implants and devices. 1st edition. Los Angeles (CA): Biomedical Research Publishing Company; 2009.

48. Yeung DK, Cheung HS, Tse GM. Human breast lesions: characterization with contrast enhanced in vivo proton MR spectroscopy-initial results. Radiology 2001;220:40–6.

49. Bartella L, Morris EA, Dershaw DD, et al. Proton MR spectroscopy with choline peak as malignancy marker improves positive predictive value for breast cancer diagnosis: preliminary study. Radiology 2006;239(3):686–92.

50. Bartella L, Thakur SB, Morris EA, et al. Enhancing nonmass lesions in the breast: evaluation with proton (1H) MR spectroscopy. Radiology 2007; 245:80–7.

51. Moy L, Do R, Salibi N, et al. Can better breast MRS be obtained at the 3T vs. 1.5T? Presented at the 92nd Annual Meeting of the Radiological Society of North America, RSNA. Chicago, IL, December 1, 2006.

52. Tsushima Y, Takahashi-Taketomi A, Endo K. Magnetic resonance (MR) differential diagnosis of breast tumors using apparent diffusion coefficient (ADC) on 1.5 T. J Magn Reson Imaging 2009; 30(2):249–55.

53. Lo GG, Ai V, Chan JK, et al. Diffusion-weighted magnetic resonance imaging of breast lesions: first experience at 3T. J Comput Assist Tomogr 2009; 33(1):63–9.

54. Bogner W, Gruber S, Pinker K, et al. Diffusion-weighted MR for differentiation of breast lesions at 3.0 T: how does selection of diffusion protocols affect diagnosis? Radiology 2009;253(2):341–51.

MR Imaging of Ductal Carcinoma In Situ

Gillian M. Newstead, MD

KEYWORDS

- DCIS • Ductal carcinoma in situ • MR imaging
- Mammography

Detection of ductal carcinoma in situ (DCIS) has increased dramatically since the advent of widespread screening for breast cancer in the early 1980s. DCIS is a preinvasive form of breast cancer whereby a clonal proliferation of malignant epithelial cells, originating in the terminal ductal lobular unit, remain confined to ducts and do not invade beyond the basement membrane into the surrounding breast tissue. Evidence suggests that approximately 30% to 50% of DCIS lesions will progress to become invasive.[1,2] DCIS may involve multiple sites separated by normal tissue contained within the same ductal system ("skip lesions") or in adjacent or remote ductal systems. DCIS, rarely diagnosed before the advent of mammographic screening, now accounts for well over 20% of malignant lesions found in screen-detected series.[3]

Early reports in the 1930s of a precursor lesion that could progress to invasion led to first use of the term "carcinoma in situ."[4,5] In the era before screening, most in situ lesions were detected clinically as a palpable mass, Paget disease, or nipple discharge. Nowadays, DCIS typically presents as a nonpalpable, 10- to 20-mm calcified lesion discovered on mammography. Calcifications predictive of DCIS are visible in up to 90% of DCIS cases diagnosed on mammography alone,[6–10] usually exhibiting a clustered, linear, or segmental distribution. The typical fine linear calcifications visible at mammography are probably caused by necrosis secondary to hypoxia occurring centrally in DCIS lesions, as blood supply by diffusion from extraductal vessels becomes inadequate due to tumor growth. Although calcified necrosis is a frequent mammographic finding in DCIS, the presenting finding may be a mass, asymmetry, or architectural distortion in approximately 10% to 20% of cases.[11–15]

The increase in rates of DCIS diagnosis in the United States is strongly associated with the concurrent increase in rates of mammography screening, and is similar to the increasing incidence of DCIS in other developed countries where breast screening programs are conducted. DCIS incidence in the United States increased sevenfold, from 1973 through the late 1990s, with the most rapid increases found among women older than 50 years. The current age-adjusted incidence rate of DCIS in the United States is 32.5 per 100,000 women; at ages 50 to 64 years, the incidence is approximately 88 per 100,000.[16] As of January 1, 2005, an estimated 500,000 United States women were living with a diagnosis of DCIS, and this number is estimated to increase to more than 1 million women by 2020, assuming constant incidence and survival rates.[16] The American Cancer Society estimates that carcinoma in situ will account for 24.5% (n = 62,280) of all breast cancer cases diagnosed in the United States in 2009.[17] Few studies have focused on risk factors for DCIS; however, it is generally agreed that the risk factors are the same as those for invasive breast cancer. These indicators include increasing age, family history of breast cancer, genetic predisposition, high mammographic density, late age at menopause, nulliparity, menopausal estrogen with progestin therapy, late age at first birth, and high postmenopausal body mass index. Mammography has proved to be uniquely successful in the identification of preinvasive cancer, resulting in highly favorable patient outcomes.

Department of Radiology, University of Chicago, 5841 South. Maryland Avenue, MC 2026, Chicago, IL 60637, USA
E-mail address: gnewstead@radiology.bsd.uchicago.edu

Magn Reson Imaging Clin N Am 18 (2010) 225–240
doi:10.1016/j.mric.2010.02.004
1064-9689/10/$ – see front matter © 2010 Elsevier Inc. All rights reserved.

BIOLOGY OF DCIS

The natural history of DCIS, and of breast cancer overall, is still poorly understood. Noninvasive cancers comprise a heterogeneous group of lesions with variable biologic, genetic, and histopathologic features, and are detected typically on x-ray mammography as microcalcifications formed inside necrotic tumors within the ducts. Tumor characteristics of in situ lesions at histology involve assessment of both qualitative and quantitative features. The qualitative features of DCIS include assessment of the architectural growth pattern, nuclear grade (high-, intermediate-, and low-grade cytologic features), and presence or absence of central necrosis. The most aggressive form of DCIS, the type that is most likely to progress to invasion, is associated with high-grade cellular and nuclear features and central necrosis "comedo type," and is associated with microcalcifications contained within the ducts.[7–10] In fact, "comedo" cancer in the 1950s and 1960s was invariably classified as an invasive cancer, because it was always diagnosed late by physical findings. Other architectural types are classified as cribriform, papillary, micropapillary, and solid types, with mixed histologic subtypes found in more than one-half of DCIS cases.[18–23]

Nuclear grading and histologic growth patterns of in situ lesions have been associated with morphologic characteristics of microcalcifications seen at mammography. There has been recent interest in the possibility that the mammographic phenotypes of breast lesions may convey important prognostic indicators or biomarkers. Women in screening mammography trials, with linear/linear-branching, or "casting" type of calcifications, have been shown to have considerably poorer survival outcome than women with amorphous or punctate calcification morphology.[24–28] Tabar and colleagues[29] have suggested that "casting" calcifications at mammography represent a "duct-forming" invasive cancer. DCIS lesions are considered to be nonobligate precursors of invasive cancer, and when progression to invasion occurs, the invasive cancers exhibit similar cytologic features, expression profiles, receptor status, and genomic characteristics. Investigations into genetic, biologic, and histopathological features of DCIS have shown many possible expressions of biochemical markers such as progesterone and estrogen receptors, Ki-67, PCN, c-erbl, and Cathepsin E. The molecular profiles of DCIS and invasive breast cancer are similar, supporting a common origin.[30–32] In general, high-grade noninvasive lesions exhibit rapid growth rates and high mitotic indices, and will almost invariably progress to an invasive cancer, whereas low-grade lesions may remain quiescent, never invade, and if they do will progress to low-grade invasive cancer.[32,33]

With increasing numbers of small cancers detected at mammography screening, breast conservation therapy is widely performed, underscoring the importance of accurate depiction of the extent of DCIS for optimal cancer staging and surgical planning. Measures of mammographic microcalcifications have been shown to significantly underestimate DCIS extent. Holland and colleagues[21] reported that discrepancies found between mammographic and histologic estimations of the extent of noninvasive cancer were related to the histologic type of DCIS, with high-grade lesion extent at mammography, more closely correlated with histologic measurements than estimates for low grade lesions. In that study, mammographically occult DCIS was present in 16% of comedo-type DCIS lesions larger than 20 mm, whereas occult disease was present in 47% of predominantly micropapillary-cribriform growth types. Standardization systems for the histopathologic classification of DCIS have been proposed by several investigators, notably the scheme introduced by Holland and colleagues[34] and the system known as the Van Nuys classification.[35,36] The Van Nuys system stratifies DCIS patients into three groups by combining high nuclear grade and "comedo-type" necrosis. In this system, low nuclear grade cases lacking comedo-type necrosis are placed into group 1, and into group 2 if necrosis is present, with all high nuclear grade cases defined as group 3.[35,36] Although mammography still remains an important method for diagnosing DCIS, it is clear that many in situ lesions may be partially or completely occult at mammography. Thus, women who undergo surgical excision of DCIS lesions diagnosed only at mammography may experience an inadequate surgical resection, with margins positive for in situ cancer, resulting in the need for reexcision surgery.

Against the background of extensive study of DCIS at mammography, including careful mammographic/histopathologic correlative investigations, additional imaging methods aimed to improve DCIS detection were sought, particularly with a view to improving the estimation of extent of disease in women with newly diagnosed breast cancer. Accurate depiction of the extent of DCIS, with or without the presence of an invasive component, is now considered essential for successful breast conservation therapy, although the original National Surgical Adjuvant Breast and Bowel Project (NSABBP) trials did not require negative margins. Noninvasive carcinoma with negative margins achieved at breast-conserving surgery results in a recurrence rate of 22.5%[1] when treated without radiation therapy. This rate increases if close or positive margins are present at surgical resection. Whole-breast radiation therapy has been shown to reduce the recurrence rate by 50%. Treatment of estrogen receptor–positive cases with tamoxifen reduces this risk by an additional 50%.[1] However, it is important that regardless of the therapeutic protocol (mastectomy, lumpectomy with radiation therapy, or wide surgical excision alone), half of the DCIS lesions are invasive when they recur, and 20% of cases present with distant metastases at 10 years.[37] Improved identification of DCIS, especially in high-risk women, could result in better patient outcome. Accordingly, further improvement in the accuracy of diagnosis of DCIS is an important goal, particularly because early diagnosis at a preinvasive stage yields excellent survival with local treatment only (surgical excision with or without radiotherapy).

MR IMAGING CHARACTERISTICS OF DCIS

Dynamic contrast-enhanced MR imaging (DCE-MRI) has been shown to visualize invasive breast cancer reliably; however, detection of in situ cancer has proved more difficult, with disappointing early reports indicating relatively low diagnostic accuracy and a variable reported sensitivity and specificity for DCIS.[38,39] Initial MR imaging screening trials reporting DCIS cases identified by mammography but occult to MR imaging supported a limited role for MR imaging in the detection of noninvasive disease.[40–42] DCE-MRI allows cancer to be distinguished from normal tissue because of the increased vascularity and capillary permeability of malignant lesions. More recent reports suggest that DCE-MRI performs as well as or better than x-ray mammography in the task of identifying DCIS lesions.[43] A study of 127 women with pure DCIS, reported in 2007 by Kuhl and colleagues,[44] reported that the sensitivity of MR imaging was vastly superior to mammography, 92% versus 56%, in the detection of DCIS. This study also showed a strong MR imaging sensitivity for high-grade lesions, 98%, compared with only 52% sensitivity for mammography. The majority of cases in this study not detected at MR imaging were low-grade lesions (87%). The improvement in DCIS detection in recent studies is likely due to improved spatial and temporal resolution made possible with modern DCE-MRI methods.

Studies have shown that enhancement kinetics, that is, the time course of the signal intensity within the lesion, can be used as an additive factor to morphology in the determination of the likelihood of malignancy for enhancing lesions visible at MR imaging. Multiple reports over the last 20 years have culminated in reproducible, routine morphologic and kinetic standards, used today in clinical practice, to distinguish benign from malignant breast lesions.[38,45–48] Improvements in the accuracy of kinetic analysis are still needed, however, as many benign and malignant lesions exhibit considerable kinetic overlap.

The BI-RADS lexicon[48] describes 3 types of enhancing lesions seen on breast MR imaging:

1. **Focus**, defined as a spot of enhancement that is too small (<5 mm) to allow confident further characterization
2. **Mass**, defined as a 3-dimensional space-occupying lesion
3. **Nonmass-like enhancement (NMLE)**, defined as enhancement of an area that is not a mass.

Although less common, NMLE is the predominant morphology pattern found in DCIS. Moreover, these lesions exhibit variable kinetic curve shapes, and may be more difficult to detect at MR imaging. Kinetic time course curves reflect perfusion and diffusion of contrast media, from blood vessels to the extracellular space, and are related to the unique physiology and vasculature of invasive, benign, and pure DCIS lesions. In a recent pilot study based on a relatively small number of patients, Jansen and colleagues[49] used an empirical mathematical model to analyze kinetic curves in NMLE versus mass lesions, and found that NMLE lesions exhibited significantly lower contrast uptake and slower washout compared with mass lesions. Furthermore, sensitivity and specificity of kinetic analysis was reduced in NMLE lesions compared with mass lesions. More specifically, it is likely that the kinetic parameters and criteria that work best to distinguish benign and malignant mass lesions may not work well with nonmass lesions, and vice versa. Others have pointed out that the considerable overlap of kinetic patterns of DCIS with benign lesions compromises its reliable identification.[50–52]

DCIS lesions often exhibit kinetic curves that persistently rise or plateau over time, a pattern not often seen with invasive malignancies. Of note, most prior studies of the kinetics of DCIS have used clinically acquired DCE-MRI data with relatively low temporal (45–90 seconds) resolution to allow for 3-dimensional whole breast imaging, and have studied contrast kinetics in one small region of interest (ROI) placed within the lesion. The kinetic curves of NMLE lesions are vulnerable to partial volume effects, as small ROIs encompassing part of the lesion also capture some of the surrounding normal tissue, diluting the reliability of the acquired enhancement data. It is understandable, therefore, that the observed differences between mass and NMLE lesions at MR imaging may be accentuated due to these partial volume effects. Although relatively sparse temporal resolution (ie, 3–6 postcontrast images) is typical for clinical breast DCE-MRI, it could be that imaging at much higher temporal resolution, with a greater number of time points, would aid substantially in lesion characterization.[53,54]

Reports correlating in situ lesions and their relationship to nuclear grade enhancement characteristics at MR imaging and mammographic findings are rare. Jansen and colleagues[55] performed a qualitative and quantitative evaluation of 82 consecutively diagnosed pure DCIS lesions on DCE-MRI and classified results according to nuclear grade and x-ray mammographic presentation. In this study, the lesion population was segmented into 4 groups according to their mammographic presentation:

1. Fine pleomorphic, fine linear, or fine linear-branching calcifications (32 of 63)
2. Amorphous or indistinct calcifications (14 of 63)
3. Noncalcified masses (8 of 63)
4. Mammographically occult cases (9 of 63).

Significant differences in the kinetic behavior of these populations were found.

Lesions with fine pleomorphic, fine linear, or fine linear-branching calcifications, and especially those presenting as masses on x-ray mammography, were more suspicious by conventional kinetic standards on MR imaging than lesions with amorphous or indistinct calcifications. In particular, lesions appearing as masses on mammography exhibited washout curves on average, whereas calcifications and occult lesions exhibited plateau curves. Nonmass, clumped enhancement in a segmental or linear distribution predominated. Pure DCIS lesions demonstrated 28% persistent, 27% plateau, and 45% washout behavior, which is similar to distributions found in other reports.[50,51] For pure DCIS lesions, the average enhancement at 1 minute (E_1) was 201%. The reported time to peak enhancement (T_{peak}) for invasive and benign lesions was 230 seconds, implying that pure DCIS lesions enhance less than invasive cancers and more than benign lesions.

It is interesting that the percent enhancement parameters (E_1 and E_{peak}) were statistically equivalent across all groups by mammographic and nuclear grade stratification. In this report, the signal enhancement ratio (SER) values were statistically equivalent for pure DCIS lesions of various grades; however, SER values varied by mammographic presentation. This finding suggests that washout as measured by SER may be a more important diagnostic parameter for assessment of in situ lesions than percent enhancement. No significant difference in enhancement kinetics among different nuclear grades of pure DCIS was found.

The findings in this article support previous reports by Viehweg and colleagues,[56] and suggest that x-ray mammographic appearance of pure DCIS may be related to its underlying physiology and vasculature in a way that nuclear grading is not. Additional reports have indicated that perfusion rates increase from benign to DCIS to invasive cancers and are correlated with microvessel density in DCIS lesions. Guidi and colleagues[57] showed an increase in vessel density around ducts with DCIS, although with variable patterns. Heffelfinger and colleagues[58,59] found that the expression of angiogenic growth factors such as vascular endothelial growth factor increases from hyperplasia to DCIS. Esserman and colleagues[60] studied the relationship between SER values of invasive tumors and tumor vascularity and histologic grade, and found that higher SER values correlate with higher vascularity and higher Scarff-Bloom-Richardson (SBR) pathologic grade.

MR IMAGING TECHNIQUE

The MR imaging protocols used in the figures shown in this article were performed using 2 1.5-Tesla imaging units (Signa: GE Healthcare, Milwaukee, WI; and Intera Achieva: Philips, the Netherlands). All patients underwent MR imaging in the prone position using parallel imaging technique. A dedicated 8-channel breast coil was used for GE Signa scanner, and a dedicated 7-channel breast coil was used for Philips Intera Achieva scanner. After obtaining bilateral nonfat-saturated T2-weighted images of the breasts, a T1-weighted 3D gradient echo sequence was performed before and 20 seconds after the injection of the contrast material. See **Table 1** at the end of this article for imaging protocols. A dynamic study in the axial plane was performed 6 times after the initiation of the intravenous injection of 0.1 mmol/kg gadodiamide (Omniscan; GE Health care) at a rate of 2 mL/s. MR imaging examinations were processed by CADstream (Confirma), and subtraction images and angiogenesis maps were obtained. The images were transferred to a workstation (Advantage Windows, software version 4.0; GE Healthcare, Milwaukee, WI, USA) for analysis.

MR IMAGING APPEARANCE OF DCIS

Pure DCIS, as discussed earlier, most often presents as nonmass-like enhancement and less commonly as a mass. DCIS can manifest in a variety of appearances, often as clumped NMLE, in a segmental, linear/ductal distribution. Kinetic features most commonly show a range of

initial contrast uptake with plateau, persistent, or washout kinetics seen in the delayed phase. Descriptors in the first edition of the BI-RADS MR imaging lexicon published in 2003[48] characterize NMLE lesions by their distribution and internal enhancement characteristics, and the kinetic pattern of initial uptake and delayed phase of contrast enhancement.

DISTRIBUTION OF NMLE

The descriptors for distribution of NMLE include Regional, Multiple Regions, Segmental, Focal (**Fig. 1**A, B) Linear/Ductal (**Fig.** 1C, D), and Diffuse.

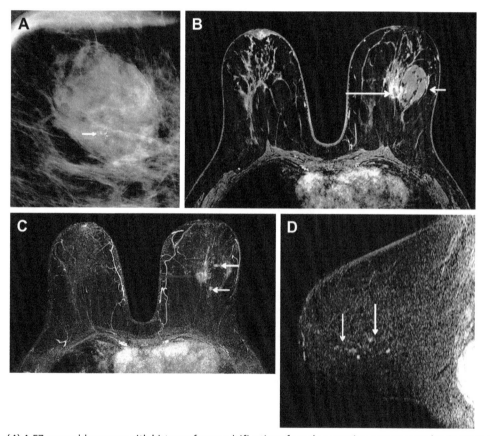

Fig. 1. (*A*) A 57-year-old woman with history of new calcifications found on routine mammography. Spot magnification view of the left breast, upper outer quadrant, shows linear and pleomorphic calcifications (*arrow*), adjacent to a known fibroadenolipoma. Stereotaxic-guided core needle biopsy with clip placement yielded DCIS, high-grade with central necrosis and solid/micropapillary type. (*B*) Staging MR imaging was performed 5 days after stereotaxic biopsy. T1-weighted axial fat suppressed image at 150 seconds post injection shows focal nonmass-like, heterogeneous enhancement at the site of prior biopsy (*long white arrow*), immediately adjacent to the medial aspect of the fibroadenolipoma (*short white arrow*). (*C*) Subtraction axial maximum intensity projection (MIP) image at 150 seconds post contrast injection shows focal heterogeneous enhancement at the biopsy site (*long red arrow*), and ductal heterogeneous enhancement anterior to the biopsy site. Two lateral foci are also seen (*white arrows*). Kinetic analysis yielded predominantly a medium initial rise with plateau enhancement in the delayed phase. (*D*) Sagittal reformatted subtraction image demonstrates NMLE enhancement anterior to the biopsy site (*white arrows*). A bracketed needle localization procedure was subsequently performed with 2 wires placed: one placed under MR imaging guidance targeting the anterior extent of the NMLE, and a second placed under radiographic guidance. Successful excision of the lesion with negative surgical margins was achieved.

Of these descriptors, segmental and linear/ductal are most commonly applied to DCIS lesions. Segmental distribution is defined as "a triangular region or cone of enhancement with apex at the nipple, which corresponds to a single duct system" (**Figs. 2** and **3**). Identification of a segmental enhancement distribution, commonly seen in DCIS, is an important tool for distinguishing malignancy from normal parenchyma. Multiplanar reformatting is essential for complete identification of the distribution of NMLE, with correlation of enhancement distribution in the axial and sagittal planes most useful (**Fig. 4**). The BI-RADS lexicon defines linear as "enhancement in a line" and ductal as "enhancement in a duct that may branch" (**Fig. 5**). Some investigators combine linear, ductal, and segmental distributions,[61,62] whereas others distinguish between segmental, ductal, and linear.[49,63] Less frequently used distributions seen in pure DCIS include regional, "enhancement that does not correspond to a single duct system; may be within multiple ducts" (**Fig. 6**), and focal area, "enhancement in a small area, in which the internal pattern can be discretely discerned" (see **Fig. 1B**).

INTERNAL ENHANCEMENT PATTERNS OF NMLE

Lexicon descriptors for internal enhancement patterns of NMLE lesions include Clumped, Heterogeneous, Homogeneous, Stippled-

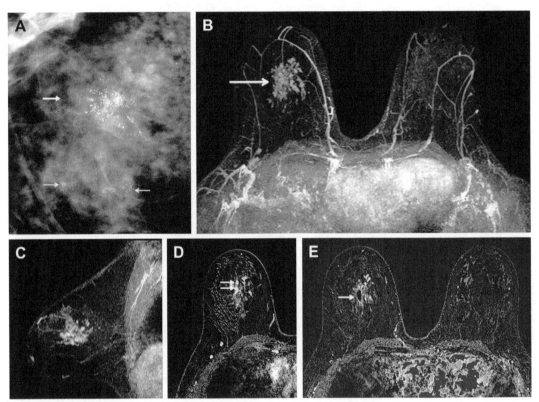

Fig. 2. (*A*) A 40-year-old woman with biopsy-proven high-grade DCIS, found on screening mammography. Spot magnification mammographic view of the right breast at 11 to 12 o'clock reveals an area of malignant pleomorphic "casting" type of calcifications spanning a distance of 5.3 cm, in a segmental distribution (*arrows*). (*B*) Staging MR imaging was obtained following stereotaxic biopsy, which yielded high-grade DCIS, solid type, with abundant necrosis. A marker clip was placed at the biopsy site. MIP image at 150 seconds post contrast injection shows a nonmass-like clumped enhancement in a segmental distribution, at the 11 to 2 o'clock position of the right breast, mid to posterior depth (*arrow*), measuring 5.3-cm AP × 2.9-cm RL × 3.6-cm craniocaudal, corresponding to the region of pleomorphic calcifications seen at mammography. (*C*) Reformatted MIP image shows to advantage the segmental distribution of the clumped NMLE. (*D*) Axial subtraction image obtained at 60 seconds post contrast injection shows a region of clustered ring enhancement (*arrows*) within the clumped NMLE. (*E*) Angiomap obtained at the second postcontrast time point with a threshold setting of 100% shows predominantly a rapid initial rise with persistent and plateau enhancement. The seroma cavity resulting from prior stereotaxic biopsy is shown (*arrow*).

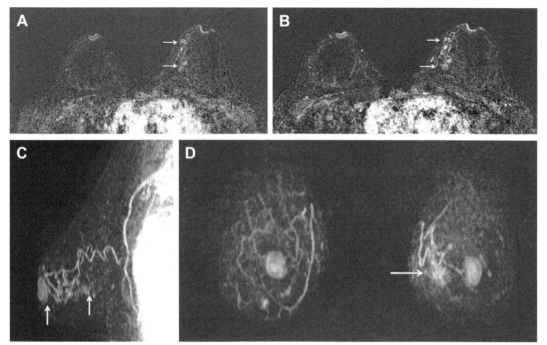

Fig. 3. (A) A 42-year-old woman underwent screening mammography, which demonstrated a 1.5-cm cluster of faint clustered punctate and amorphous microcalcification in the left breast at 8 o'clock, posterior depth. Stereotaxic biopsy yielded low- to intermediate-grade DCIS, micropapillary and cribriform type. Axial subtraction MR image at 75 seconds post contrast injection demonstrates a segmental NMLE with heterogeneous internal enhancement (arrows), extending anteriorly from the prior biopsy site, spanning a distance of 5.5 cm, suggesting a more extensive lesion than evidenced by the mammographic findings. (B) Axial subtracted image at 150 seconds post contrast injection shows increasing segmental enhancement (arrows), with a slow initial rise and a persistent time course curve. (C) Sagittal reformatted MIP image obtained at 150 seconds post contrast injection shows a segmental NMLE representing DCIS (right arrow). Note normal nipple enhancement (left arrow). (D) Coronal reformatted MIP image obtained at 150 seconds post contrast injection shows the segmentally distributed NMLE representing DCIS.

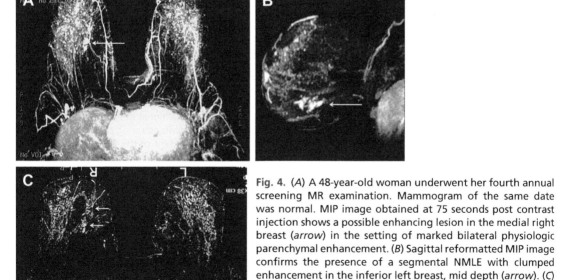

Fig. 4. (A) A 48-year-old woman underwent her fourth annual screening MR examination. Mammogram of the same date was normal. MIP image obtained at 75 seconds post contrast injection shows a possible enhancing lesion in the medial right breast (arrow) in the setting of marked bilateral physiologic parenchymal enhancement. (B) Sagittal reformatted MIP image confirms the presence of a segmental NMLE with clumped enhancement in the inferior left breast, mid depth (arrow). (C) Axial angiomap image obtained at 150 seconds, with a 100% threshold setting, shows the enhancing NMLE with rapid enhancement and washout, and plateau-type enhancement in the delayed phase (arrows). There is diffuse bilateral parenchymal enhancement, exhibiting rapid initial rise and a persistent enhancement in the delayed phase.

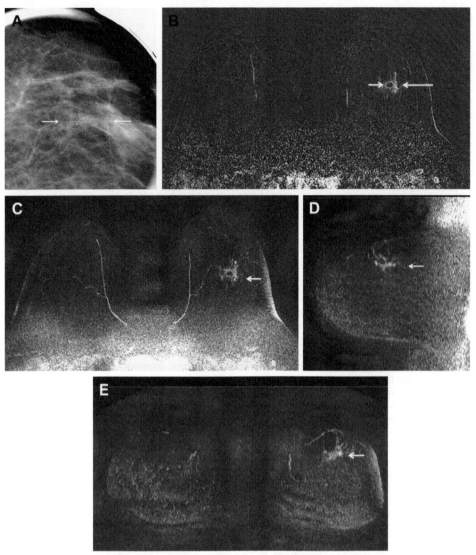

Fig. 5. (*A*) A 68-year-old woman presented for staging MR imaging. Screening mammographic examination revealed a suspicious 2.1-cm cluster of punctate and pleomorphic calcifications in the left breast at 2 o'clock (*arrows*); stereotaxic biopsy yielded intermediate-grade DCIS. (*B*) Axial subtraction image obtained at 75 seconds post contrast injection shows a postbiopsy seroma with surrounding NMLE ductal/linear heterogeneous enhancement at 2 o'clock (*arrows*), measuring 3.9 × 3.4 × 2.5 cm (craniocaudal) and demonstrating rapid initial rise and plateau delayed phase kinetics. (*C*) Axial MIP image shows to advantage the extent of the NMLE (*arrow*), which proved to be unifocal. The remainder of the left breast and the right breast were normal. (*D*) Sagittal MIP reformatted image shows ductal/linear NMLE (*arrow*). (*E*) Coronal MIP reformatted image showing NMLE extent (*arrow*). The 3-dimensional visualization of DCIS is better appreciated with multiplanar reconstruction postprocessing.

Punctate, and Reticulo-dendritic. The most common internal enhancement pattern found in pure DCIS is clumped, or "scattered and occasionally confluent regions of enhancement, an aggregation or cluster of enhancing foci in a cobblestone pattern" (see **Fig. 2**). Heterogeneous internal enhancement pattern, or "confluent, nonuniform enhancement variable in signal intensity" (see **Fig. 1**C,D), is also common, with the other patterns less frequently seen. Not included in the current lexicon is the descriptor "clustered ring enhancement," described in an article by Tozaki and colleagues[64] as a finding in which minute ring enhancements are clustered.

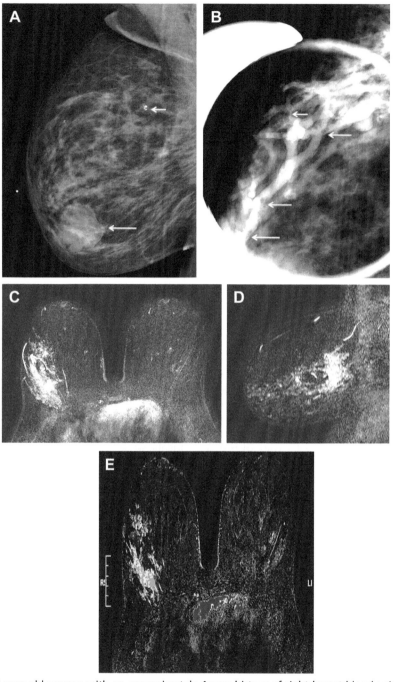

Fig. 6. (*A*) A 38 year-old woman with an approximately 4-year history of right breast bloody nipple discharge. Mediolateral oblique view mammogram shows a fibroadenoma in the anterior breast (*long arrow*), and a benign posterior calcification (*short arrow*). No suspicious calcifications were visible and no palpable mass was present. Ultrasound (not shown) revealed extensive ductal dilatation at the 9 o'clock location of the right breast. (*B*) Spot magnified view obtained during ductography, shows dilated ducts at 9 o'clock varying in caliber and multiple internal microlobulated mural-based filling defects (*arrows*). (*C*) MIP image obtained at 75 seconds following contrast injection shows extensive NMLE in a regional distribution with clumped internal enhancement. (*D*) Sagittal reformatted MIP image shows NMLE extending from the posterior breast to the nipple. (*E*) Axial angio-map view obtained at 150 seconds post contrast injection shows extensive heterogeneous internal enhancement, with rapid initial rise and washout kinetics in the delayed phase. Percutaneous ultrasound-guided biopsy yielded intraductal papillary and micropapillary carcinoma of intermediate grade.

In that report, 2 types of enhancement are described: "heterogeneous enhancement inside of which minute ring enhancements are seen clustered," and less frequently seen, "a clumped enhancement with the enhancing masses or foci constituting a ring-like enhancement pattern" (see **Fig. 2**D,E). In his study of 61 patients presenting with NMLE, the presence of clustered ring enhancement was found in 63% (22/35) of malignant lesions and only 4% of benign lesions (1/26). The investigators propose that clustered ring enhancement is a reflection of in situ carcinoma with an abundant blood supply, exhibiting a washout enhancement pattern, and that the ring pattern of enhancement is explained by contrast medium accumulating in the periductal stroma or ductal wall. With high spatial and temporal resolution techniques now available at MR imaging, this internal enhancement pattern is more frequently observed than with older techniques.

KINETIC PATTERNS

The kinetic curve shape is created by perfusion and diffusion of contrast material from the blood vessels into the extracellular space. With today's MR imaging techniques, a temporal resolution of 60 to 120 seconds will not image perfusion of the contrast material into a lesion but rather captures diffusion of contrast material. The BI-RADS lexicon[48] describes the initial phase of enhancement as Fast, Medium, or Slow, and the delayed phase as Persistent, Plateau, or Washout. The initial phase characterizes the percentage of initial wash-in of contrast (enhancement pattern within 2 minutes or when the shape of the kinetic curve starts to change), and the delayed phase (enhancement pattern after 2 minutes or after the curve starts to change). Time course curves may be classified as either persistent (type I), continued increase in signal over time; plateau (type II), signal intensity does not change over time after initial rise; or washout (type III), signal intensity decreases from the highest point after an initial rise.

INTERPRETATION CHALLENGES

Recognition of DCIS lesions at breast MR imaging often presents a diagnostic challenge for the radiologist. Unlike many breast masses, DCIS is not usually visible on T2-weighted sequences, neither with or without fat nulling, nor on unenhanced T1-weighted images, because the lesions may be indistinguishable from normal breast parenchyma, particularly if the lesion extent is small. As discussed earlier, the pharmacokinetic time or signal intensity time course curves associated with pure DCIS are variable. In the initial phase, rapid uptake, greater than the surrounding breast parenchyma, is usually seen; in the delayed phase, persistent, plateau, and washout kinetics have all been described. Given that with current MR protocols as many as 30% of DCIS cases show the least suspicious pattern, that of persistent enhancement, interpretation considerations are benefited by emphasizing morphology, particularly distribution parameters, rather than kinetic characteristics. The distinctive morphology of DCIS and the variable kinetic patterns discussed here may prompt some to suggest that MR acquisitions that emphasize spatial over temporal resolution are more sensitive to DCIS. Although spatial resolution is important,[52] sufficient temporal resolution is also needed to distinguish the more slowly and moderately enhancing pure DCIS lesions from enhancing parenchyma. Normal tissue enhancement is usually slower than lesion contrast uptake, and usually increases persistently over time. Creation of thin maximum intensity projection images and multiplanar reconstruction images of areas of questionable NMLE at the physician interpretation workstation, rather than reading planar stacks of images, may accentuate the enhancement distribution of DCIS and aid in distinguishing in situ lesions from parenchyma (see **Fig. 4**). Similarly, review of the source (nonsubtracted) datasets, where both the enhancing and nonenhancing parenchyma are visible, may aid the radiologist in distinguishing, for example, segmental distribution of DCIS from patchy parenchymal enhancement. Recognition and understanding of the unique morphology and kinetic characteristics of pure DCIS on MR imaging may improve the detection of early breast cancer.

COMPUTER-AIDED DIAGNOSIS

The kinetic parameters in routine clinical MR scans are calculated from signal intensity rather than contrast concentration, which can lead to errors due to the variability of the native T_1 of the tissue. In addition, various institutions use different scanners, imaging protocols and pulse sequences, with resultant variability in computer-aided diagnosis (CAD) output across different manufacturers' platforms, compounding the difficulties in comparing studies obtained at different locations over time.[65]

DCIS enhancement rates will often remain below the typical enhancement thresholds of invasive cancers, and this means that for diagnosing DCIS, current criteria related to enhancement kinetics are probably not useful, and current CAD software systems calibrated to the enhancement pattern of invasive cancers, typically 80% or thereabouts, will likely consistently fail to highlight DCIS. This observation may be useful for improving CAD systems, suggesting that if kinetic classifiers are trained separately for lesions based on type of enhancement (mass or nonmass-like), diagnostic accuracy might be improved. Perhaps CAD kinetic analysis should be performed after lesions have been classified as exhibiting mass, nonmass-like, or focus type enhancement. Several potential avenues can be explored to improve diagnostic accuracy for NMLE lesions at DCE-MRI. For example, using an automated algorithm to select a representative kinetic curve or applying measures of kinetic heterogeneity may be useful.[66] Some have also suggested that using spectroscopic techniques may increase specificity for nonmass lesions.[67] Consideration of the longer time to peak enhancement of pure DCIS lesions should be taken into account in cases where CAD schemes have thresholds that may be set too high and too early, and possibly run the risk of a false-negative diagnosis. In contrast, if thresholds are set too low, more false-positive diagnoses may result, prompting an increased number of benign biopsies.

IMPACT ON PATIENT MANAGEMENT

It is clear that identification of mammographically occult DCIS at MR imaging, especially for the patient undergoing staging of an index cancer, has changed surgical management. The questions can be posed: to what degree does the improved sensitivity of breast MR imaging inform treatment decisions and improve patient outcomes? How does preoperative MR imaging affect the rates of breast biopsy and subsequent treatment involving needle localization procedures with excision, local excision with radiotherapy, and mastectomy? It is generally acknowledged that disease-free surgical margins are associated with a decreased risk of local recurrence, but there is no widespread agreement as to the optimal margin size, or, perhaps more importantly, the effect on survival. Tumor characteristics associated with recurrence following breast-conserving surgery include high nuclear grade, presence of comedo-necrosis and/or microinvasion, large size, and adequacy of the surgical resection. Preoperative mapping of MR visible, mammographically occult DCIS often requires MR-guided biopsy (or biopsies) and clip placement(s) to document lesion extent. Multiple-wire placement bracketing imaging findings results in complex surgical excisions, necessitating close communication between the surgeon and radiologist for successful outcome. Despite improved tumor mapping with MR imaging, some reports suggest that this capability does not always translate to a decrease in the number of patients with positive margins at surgical excision.[68] One explanation might be that breast surgery is performed with the patient in the supine position and correlation of lesion(s) location with prone MR images is challenging for the surgeon, particularly for successful resection of multifocal disease associated with DCIS. Another might be that current surgery is most often oriented orthogonally to the length of target DCIS lesions, making surgical extirpation less facile even when the lesions are reasonably bracketed. Ongoing research into tumor ablation methods using MR guidance may ultimately allow successful treatment in the prone position, where online monitoring of tumor margins may decrease morbidity and reoperation rates.

FUTURE RESEARCH: HIGH TEMPORAL RESOLUTION IMAGING

Several prior reports have investigated contrast uptake of breast lesions at high temporal resolution, indicating improved diagnostic accuracy.[23,53] Increased capillary cuffing has been observed around ducts containing high-grade DCIS. In a recent report, Veltman and colleagues[69] calculated pharmacokinetic parameters from fast imaging acquisition during initial enhancement, and found that combining high temporal analysis with low temporal analysis improved lesion classification. Such studies have demonstrated the potential for high *temporal* resolution imaging improving diagnostic accuracy, but they have not included as yet a detailed analysis of in situ lesions. The kinetics of DCIS, have been typically studied using conventionally acquired low temporal resolution data, usually with qualitative or semiquantitative analysis. Quantitative mathematical modeling of high temporal resolution kinetic data for evaluation of noninvasive cancer, including analysis of internal lesion heterogeneity and assessment of washout beyond the initial enhancement phase of 90 seconds, could provide important further insights that ultimately result in improved diagnosis. Investigation into the correlations between established lesion biomarkers, such as microvessel density and estrogen receptor status, and quantitative MR enhancement characteristics, may yield surrogate imaging parameters that could distinguish between pathologic subtypes and provide prognostic indicators for both preinvasive and invasive malignancies. These prognostic biomarkers might provide patient selection criteria, for example, indicating which patients with a new DCIS diagnosis could be spared sentinel node biopsy from those patients who would be better served by undergoing this invasive procedure. It would ideally be preferable to acquire DCE-MRI data with both high spatial and high temporal resolution, especially during the first pass of the contrast media bolus, so that lesion morphology and physiology could be accurately assessed. Early contrast media uptake is approximately proportional to the product of vascular permeability and perfusion rate, which are closely linked to tumor grade and prognosis. Previous research has demonstrated the potential value of analyzing early lesion enhancement with high temporal resolution, and results from Oshida and colleagues[70] suggest that functional MR imaging–based parameters derived from moderately high (30 seconds) temporal resolution DCE-MRI are linked to histologic findings.

FUTURE RESEARCH: MOUSE MODELS OF DCIS

Marked morphologic and kinetic differences exist among focus, mass, and nonmass-like lesions, and it is likely that these differing types of enhancement reflect fundamental differences in lesion physiology. The actual pathophysiologic correlate of MR imaging contrast enhancement of DCIS is completely unknown. There is no blood vessel infiltration into ducts containing DCIS. What, therefore, is the underlying mechanism for DCIS enhancement at MR imaging? In an attempt to answer this question, Jansen and colleagues[71] showed that following intravenous injection of gadolinium (Gd)-chelate–containing contrast agents, murine DCIS consistently exhibits enhancement on DCE-MRI and in addition, as demonstrated by x-ray fluorescence microscopy (XFM) techniques, showed that Gd selectively accumulates within the DCIS-containing ducts. Studies of XFM for iron excluded the presence of red blood cells in the ROI, confirming that Gd was indeed present inside the extravascular/extracellular space of the ducts and not contained within blood vessels. These results (DCE-MRI and XFM) were shown to be concordant in that there was no relevant Gd uptake in normal mammary gland ducts. The mechanism of enhancement in DCIS as indicated by Jansen's results, shows that Gd diffuses from the intravascular to the extravascular, interstitial space and then from the extravascular to the intraductal space.

This study prompts several questions. Does DCE-MRI reflect a biologic or a structural difference between normal ducts and ducts containing DCIS? Do these findings support the conclusion that there is an increased permeability of the basement membrane of DCIS-containing ducts, which allows Gd or Gd chelates to penetrate the membrane and accumulate within DCIS-filled ducts? The increased ductal permeability suggested by this study is probably explained by an increase in protease activity induced by the intraductal cancer cells. Could this protease activity constitute a first step toward progression to invasive cancer? Could the resultant pattern of enhancement at DCE-MRI reflect the biologic growth patterns reflected in differing DCIS architecture? These new observations demonstrate that Gd within the mammary ducts is imaged directly at MR imaging and that in situ carcinoma is visualized in accordance with the appearance of DCIS on clinical MR imaging examinations, that is, visualization of ductal enhancement or, in the case of more extensive DCIS, segmental enhancement. Further research is needed to corroborate these findings and to investigate DCIS enhancement in both murine and human subjects.

It has been reported that the sensitivity of MR imaging for detection of DCIS increases with higher nuclear grades of DCIS, which in turn have been shown to be associated with likelihood of progression to invasive cancer.[44] Will MR imaging be able to visualize preferentially the "aggressive and therefore prognostically important" DCIS lesions that indeed have the potential to progress to invasive cancer? There is strong evidence to suggest that the imaging phenotype of DCIS lesions based on their appearance at mammography and MR imaging conveys important biologic information that will be useful for clinical patient management, and could provide a biomarker analog that would help to predict the natural behavior of DCIS. Despite available research to date, we are currently unable to identify with certainty which cases of DCIS will progress to invasion, or to predict recurrence probability, or therapeutic response. At the present time, our knowledge is limited to the identification of surrogate markers for clinical behavior and patient outcome, such as survival, local recurrence, and risk of development of invasive breast cancer. Further understanding of tumor biology is clearly needed, but at present there are insufficient reliable models representing human DCIS or understanding of its natural history to support the comprehensive investigations into cellular and molecular alterations in the epithelium and microenvironment necessary to answer some of these crucial questions.

Table 1
MR Imaging Protocols

Bilateral Nonfat-saturated T2-weighted images

	TR/TE
Signa	5000 ms/103.5 ms
Intera Achieva	16,907 ms/120 ms

T1-weighted 3D gradient echo sequence

	TR/TE	Flip Angle	Field of View	Matrix	Section Thickness	Acquisition Time
Signa	4.6 ms / 2.2 ms	10°	34 x 34 cm	320 x 320	2 mm	75 seconds
Intera Achieva	7.9 ms / 3.9 ms	10°	48 x 48 cm	352 x 352	2 mm	75 seconds

SUMMARY

DCE-MRI of the breast is complementary to mammography in the detection of DCIS, because enhancement may be visible in areas of calcified as well as noncalcified noninvasive carcinoma, allowing detection of even mammographically occult disease. A larger percentage of in situ disease, therefore, should be detected at MR imaging than at mammography, in both breast cancer screening and diagnostic studies. MR imaging thus has the potential to prevent development of some invasive cancers, and also provide more accurate tumor mapping for cancer treatment. There are increasing concerns that mammographic screening causes overdiagnosis and subsequent overtreatment of biologically insignificant DCIS, which may never become life threatening. Accordingly, we must consider to what degree might breast MR imaging result in overdetection of biologically insignificant DCIS, or other proliferative lesions. What are the psychological, physical, medical, and economic costs associated with overdetection by both mammography and MR imaging? There is nonetheless the intriguing possibility that MR imaging phenotypes may convey important prognostic information, allowing further differentiation of biologically relevant DCIS from biologically inert DCIS. It is hoped that with future research, we may be able to identify MR imaging features that, combined with clinical, mammographic, and biologic characteristics, improve risk stratification for patients diagnosed with DCIS, and ultimately further decrease the mortality toll of breast cancer. It is possible, perhaps, that given the higher overall increased sensitivity obtained by MR imaging, and the likelihood that MR imaging may identify prognostically relevant disease, overall patient outcomes will be improved over the current clinical practice that primarily relies on the proven benefits of mammography.

REFERENCES

1. Leonard GD, Swain SM. Ductal carcinoma in situ, complexities and challenges. J Natl Cancer Inst 2004;96:906–20.
2. Page DL, DuPont WD, Rogers LW, et al. Intraductal carcinoma of the breast. Follow-up after biopsy only. Cancer 1982;49:751–8.
3. Ernster VL, Ballard-Barbash R, Barlow WE, et al. Detection of ductal carcinoma in situ in women undergoing screening mammography. J Natl Cancer Inst 2002;94:1546–54.
4. MacCarty WC. The histogenesis of cancer (carcinoma) of the breast and its clinical significance. Surg Gynecol Obstet 1913;17:441–59.
5. Broders AC. Carcinoma in situ contrasted with benign penetrating epithelium. JAMA 1932;99:1670–4.
6. Dershaw DD, Abramson A, Kinne DW. Ductal carcinoma in situ: mammographic findings and clinical implications. Radiology 1989;170:411–5.
7. Homer MJ, Safaii H, Smith JJ, et al. The relationship of mammographic microcalcification to histologic malignancy: radiologic-pathologic correlation. AJR Am J Roentgenol 1989;153:1187–9.
8. Bassett LW. Mammographic analysis of calcifications. Radiol Clin North Am 1992;30:93–105.
9. Stomper PC, Connolly JL, Meyer JE, et al. Clinically occult ductal carcinoma in situ detected with mammography: analysis of 100 cases with radiologic-pathologic correlation. Radiology 1989;172(1):235–41.
10. Lafontan B, Daures JP, Salicru B, et al. Isolated clustered microcalcifications: diagnostic value of mammography—series of 400 cases with surgical verification. Radiology 1994;190:479–83.

11. Ikeda DM, Andersson I. Ductal carcinoma in situ: atypical mammographic appearances. Radiology 1989;172:661–6.

12. Koerner FC. A brief historical perspective on the pathology of the breast: from Cheatle to Azzopardi and beyond. Semin Diagn Pathol 2004;21(1):3–9.

13. Finney JM. Joseph Colt Bloodgood 1867–1935. Ann Surg 1937;105(91):150–1.

14. Mitnick JS, Roses DF, Harris MN, et al. Circumscribed intraductal carcinoma of the breast. Radiology 1989;170:423–5.

15. Farshid G, Downey P, Gill PG. Atypical presentations of screen-detected DCIS: implications for pre-operative assessment and surgical intervention. Breast 2007;16:161–71.

16. The National Cancer Institute (NCI). Overview of the SEER Cancer Statistics Review 1975–2005. Available at: http://seer.cancer.gov/csr/1975_2005/results_single/sect_01_intro.28pgs.pdf. Accessed February 5, 2010

17. American Cancer Society. Cancer facts and figures 2009. Atlanta (GA): American Cancer Society; 2009. p. 3–11.

18. Davis R, Stacey AJ. The detection and significance of calcifications in the breast: a radiologic and pathologic study. Br J Radiol 1976;49:12–26.

19. Dongen J, Harris JR, Peterse JL, et al. In situ breast cancer: the EORTC consensus meeting. Lancet 1989;8653:25–7.

20. Dongen JA, Holland R, Peterse JL, et al. Ductal carcinoma in-situ of the breast; second EORTC consensus meeting [review]. Eur J Cancer 1992;28(2):626–9.

21. Holland R, Hendriks JH, Verbeek AL, et al. Extent, distribution, and mammographic/histologic correlations of breast ductal carcinoma in situ. Lancet 1990;335:519–22.

22. Stomper PC, Connolly JL. Ductal carcinoma in situ of the breast: correlation between mammographic calcification and tumor subtype. Am J Roentgenol 1992;159:483–5.

23. Tabar L. Ductal carcinoma in situ. Mod Pathol 1990;3(4):440.

24. James JJ, Evans AJ, Pinder SE, et al. Is the presence of mammographic comedo calcification really a prognostic factor for small screen-detected invasive breast cancers? Clin Radiol 2003;58(1):54–62.

25. Peacock C, Given-Wilson RM, Duffy SW. Mammographic casting-type calcification associated with small screen-detected invasive breast cancers: is this a reliable prognostic indicator? Clin Radiol 2004;59(2):165–70 [discussion: 163–4].

26. Tabar L, Chen HH, Yen AM, et al. Mammographic tumor features can predict long-term outcomes reliably in women with 1-14-mm invasive breast carcinoma. Cancer 2004;101(8):1745–59.

27. Thurfjell E, Thurfjell MG, Lindgren A. Mammographic finding as predictor of survival in 1-9 mm invasive breast cancers. Worse prognosis for cases presenting as calcifications alone. Breast Cancer Res Treat 2001;67(2):177–80.

28. Zunzunegui RG, Chung MA, Oruwari A, et al. Casting-type calcifications with invasion and high-grade ductal carcinoma in situ: a more aggressive disease? Arch Surg 2003;138(5):537–40.

29. Tabar L, Tot T, Dean PB. Breast cancer: early detection with mammography. Stuttgart (Germany): Georg Thieme Verlag; 2007. 129–72.

30. Hieken TJ, Farolan M, D'Alessandro S, et al. Predicting the biologic behavior of ductal carcinoma in situ: an analysis of molecular markers. Surgery 2001;130:593–600.

31. Ringberg A, Anagnostaki L, Anderson H, et al. South Sweden Breast Cancer Group. Cell biological factors in ductal carcinoma in situ (DCIS) of the breast-relationship to ipsilateral local recurrence and histopathological characteristics. Eur J Cancer 2001;37:1514–22.

32. Bobrow GL, Happerfield LC, Gregory WM, et al. The classification of ductal carcinoma in situ and its association with biological markers. Semin Diagn Pathol 1994;11:199–207.

33. Recht A, Rutgers EJ, Fentiman IS, et al. The fourth EORTC DCIS consensus meeting (Chateau Marquette, Heemskerk, The Netherlands, 23-24 January 1998)—conference report. Eur J Cancer 1998;34:1664–9.

34. Holland H, Peterse JL, Millis RR, et al. Ductal carcinoma in situ: a proposal for a new classification. Semin Diagn Pathol 1994;11:167–80.

35. Silverstein MJ, Poller DN, Waismann JR, et al. Prognostic classification of breast ductal carcinoma-in-situ. Lancet 1995;345:1154–7.

36. Silverstein MJ, Lagios MD, Craig PH, et al. A prognostic index for ductal carcinoma in situ of the breast. Cancer 1996;77:2267–74.

37. Bijker N, Peterse JL, Duchateau L, et al. Risk factors for recurrence and metastasis after breast-conserving therapy for ductal carcinoma-in-situ: analysis of European Organization for Research and Treatment of Cancer Trial 10853. J Clin Oncol 2001;19:2263–71.

38. Kuhl CK, Mielcareck P, Klaschik S, et al. Dynamic breast MR imaging: are signal intensity time course data useful for differential diagnosis of enhancing lesions? Radiology 1999;211(1):101–10.

39. Boetes C, Strijk SP, Holland R, et al. False negative MR imaging of malignant breast tumors. Eur Radiol 1997;7(8):1231–4.

40. Kriege M, Brekelmans CT, Boetes C, et al. Efficacy of MRI and mammography for breast-cancer screening in women with a familial or genetic predisposition. N Engl J Med 2004;351:427–37.

41. Warner E, Plewes DH, Hill KA, et al. Surveillance of BRCA 1 and BRCA 2 mutation carriers with magnetic resonance imaging, ultrasound, mammography and clinical breast examination. JAMA 2005;292:1317–25.

42. Leach MO, Boggis CR, Dixon AK, et al. MARIBS study group. Screening with magnetic resonance imaging and mammography of a UK population at high familial risk of breast cancer: a prospective multicentre cohort study (MARIBS). Lancet 2005; 365(9473):1769–78.

43. Morris E, Liberman L. Ductal carcinoma in situ. In: Morris EA, Liberman L, editors. Breast MRI: diagnosis and intervention. Philadelphia: Springer; 2004. p. 164–72.

44. Kuhl CK, Schrading S, Bieling H, et al. MRI for diagnosis of pure ductal carcinoma in-situ; a prospective observational study. Lancet 2007;370:485–92.

45. Kaiser WA, Zeitler E. MR imaging of the breast: fast imaging sequences with and without GD-TPA. Radiology 1989;170:681–6.

46. Orel SG. High-resolution MR imaging for the detection, diagnosis and staging of breast cancer. Radiographics 1998;18:903–12.

47. Heywang-Kobrunner SH, Viehweg P, Heinig A, et al. Contrast-enhanced MRI of the breast: accuracy, value, controversies, solutions. Eur J Radiol 1997; 24:94–108.

48. ACR. American College of Radiology (ACR) breast imaging reporting and data system atlas (BIRADS). Reston (VA): ACR; 2003.

49. Jansen SA, Fan X, Karczmar GS, et al. DCEMRI of breast lesions: is kinetic analysis equally effective for both mass and non-mass-like enhancement? Med Phys 2008;35(7):3102–9.

50. Neubauer H, Li M, Kuehne-Heid R, et al. High grade and non-high grade ductal carcinoma in situ on dynamic MR mammography: characteristic findings for signal increase and morphological pattern of enhancement. Br J Radiol 2003;76:3–12.

51. Van Goethem M, Schelfout K, Kersschot E, et al. Comparison of MRI features of different grades of DCIS and invasive carcinoma of the breast. JBR-BTR 2005;88:225–32.

52. Harms SE. The use of breast magnetic resonance imaging in ductal carcinoma in situ. Breast J 2005; 11:379–81.

53. Boetes C, Barentsz JO, Mus RD, et al. MR characterization of suspicious breast lesions with a gadolinium-enhanced TurboFLASH subtraction technique. Radiology 1994;193:777–81.

54. Sardanelli F, Rescinito G, Giordano GD, et al. MR dynamic enhancement of breast lesions: high temporal resolution during the first-minute versus eight-minute study. J Comput Assist Tomogr 2000; 24:724–31.

55. Jansen SA, Newstead GM, Abe H, et al. Pure ductal carcinoma in situ: kinetic and morphologic MR characteristics compared with mammographic appearance and nuclear grade. Radiology 2007; 245:684–91.

56. Viehweg P, Lampe D, Buchmann J, et al. In situ and minimally invasive breast cancer: morphologic and kinetic features on contrast-enhanced MR imaging. MAGMA 2000;11(3):129–37.

57. Guidi AJ, Schnitt SJ, Fischer L, et al. Vascular permeability factor (vascular endothelial growth factor) expression and angiogenesis in patients with ductal carcinoma in situ of the breast. Cancer 1997;80:1945–53.

58. Heffelfinger SC, Miller MA, Yassin R, et al. Angiogenic growth factors in preinvasive breast disease. Clin Cancer Res 1999;5(10):2867–76.

59. Heffelfinger SC, Yassin R, Miller MA, et al. Vascularity of proliferative breast disease and carcinoma in situ correlates with histological features. Clin Cancer Res 1996;2(11):1873–8.

60. Esserman L, Hylton N, George T, et al. Contrast-enhanced magnetic resonance imaging to assess tumor histopathology and angiogenesis in breast carcinoma. Breast J 1999;5(1):13–21.

61. Menell JH, Morris EA, Dershaw DD, et al. Determination of the presence and extent of pure ductal carcinoma in situ by mammography and magnetic resonance imaging. Breast J 2005;11:382–90.

62. Morakkabati-Spitz N, Leutner C, Schild H, et al. Diagnostic usefulness of segmental and linear enhancement in dynamic breast MRI. Eur Radiol 2005;15:2010–7.

63. Rosen EL, Smith-Foley SA, DeMartini WB, et al. BIRADS MRI enhancement characteristics of ductal carcinoma in situ. Breast J 2007;13:545–50.

64. Tozaki M, Igarashi T, Fukuda K. Breast MRI using the VIBE sequence: clustered ring enhancement in the differential diagnosis of lesions showing non-mass-like enhancement. AJR Am J Roentgenol 2006; 187(2):313–21.

65. Jansen SA, Shimauchi A, Zak L, et al. Kinetic curves of malignant lesions are not consistent across MR systems: the need for improved standardization of breast DCEMRI acquisitions. AJR Am J Roentgenol 2009;193(3):832.

66. Williams TC, DeMartini WB, Partridge SC, et al. Breast MR imaging: computer-aided evaluation program for discriminating benign from malignant lesions. Radiology 2007;244:94–103.

67. Bartella L, Thakur SB, Morris EA, et al. Enhancing non-mass lesions in the breast: evaluation with proton (1H) MR spectroscopy. Radiology 2007;245:80–7.

68. Bleicher RJ, Ciocca RM, Egleston BL, et al. Association of routine pretreatment magnetic resonance imaging with time to surgery, mastectomy rate, and margin status. J Am Coll Surg 2009;209:180–7, © 2009.

69. Veltman J, Stoutjesdijk M, Mann R, et al. Contrast-enhanced magnetic resonance imaging of the

breast: the value of pharmacokinetic parameters derived from fast dynamic imaging during initial enhancement in classifying lesions. Eur Radiol 2008;18(6):1123–33.

70. Oshida K, Nagashima T, Ueda T, et al. Pharmacokinetic analysis of ductal carcinoma in situ of the breast using dynamic MR mammography. Eur Radiol 2005;15(7):1353–60.

71. Jansen SA, Paunesku T, Fan X, et al. X-ray fluorescence microscopy and dynamic contrast enhanced MR imaging of gadolinium uptake within the mammary ducts. Radiology 2009;253(2):399–406.

Update on Screening Breast MRI in High-Risk Women

C. Boetes, MD, PhD

KEYWORDS

• Breast • Cancer • Screening • Increased risk • MRI

Breast cancer is a major health problem in Europe and the United States. At the moment, 1 in 8 women in the Western European countries develops breast cancer during her lifetime, and approximately 30% of these women die of the disease. Although a nationwide screening program for breast cancer has shown a mortality reduction of approximately 1.2% annually in the Netherlands, mammography has a limited sensitivity especially in the dense breast, and cancers are missed at screening.[1,2]

In women with an increased risk for breast cancer, mammographic results are even more disappointing because in many cases these women are young, and younger women have often more dense breasts than postmenopausal women.

The first results regarding breast cancer screening with MRI were published by Tilanus-Linthorst and colleagues[3] in 2000. In this series, MRI detected, in 3% of the cases, a malignancy not seen on conventional imaging. After that publication, many studies were published showing the value of screening with MRI and mammography compared with screening with mammography alone in the group of women with an increased risk for breast cancer.

GENETIC COUNSELING

There are many factors that influence a woman's risk of developing breast cancer. Family history and increasing age are among the most significant risk factors. Approximately 20% to 30% of all women who have breast cancer have a relative with breast cancer.[4] Five percent to 10% of all breast cancer cases are truly hereditary.

In performing risk assessment, family history is important as is the ethnic background of a patient. For instance, women of Ashkenazi Jewish origin have an increased risk of being BRCA1 or BRCA2 carriers compared with other ethnic groups.[5] It is recommended that women with a likelihood of at least 10% of being a gene mutation carrier be referred for genetic counseling and testing (**Table 1**).[6,7]

There are different models used for risk assessment. The Cancer and Steroid Hormone Study is a population-based case-control study, often referred as the Claus model,[8] that fits genetic models to derive age-specific breast cancer risk assessment for women with a first-degree relative with breast cancer. The assessment of risk is based on the relative's age at diagnosis and the degree of relationship of these relatives.

Another often-used model is Gail and colleagues' model.[9] This model uses the following risk factors: age at menarche, age at first live birth, number of previous biopsies, presence of atypical hyperplasia, and number of first-degree relatives with breast cancer. There are some limitations to this model, for instance, the number of biopsies and the exclusion of more extended information about the family history. Evaluating a woman with both risk models in many cases gives discordant results.

BRCAPRO is a pedigree-based risk assessment model. BRCAPRO, however, only considers first- and second-degree family members.[10]

Department of Radiology, Maastricht University Medical Center, P.O. Box 5800, 6202 AZ Maastricht, the Netherlands
E-mail address: c.boetes@mumc.nl

Magn Reson Imaging Clin N Am 18 (2010) 241–247
doi:10.1016/j.mric.2010.02.003

Table 1
Criteria for referral for genetic consulting

1. One first-degree member

Breast cancer (BC) < 35
Bilateral or multicentric tumor, first tumor < 50
Ovarian cancer and BC < 70
Ovarian cancer < 50
Male BC
Breast cancer

2. Two or more relatives in the same side

Two first-degree with BC < 50
BC < 50 and ovarian cancer at any age
Prostate cancer < 60 and first-degree BC < 50
Two relatives with ovarian cancer
Three or more first-degree relatives, one < 50

INDICATIONS FOR PERFORMING MRI SCREENING

Different guidelines have been published in the past decade providing indications for breast MRI in women with an increased risk for the development of breast cancer.

In the 1990s the first nonrandomized studies were initiated in the Netherlands, the United Kingdom, Canada, the United States, Italy, and Germany to determine the additional value of breast MRI to mammography in women who are BRCA1 or -2 carriers or have a lifetime risk of at least 20% to 25% for developing breast cancer. On the basis of these various retrospective studies, the American Cancer Society recommends annual MRI examination for all women with a lifetime risk of more than 20% to 25%.[11] These guidelines are completely incorporated in the guidelines of the European Society of Breast Imaging,[12] which describe in detail which groups of women should undergo breast MRI (**Box 1**).

Box 1
Recommendations for MRI screening together with mammography

1. BRCA mutation
2. First-degree untested relative of BRCA carrier
3. Radiation to chest wall between ages 10 and 30
4. Li-Fraumeni syndrome and first-degree relatives
5. Cowden syndrome and first-degree untested relatives

BRCA1 AND -2 MUTATION CARRIERS

A BRCA1 mutation carrier has a lifetime risk, according the Breast Cancer Linkage Consortium (BCLC), of 87% for getting breast cancer.[13] Brose and colleagues[14] calculated a lower lifetime risk of approximately 73%. In the Ashkenazi Jewish women who are BRCA1 carriers, the lifetime risk is slightly lower, between 40% and 60%.[15]

In the group of BRCA1 mutation carriers, other cancers are also more frequently detected. BRCA1 carriers have a 40% to 65% cumulative risk of getting a contralateral breast cancer and a 20% to 45% risk of developing ovarian cancer.[16] Prostate cancer is probably also one of the malignancies associated with BRCA1, although less frequent than in BRCA2.[17] Male breast cancer is also seen in BRCA1 families as well as pancreatic cancer.[18] The lifetime risk for developing breast cancer in BRCA2 mutation carriers is slightly lower than in BRCA1 groups. The age at onset is slightly later.[19] According to the BCLC, the lifetime risk in BRCA2 is 84%. A large meta-analysis pooled pedigree data, however, that included more than 8000 women revealed an average cumulative breast cancer risk to age 70 in BRCA1 carriers of 65% versus 45% in BRCA2 carrier groups.[20] BRCA2 mutation carriers also have an increased risk for getting other cancers (similar to those described previously).

BRCA1-associated breast cancers are more frequently high grade and receptor status negative.[21,22] Moreover, lymphocytic infiltration is seen more often. The tumors, even when small in size, are often growing with pushing borders.[23] In contradistinction, BRCA2 breast cancer behaves more like the group of sporadic breast cancers. BRCA1 tumors often have medullary or atypical medullary features. Although *ductal carcinoma in situ* (DCIS) in and around the invasive ductal cancer is also detected in BRCA1 mutation carriers, it is less frequent than in sporadic invasive ductal cancers.[21] Unlike sporadic breast cancers where the size of the tumor is a predictor for lymph node invasion, this is not the case in BRCA1 mutation carriers.[24] Although the tumor characteristics of the BRCA1 carriers show unfavorable signs, currently there is no difference in survival between this group of women and women with a sporadic breast cancer.

SPORADIC HEREDITARY BREAST CANCER SYNDROMES

There are other, more sporadic hereditary diseases that have an increased risk for breast cancer. The Li-Fraumeni syndrome is an autosomal dominant disease causing an increased risk for developing different kinds of cancers, such as sarcoma, leukemia, and breast carcinoma. Approximately 30% of all malignancies in this syndrome develop before the age of 15, and by the age of 70 approximately 90% of the malignancies have occurred.[25,26] The Li-Fraumeni syndrome germline TP53 mutation has an unusual high prevalence in parts of Brazil. The incidence there is 1: 300 individuals.[27] Early breast cancer before age of 40 is often seen in this group of patients.

Cowden disease (multiple hamartoma syndrome) is also a rare genetic disease with an increased risk for developing breast cancer and for thyroid cancer (**Fig. 1**).[28]

Peutz-Jeghers syndrome is characterized by hamartomatous polyps in the small bowel and also malignancies of the gastrointestinal tract and breast.[29] In Peutz-Jeghers syndrome, the lifetime risk for developing colon cancer is approximately 40%, for pancreatic cancer 35%, and for stomach cancer 30%. The risk for developing breast cancer is approximately 55%.

Muir-Torre syndrome is a variant of the hereditary nonpolyposis colon cancer. Women affected with this syndrome also have an increased risk for developing breast and endometrial cancer.

Ataxia telangiectasia is an autosomal recessive condition. Patients with this syndrome have immunodeficiency, cerebellar degeneration, and an increased risk for developing solid tumors, leukemia, and malignant lymphoma. They also have an increased risk for developing breast cancer.[30]

Patients with a family history of breast cancer tend to develop breast carcinoma at a younger age than women with no family history. The prevalence of bilateral breast cancer is also higher than seen in sporadic cases.

INDIVIDUAL INCREASED RISK

Women who received irradiation to the chest in their second or third decade of life, most for treatment of a malignant lymphoma, have a 4- to 5-fold increased risk for the development of breast cancer. In most cases, breast cancer develops approximately 20 years after the irradiation.[31] There are several other factors that increase the risk of breast cancer, such as a diagnosis of lobular carcinoma in situ (LCIS). The lifetime risk in this group of patients may exceed 20%, but only 1 publication shows some benefit in performing breast MRI in this group of patients.[32]

In the group of patients with a diagnosis of LCIS, other risk factors, such as family history, age, and breast density, also should be considered in the decision for performing breast MRI.

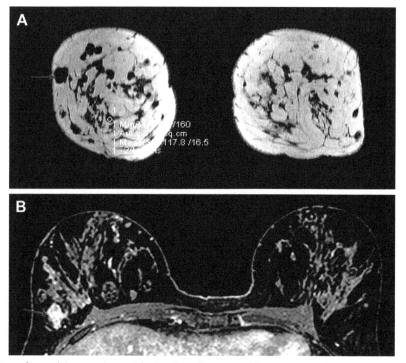

Fig. 1. (A) MRI performed in a patient with Cowden disease and breast cancer (*arrow*). (B) MRI performed in a patient with Cowden disease and breast cancer (*arrow*).

A high breast density is also a risk factor for breast cancer; however, until now no data regarding the additional value of MRI in this group of women are available.

In a study published by Morris and colleagues,[33] MRI detected more mammographically occult tumors in women with a family history and a personal history for breast cancer.

Although women with a personal history of breast cancer have an increased risk, there is no sufficient evidence in support of performing MRI in this group.

TREATMENT OPTIONS

Prevention

   Prophylactic mastectomy reduces the risk for developing breast cancer by at least 90%. In this group of women, subcutaneous mastectomy is not the procedure of choice because a considerable amount of glandular tissue, especially around the nipple, is not removed. A total mastectomy is the best prevention.[34]

   Prophylactic oophorectomy reduces the risk for breast cancer in BRCA1 and BRCA2 gene carriers by approximately 50% in premenopausal women. It also reduces the risk for ovarian cancer. If prophylactic oophorectomy is performed premenopause, however, there is an increased risk for cardiovascular diseases and osteoporosis.[35]

   Chemoprevention with tamoxifen reduces the risk for breast cancer by approximately 50% but only for receptor-positive tumors.[36] The risk for receptor-negative tumors is not diminished by tamoxifen. The effect of the use of hormonal replacement therapy in BRCA1 and -2 mutation carriers is not clear.

RESULTS OF SCREENING

The first results regarding the value of screening with MRI in women with an increased risk for breast cancer were published approximately a decade ago.

Stoutjesdijk and colleagues[37] published the first results of a cohort of 179 women with a lifetime risk of 15% or more. In this series, 13 breast cancers were detected; 7 cancers were not seen on mammography, but MRI detected them all.

At the same time, Tilanus-Linthorst and colleagues[3] published the results of MRI screening in a group of 109 women with a lifetime risk of more than 25% and a breast density of more than 50%. MRI detected 3 cancers occult at mammography. In the Netherlands, approximately 20% of familial breast cancer is caused by BRCA1, 5% by BRCA2, and approximately 75% is non-BRCA1 or non-BRCA2.

The first large published study that reported on the value of MRI screening was the Dutch Magnetic Resonance Imaging Screening (MRISC) study in 2004.[38] Although the best study design would have been a randomized controlled trial with a study group of high-risk women who were screened and a control group of high-risk women who were not screened, most women will not consent to randomization. Therefore, the results from this screening study of the high-risk women were compared with a control group of nonscreened women from an external source.

This multicenter study included 1909 women: 358 women were gene carriers, 1052 women had a lifetime risk of 30% to 50% (high risk), and 499 women had a lifetime risk between 15% and 30%. Participants visited the family cancer clinic twice a year. Visit A consisted of a clinical breast examination and visit B a clinical breast examination, mammography, and MRI.

MRI was performed in premenopausal women between days 5 and 15 of the menstrual cycle to minimize glandular tissue enhancement. Inclusion criteria included a cumulative lifetime risk of 15% or more. The women in the study were divided into 3 groups depending on their lifetime risk for breast cancer: group 1 were BRCA1 or -2 mutation carriers with an assumed lifetime risk of 60% or more; group 2 had a lifetime risk of between 30% and 50%; and group 3 had a moderate risk of between 15% and 30%. The risk assessment was performed according the Claus tables. The age range of the women included in the study was between 25 and 70 years.

In the group of mutation carriers, 19 malignancies were detected, 16 invasive and 3 DCIS. In the high-risk group, 15 invasive malignancies were seen and no DCIS. In the moderate-risk group, 11 malignancies were found, of which 8 were invasive. In this study, the sensitivity of MRI for invasive cancer was 79.5% and of mammography was 33.3% (**Fig. 2**). The characteristics of the breast tumors detected in the study group were compared with those of 2 control groups.

The first control group was extracted from a population study investigating the frequency of BRCA mutations in a group of unselected symptomatic patients with primary breast cancer. The second group consisted of nonscreened family members with breast cancer of the participating women. The tumors in the study group were significantly smaller than in the control groups and were less likely to be node positive.

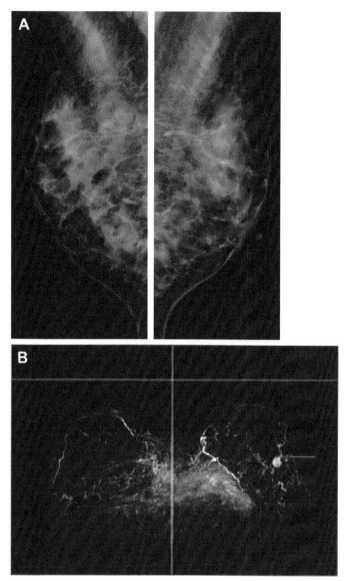

Fig. 2. (*A*) BRCA1 mutation carrier, dense mammography, no abnormalities. (*B*) MRI revealed invasive ductal carcinoma (*arrow*) in the left breast.

In 2005, the results of the Magnetic Resonance Imaging Breast Screening (MARIBS) trial were revealed.[39] This was also a prospective multicenter study of 649 women. Included were all gene mutation carriers and women with an annual risk of breast cancer of at least 0.9%. In this study, mammography had a sensitivity of 40% and MRI of 77%. The combined sensitivity was 94%. Therefore, annual screening with mammography and MRI detects most cancers in this group of women with a high increased risk.

At the same time, the results of a Canadian screening study were published. This study included only BRCA1 and BRCA2 mutations[40];

236 women were included in this ultrasound investigation and 22 cancers were detected. Mammography had a sensitivity of 36%, ultrasound of 33%, and MRI of 77%. These study results also showed the superior sensitivity of MRI compared with mammography and ultrasound.

In 2007, the results from the High Breast Cancer Risk Italian Trial (HIBCRIT) were published.[41] This study included 278 women, all BRCA1 and BRCA2 carriers. Also, the sensitivity of MRI was the highest, 94% compared with the sensitivity of mammography of 59%.

Lastly, a screening study published in 2009[42] evaluated 609 high-risk women with

Table 2
Results of different screening trials

	Dutch MRISC Study, Kriege et al, 2004	Toronto, Canada, Warner et al, 2004	MARIBS	HIBCRIT Study, Sardanelli et al, 2007	Weinstein et al, 2009
CE MRI sensitivity (95% CI)	71.1% (55.7–83.6)	77.3% (54.6–92.2)	77% (60–90)	93.8% (71.7–98.9)	71.0%
XRM sensitivity	40.0% (25.7–55.7)	36.4% (17.2–59.3)	40% (24–58)	58.8% (36.0–78.4)	39.0%
CE MRI specificity	89.8% (88.9–90.7)	95.4 (93.0–97.2)	81% (80–83)		79.0%
XRM specificity	95.0% (94.3–95.6)	99.8% (98.7–100)	93% (92–95)		91.0%

Abbreviations: CE, contrast-enhanced; XRM, x-ray mammography.

mammography, whole breast ultrasound, and MRI. Film-screen mammography revealed a sensitivity of 33%, digital mammography 39%, and whole breast ultrasound 17%. The sensitivity of MRI was 71%. It can be concluded from this study that the addition of MRI to mammography in this group of patients provides the greatest potential to detect malignant tumor foci.

SUMMARY

It can be concluded that a screening MRI in asymptomatic, high-risk women plays an important role for detection of malignant tumors with an overall sensitivity of more than 70% compared with a lower sensitivity of 35% for mammography alone. The combination of mammography and MRI has the highest sensitivity (**Table 2**).

REFERENCES

1. Fracheboud J, Otto SJ, van Dijck JA, et al. Decreased rates of advanced breast cancer due to mammography screening in The Netherlands. Br J Cancer 2004;91(5):861–7.
2. Kerlikowske K, Grady D, Barclay J, et al. Effect of age, breast density, and family history on the sensitivity of first screening mammography. JAMA 1996; 276(1):33–8.
3. Tilanus-Linthorst MM, Obdeijn IM, Bartels KC, et al. First experiences in screening women at high risk for breast cancer with MR imaging. Breast Cancer Res Treat 2000;63(1):53–60.
4. Claus EB, Schildkraut JM, Thompson WD, et al. The genetic attributable risk of breast and ovarian cancer. Cancer 1996;77(11):2318–24.
5. Struewing JP, Hartge P, Wacholder S, et al. The risk of cancer associated with specific mutations of BRCA1 and BRCA2 among Ashkenazi Jews. N Engl J Med 1997;336(20):1401–8.
6. American Society of Clinical Oncology. American Society of Clinical Oncology policy statement update: genetic testing for cancer susceptibility. J Clin Oncol 2003;21(12):2397–406.
7. Statement of the American Society of Clinical Oncology: genetic testing for cancer susceptibility, Adopted on February 20, 1996. J Clin Oncol 1996; 14(5):1730–6 [discussion: 37–40].
8. Claus EB, Risch N, Thompson WD. Autosomal dominant inheritance of early-onset breast cancer. Implications for risk prediction. Cancer 1994;73(3):643–51.
9. Gail MH, Brinton LA, Byar DP, et al. Projecting individualized probabilities of developing breast cancer for white females who are being examined annually. J Natl Cancer Inst 1989;81(24):1879–86.
10. Euhus DM, Smith KC, Robinson L, et al. Pretest prediction of BRCA1 or BRCA2 mutation by risk counselors and the computer model BRCAPRO. J Natl Cancer Inst 2002;94(11):844–51.
11. Saslow D, Boetes C, Burke W, et al. American Cancer Society guidelines for breast screening with MRI as an adjunct to mammography. CA Cancer J Clin 2007;57(2):75–89.
12. Mann RM, Kuhl CK, Kinkel K, et al. Breast MRI: guidelines from the European Society of Breast Imaging. Eur Radiol 2008;18(7):1307–18.
13. Ford D, Easton DF, Stratton M, et al. Genetic heterogeneity and penetrance analysis of the BRCA1 and BRCA2 genes in breast cancer families. The Breast Cancer Linkage Consortium. Am J Hum Genet 1998; 62(3):676–89.
14. Brose MS, Rebbeck TR, Calzone KA, et al. Cancer risk estimates for BRCA1 mutation carriers identified in a risk evaluation program. J Natl Cancer Inst 2002;94(18):1365–72.
15. Warner E, Foulkes W, Goodwin P, et al. Prevalence and penetrance of BRCA1 and BRCA2 gene

mutations in unselected Ashkenazi Jewish women with breast cancer. J Natl Cancer Inst 1999;91(14): 1241–7.

16. Easton DF, Ford D, Bishop DT. Breast and ovarian cancer incidence in BRCA1-mutation carriers. Breast Cancer Linkage Consortium. Am J Hum Genet 1995;56(1):265–71.

17. Edwards SM, Kote-Jarai Z, Meitz J, et al. Two percent of men with early-onset prostate cancer harbor germline mutations in the BRCA2 gene. Am J Hum Genet 2003;72(1):1–12.

18. Ozcelik H, Schmocker B, Di Nicola N, et al. Germline BRCA2 6174delT mutations in Ashkenazi Jewish pancreatic cancer patients. Nat Genet 1997;16(1): 17–8.

19. Frank TS, Deffenbaugh AM, Reid JE, et al. Clinical characteristics of individuals with germline mutations in BRCA1 and BRCA2: analysis of 10,000 individuals. J Clin Oncol 2002;20(6):1480–90.

20. Antoniou A, Pharoah PD, Narod S, et al. Average risks of breast and ovarian cancer associated with BRCA1 or BRCA2 mutations detected in case Series unselected for family history: a combined analysis of 22 studies. Am J Hum Genet 2003; 72(5):1117–30.

21. Pathology of familial breast cancer: differences between breast cancers in carriers of BRCA1 or BRCA2 mutations and sporadic cases. Breast Cancer Linkage Consortium. Lancet 1997; 349(9064):1505–10.

22. Lakhani SR, Van De Vijver MJ, Jacquemier J, et al. The pathology of familial breast cancer: predictive value of immunohistochemical markers estrogen receptor, progesterone receptor, HER-2, and p53 in patients with mutations in BRCA1 and BRCA2. J Clin Oncol 2002;20(9):2310–8.

23. Tilanus-Linthorst M, Verhoog L, Obdeijn IM, et al. A BRCA1/2 mutation, high breast density and prominent pushing margins of a tumor independently contribute to a frequent false-negative mammography. Int J Cancer 2002;102(1):91–5.

24. Foulkes WD, Brunet JS, Stefansson IM, et al. The prognostic implication of the basal-like (cyclin E high/p27 low/p53+/glomeruloid-microvascular-proliferation+) phenotype of BRCA1-related breast cancer. Cancer Res 2004;64(3):830–5.

25. Li FP, Fraumeni JF Jr, Mulvihill JJ, et al. A cancer family syndrome in twenty-four kindreds. Cancer Res 1988;48(18):5358–62.

26. Nichols KE, Malkin D, Garber JE, et al. Germ-line p53 mutations predispose to a wide spectrum of early-onset cancers. Cancer Epidemiol Biomarkers Prev 2001;10(2):83–7.

27. Achatz MI, Hainaut P, Ashton-Prolla P. Highly prevalent TP53 mutation predisposing to many cancers in the Brazilian population: a case for newborn screening? Lancet Oncol 2009;10(9):920–5.

28. Eng C. Genetics of Cowden syndrome: through the looking glass of oncology. Int J Oncol 1998;12(3): 701–10.

29. Giardiello FM, Brensinger JD, Tersmette AC, et al. Very high risk of cancer in familial Peutz-Jeghers syndrome. Gastroenterology 2000;119(6):1447–1453.

30. Athma P, Rappaport R, Swift M. Molecular genotyping shows that ataxia-telangiectasia heterozygotes are predisposed to breast cancer. Cancer Genet Cytogenet 1996;92(2):130–4.

31. Wolden SL, Hancock SL, Carlson RW, et al. Management of breast cancer after Hodgkin's disease. J Clin Oncol 2000;18(4):765–72.

32. Arpino G, Laucirica R, Elledge RM. Premalignant and in situ breast disease: biology and clinical implications. Ann Intern Med 2005;143(6):446–57.

33. Morris EA, Liberman L, Ballon DJ, et al. MRI of occult breast carcinoma in a high-risk population. AJR Am J Roentgenol 2003;181(3):619–26.

34. Hartmann LC, Sellers TA, Schaid DJ, et al. Efficacy of bilateral prophylactic mastectomy in BRCA1 and BRCA2 gene mutation carriers. J Natl Cancer Inst 2001;93(21):1633–7.

35. Kurian AW, Sigal BM, Plevritis SK. Survival analysis of cancer risk reduction strategies for BRCA1/2 mutation carriers. J Clin Oncol 2010;28(2):222–31.

36. Hemann MT, Rudolph KL, Strong MA, et al. Telomere dysfunction triggers developmentally regulated germ cell apoptosis. Mol Biol Cell 2001;12(7):2023–30.

37. Stoutjesdijk MJ, Boetes C, Jager GJ, et al. Magnetic resonance imaging and mammography in women with a hereditary risk of breast cancer. J Natl Cancer Inst 2001;93(14):1095–102.

38. Kriege M, Brekelmans CT, Boetes C, et al. Efficacy of MRI and mammography for breast-cancer screening in women with a familial or genetic predisposition. N Engl J Med 2004;351(5):427–37.

39. Leach MO, Boggis CR, Dixon AK, et al. Screening with magnetic resonance imaging and mammography of a UK population at high familial risk of breast cancer: a prospective multicentre cohort study (MARIBS). Lancet 2005;365(9473): 1769–78.

40. Warner E, Plewes DB, Hill KA, et al. Surveillance of BRCA1 and BRCA2 mutation carriers with magnetic resonance imaging, ultrasound, mammography, and clinical breast examination. JAMA 2004;292(11): 1317–25.

41. Sardanelli F, Podo F, D'Agnolo G, et al. Multicenter comparative multimodality surveillance of women at genetic-familial high risk for breast cancer (HIBCRIT study): interim results. Radiology 2007;242(3): 698–715.

42. Weinstein SP, Localio AR, Conant EF, et al. Multimodality screening of high-risk women: a prospective cohort study. J Clin Oncol 2009;27(36):6124–8.

Role of Breast MR Imaging in Neoadjuvant Chemotherapy

H. Carisa Le-Petross, MD, FRCPC[a], Nola Hylton, PhD[b],*

KEYWORDS

- Breast cancer treatment • Neoadjuvant chemotherapy
- MR imaging • Breast neoplasm • Treatment response

Neoadjuvant chemotherapy (NAC) or primary systemic therapy given before surgery is now widely used as an alternative to the traditional approach of postoperative adjuvant chemotherapy in patients with breast cancer. Neoadjuvant chemotherapy is as effective as chemotherapy after surgery.[1–3] Neoadjuvant chemotherapy is most often used in the treatment of patients with locally advanced breast cancer (LABC) because of the poor prognosis associated with this disease. The combination of NAC and surgery offers better local disease control and overall survival than surgery alone in patients with breast cancer, especially those with LABC.[4,5] Moreover, NAC may allow the conversion of non-operable to operable disease or permit breast conservation therapy in patients who otherwise would have required mastectomy. However, a complete pathologic response to NAC does not occur in all patients. Therefore, it is important to identify early in the course of therapy which patients are likely to have a complete response to therapy and which patients are not. This information allows the physicians to tailor disease management and may improve patients' outcomes and prolong survival.

It is imperative, therefore, that we identify the most accurate early predictor of response to therapy. Physical examination, mammography, and sonography (US) have all been used to assess response to NAC, but each of these approaches has limitations. Physical examination, though widely used for this indication, is unreliable and subjective, relying on the physician's experience. Furthermore, physical examination cannot differentiate posttreatment fibrosis or residual necrotic tissue from residual viable tumor mass. Feldman and colleagues[4] reported that 45% of complete clinical responders had macroscopic tumor at histologic examination, whereas 60% of patients without histologic gross residual tumor had an incomplete clinical response. In another series of 49 subjects, physical examination overestimated tumor regression in 23% of cases and underestimated response in 9%.[6] Mammography may overestimate residual disease because of its inability to detect changes in the microcalcifications associated with the malignancy. Early series evaluating the role of US reported that US tends to underestimate residual tumor size and is actually less accurate than physical examination.[7–9]

MR imaging is the first breast imaging modality that not only allows detailed visualization of the anatomy but also, when an intravenous contrast agent is administered or advanced sequences (eg, diffusion-weighted imaging or spectroscopy) are used, provides functional information. This article reviews the published data on the role of breast MR imaging in assessing tumor response in women receiving neoadjuvant chemotherapy.

[a] Department of Radiology, The University of Texas M.D. Anderson Cancer Center, 1515 Holcombe Boulevard, Unit 1350, Houston, TX 77030, USA
[b] Department of Radiology and Biomedical Imaging, University of California San Francisco, 1600 Divisadero Street, Box 1667, San Francisco, CA 94143-166, USA
* Corresponding author.
E-mail address: nola.hylton@radiology.ucsf.edu

Magn Reson Imaging Clin N Am 18 (2010) 249–258
doi:10.1016/j.mric.2010.02.008
1064-9689/10/$ – see front matter © 2010 Published by Elsevier Inc.

Table 1
Reported sensitivity and specificity of MR imaging in assessing response to NAC

Authors	No. of pts	NAC	Sensitivity (%)	Specificity (%)
Abraham et al[12]	39	B, A	97	—
Belli et al[50]	45	B, D	90	100
Bhattacharyya et al[48]	32	B, A	88	50
Choi et al[49]	41	B, A	71	95
Warren et al[47]	67	B, A	100	80

Abbreviations: A, after; B, before; D, during.

MR IMAGING

Breast MR imaging has a reported sensitivity of 95% to 97% for the detection of invasive breast cancer and 50% to 100% for the assessment of response to NAC (**Table 1**). This high sensitivity is dependent on the ability of MR imaging to differentiate untreated hypervascular tumor from the background enhancing fibroglandular tissue or breast tissue. In patients undergoing neoadjuvant chemotherapy, the antiangiogenic effect of cytotoxic chemotherapy agents reduces the vascularity of the tumor mass. This decrease in tumor vascularity would be expected to be associated with a decrease in enhancement of that lesion on MR imaging (**Fig. 1**). This dampening effect of chemotherapy on enhancement of the lesion may compromise the ability to visualize residual viable tumor. However, the alteration of tumor vascularity or other MR characteristics can help identify predictive features to differentiate patients whose cancer is likely to respond to the chemotherapy from those whose cancer would not respond

(**Fig. 2**). Since 1996, at least 37 studies have been published on the use of MR imaging in identifying such predictors.[3,7,10–47] Many of these studies are single-institution trials with small sample sizes, ranging from 13 to 73 subjects. The studies vary in the criteria used for distinguishing complete responders from partial responders or non-responders. The MR imaging examinations performed in each trial are not standardized with regards to type of scanners, Tesla strength of the scanners, number and type of MR imaging sequences performed for each examination, number of post-contrast sequences performed, or timing of post-contrast sequences. Despite these differences, many of the observations from the studies were similar and are discussed in further detail later in this article.

MR IMAGING ASSESSMENT OF TUMOR SIZE

Accurate measurement of tumor size, before neoadjuvant chemotherapy, is important for staging, treatment monitoring, and determining prognosis.

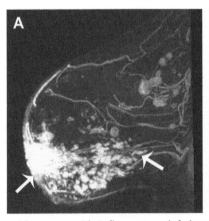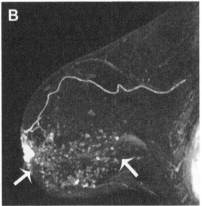

Fig. 1. 69-year-old woman with inflammatory left breast carcinoma who received MR imaging examinations before (*A*) and while undergoing neoadjuvant chemotherapy (NAC) (*B*). (*A*) Maximum intensity projection before initiation of NAC demonstrates a 14 cm area of abnormal enhancement (*arrows*) from multicentric disease and associated axillary adenopathy. (*B*) Maximum intensity projection after four cycles of NAC demonstrates overall decrease in enhancement and intensity of the multicentric disease, with scattered residual enhancing foci within the same 14 cm area.

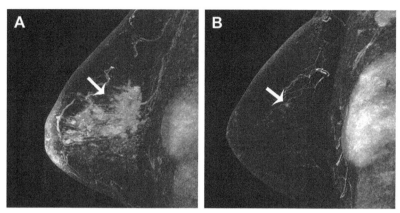

Fig. 2. 54-year-old woman with a diagnosis of left breast invasive ductal carcinoma who received neoadjuvant chemotherapy, with complete clinical response to therapy. (*A*) Maximum intensity projection image, obtained before treatment, demonstrates an 8.5 cm enhancing biopsy proven carcinoma (*arrow*). (*B*) Maximum intensity projection image, obtained after eight cycles of NAC, demonstrates a tiny 5 mm enhancing focus (*arrow*) at the site of prior 8.5 cm enhancing mass. The MR finding is consistent with clinical and pathologic complete response to therapy.

Tumor size has been known to predict patient survival and is the basis of most disease-staging systems.[7] Studies have shown that imaging-based measurements are superior to clinical palpation in determining tumor size and predicting pathologic complete response.[10,11] MR imaging more accurately reflects true pathologic tumor size and is more reliable than physical examination, mammography, or US in predicting the amount of residual disease after neoadjuvant chemotherapy (**Fig. 3**).[12–17] In one study, MR imaging measured the final tumor size accurately, to be within 1 cm of the final tumor size determined by gross histologic examination (**Fig. 4**).[18] In another trial of only 15 subjects, MR imaging over-estimated main lesion diameter by only 3.4 mm, and this difference was not statistically significant.[19] Several studies have shown that MR imaging prediction of tumor response to NAC correlates well with pathology, with the correlation coefficient (r) between MR imaging and histology ranging between 0.6 and 0.9.[13,18–23,47] In one series, MR imaging correctly assessed the residual disease in 83% of the cases, with only one false negative case in which a 2 mm residual invasive carcinoma was not detected.[25] MR imaging can underestimate residual disease in 2% to 10% of cases, especially if the tumor shrinkage pattern from the chemotherapy is patchy with areas of necrosis between nests of viable tumor or tiny tumor foci scattered over a large area.[18,21,26,47] In a trial of 40 subjects with LABC, the underestimation was seen more frequently in patients treated with docetaxel-based chemotherapy than in those treated with

5-fluoro-uraci-epirubicin regimens.[24] Overestimation of tumor size after neoadjuvant chemotherapy was reported in as many as 6% to 33% of the cases.[17,18,23] These contradicting observations of underestimation and overestimation by MR imaging are derived from single institutional trials with small sample sizes; validation studies are needed with larger sample sizes and standardization chemotherapy regimens.

Some investigators have used tumor-volume calculations, in combination with largest tumor diameter to assess response to neoadjuvant chemotherapy. Some observed that a change in the initial and final tumor volume measurements by MR imaging had a stronger association with recurrence-free survival in those who received NAC compared with other prognostic indicators, such as largest tumor diameter.[22] This volume change can be observed after only one cycle of chemotherapy and is suggested to be associated with recurrence-free survival. Other investigators compared the largest tumor size with tumor volume as possible predictors for response to therapy and noted that a tumor volume reduction of more than 65% after two cycles of chemotherapy was the most predictive value for predicting histologic response.[23] Defining the margins of the breast tumors to accurately measure the largest diameter or calculate the tumor volume can be challenging during and after neoadjuvant chemotherapy.[19,22,23] Additional information on tumor vascularity from contrast-enhanced MR imaging may be beneficial when combined with the morphologic assessment and size or volume change from NAC.

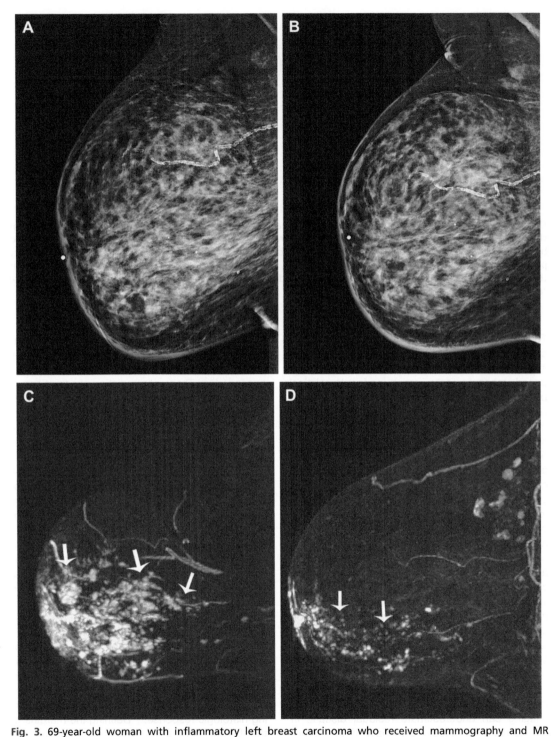

Fig. 3. 69-year-old woman with inflammatory left breast carcinoma who received mammography and MR imaging examinations before (*A, C*) and while undergoing neoadjuvant chemotherapy. (*B, D*). Minimal improvement is noted between the mammogram performed before initiation of chemotherapy (*A*) and during chemotherapy. (*B*) However, the MR imaging performed during chemotherapy (*D*) demonstrates a more dramatic decreased in tumor burden compared with the MR imaging performed before chemotherapy (*C*) than mammography.

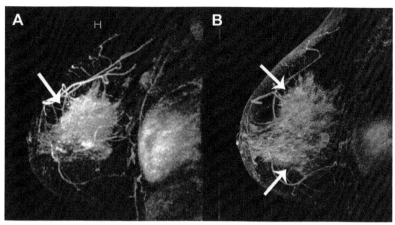

Fig. 4. 45-year-old woman with a diagnosis of invasive ductal carcinoma and ipsilateral nodal metastasis who had partial clinical response after eight cycles of neoadjuvant chemotherapy. (*A*) Maximum intensity projection image demonstrates a 6.1 cm enhancing mass (*arrow*) in the left breast before NAC. (*B*) Maximum intensity projection image is performed after NAC, which demonstrates an 8 cm area of enhancement (*arrow*). This area has increased in size since the pretreatment MR imaging, compatible with no response to therapy. Final pathology at mastectomy revealed a 9 cm carcinoma, comprising of 40% viable tumor, with therapy effect. MR imaging measurement of residual disease is within 1 cm of the final tumor size by gross pathology.

MR IMAGING ASSESSMENT OF TUMOR ENHANCEMENT

Even though the widely used Response Evaluation Criteria In Solid Tumors (RECISTS) is based on the largest diameter of the cancer, alteration of tumor enhancement by chemotherapy caused by changes in the microvascular density of the cancer can be a prognostic factor in predicting response to NAC. Tumor enhancement is characterized as very early phase (0 to 60 seconds), initial enhancement (60 to 120 seconds) of the dynamic series, or delayed phase (more than 120 seconds) after injection of a gadolinium-based intravenous contrast. Balu-Maestro and colleagues[14] reported the disappearance of early or initial abnormal enhancement in five cases of complete histologic response. Rieber and colleagues[24] found that flattening of the time-intensity curve or disappearance of the washout segment of the kinetic curve after one course of chemotherapy and absence of contrast uptake after four courses predict complete pathologic response. Other investigators observed decreases in the rate and magnitude of contrast enhancement within the tumor mass in patients whose disease responded to chemotherapy, and an increase or no change in patients whose disease responded poorly to therapy (**Fig. 5**).[25–28] In a study of 54 subjects who had breast MR imaging examinations before and after two cycles of chemotherapy, the change in the largest diameter of late enhancement during chemotherapy was the most predictive MR imaging characteristic for tumor response;

a decrease less than 25% in largest diameter of late enhancement was indicative of residual tumor at final pathologic examination.[29] A feasibility study in 19 women of tumor washout volume during the late enhancement phase demonstrated a significant reduction of the washout volume after two cycles of chemotherapy.[30] The tumor volume reduction by more than 65% (after two cycles of chemotherapy) was also demonstrated in a larger trial of 30 subjects to be a stronger predictor of histopathological response than early enhancement ratio.[23] When combined with tumor size measurement, the change in overall tumor volume and voxel analysis of contrast enhancement time curves may improve the specificity of diagnosis and produce information about tumor heterogeneity, permeability, and vascularity.

FUNCTIONAL MR IMAGING ASSESSMENT

Contrast-enhanced MR imaging is valuable in monitoring residual tumor because this imaging modality allows excellent correlation of MR imaging detected size and volume with gross histologic tumor size. The pathologic size, a widely used reference standard, is a unidimensional measurement and many times is obtained in a different plane than that used to identify the largest diameter on MR imaging. Volumetric acquisition on MR imaging can be easily obtained with emerging computer-assisted software but it is more difficult to accomplish volume acquisition with pathologic specimens, especially for diffuse residual disease. Additional parameters, such as

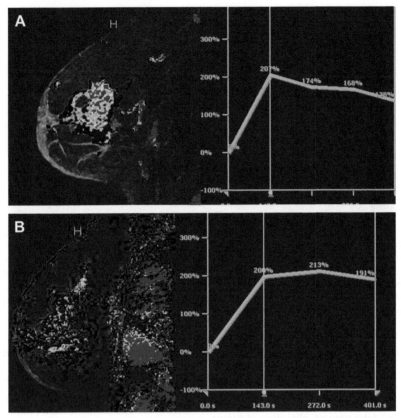

Fig. 5. 44-year-old woman with diagnosis of locally advanced breast carcinoma who underwent neoadjuvant chemotherapy, with partial response at early stage of therapy follow by disease progression. (*A*) The colorized image (*left*) with the corresponding time signal intensity curve (*right*) demonstrates the peak enhancement of 207% above baseline with delay washout curve shape. (*B*) After one cycle of chemotherapy, the colorized image (*left*) with the corresponding time-intensity curve (*right*) demonstrates no decrease in the magnitude of the peak enhancement at 200% above baseline with delayed plateau curve shape.

functional MR measurements (K^{trans}, v_e, apparent diffusion coefficient, and choline concentration), have been studied and shown by several investigators to improve the sensitivity and specificity of breast MR imaging when coupled with size and volumetric data. Successful chemotherapy is hypothesized to cause a reduction in the tumor angiogenic factors, such as vascular endothelial growth factor, a strong stimulus of tumor neo-angiogenesis and a potent tissue permeability factor in breast cancer, and subsequent cell death. A change in the tissue permeability factor would be reflected in a reduction in the volume transfer constants or K^{trans}. The volume transfer constants of gadolinium-based contrast between blood plasma and the extravascular extracellular space were evaluated in an initial clinical trial of 25 subjects. Padhani and colleagues[31] showed that size and transfer constant range were equally accurate in predicting the absence of pathologic response after two cycles of treatment.

FUNCTIONAL MR IMAGING ASSESSMENT: SPECTROSCOPY

Even though changes in tumor size during NAC is a good predictor of the final response to NAC, additional functional parameters, such as Proton (1H) MR spectroscopy (MRS), may allow prediction of responders from non-responders even before the tumor shrinks. MR spectroscopy allows the detection of peak resonance from metabolic compounds, such as choline-containing compounds (tCho) (**Fig. 6**). This technique became of interest in breast imaging because tCho was commonly present in malignant breast lesions but not in benign or normal tissues. Changes in the intracellular metabolism between the pretreatment and after treatment may be detected before any gross morphologic change can be detected. MRS was reported to have a sensitivity of 100% and a specificity of 85% for the detection of malignancy in enhancing

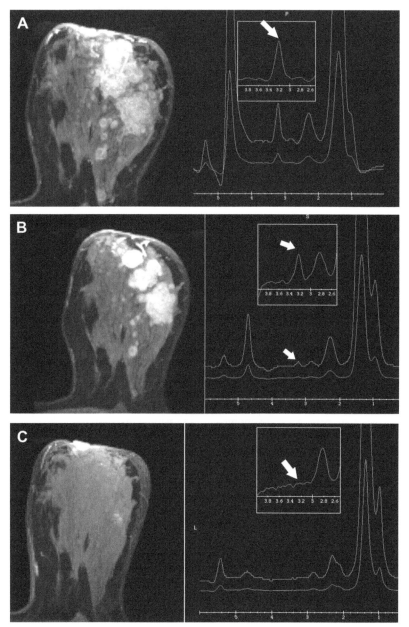

Fig. 6. 35-year -old woman with locally advanced invasive ductal carcinoma who had MR imaging with spectroscopy before initiation of NAC, during, and after completion of NAC. (*A*) Before treatment, the multicentric carcinoma is 12 cm (*left*); tCho peak (*arrow*) is visible at 3.22 ppm in water-fat suppressed spectrum (*right*). (*B*) After once cycle of NAC, the multicentric carcinoma decreased to 8 cm (*left*); tCho peak (*arrow*) also decreased in magnitude, relative to background (*right*). (*C*) After completion of NAC, the residual carcinoma is 1 cm (*left*); no detectable tCho peak above background (*right*). Final pathology of the left mastectomy specimen showed a residual 3 cm area of fibrosis with 2% residual viable tumor.

non-mass lesions.[32] In 67 subjects with invasive carcinoma and receiving NAC, the sensitivity and specificity of MRS were 78% and 86%, respectively. In this study, the absence or reduction in choline peak occurred in 89% of the subjects.[33] Meisamy and others also reported a change in tCho, as early as 24 hours after the first dose of chemotherapy in 13 subjects.[34] The changes were statistically significant between responders and non-responders. In a more recent study of 35 subjects with breast cancer who consented for MRS examination before treatment, during and after completing NAC, the change in tumor size and tCHo were found to significantly differentiate between the responders and the non-responders only at the second follow-up studies but not at the first follow-up studies. The change in tumor size during NAC was actually a more accurate predictor of complete pathologic response than MRS.[35]

FUNCTIONAL MR IMAGING ASSESSMENT: DIFFUSION-WEIGHTED MR IMAGING

Diffusion-weighted imaging (DWI) can be used to characterize cellular edema and density by providing a method to assess the movement of water molecules. Diffusion is restricted or decreased in tissues with high cellularity, such as malignant tumors, compared with benign lesions or cystic lesions. This functional information is described as the apparent diffusion coefficient (ADC) of water molecules in a lesion. The ADC correlates inversely with the tissue cellularity. Quantitative analyses are employed to distinguish between zones of viable cells, edema, and necrosis for treatment planning. Serial changes in tissue cellularity in response to therapy are measurable by diffusion using various quantitative methods that include whole-tumor ADC average, histogram analysis, and pretreatment versus posttreatment voxel-based differences.

Limited published data are available on the use of DWI in assessing response to neoadjuvant chemotherapy in breast cancer. In one series of subjects with breast cancer and liver metastases, increases in tumor ADC value and decreases in tumor enhancement were observed earlier than changes in tumor size.[36] In another series of 47 women with LABC who received NAC, the sensitivity and negative predictive value were improved significantly when DWI was added to contrast-enhanced dynamic MR imaging. However, the specificity of DWI and contrast-enhanced dynamic MR imaging remained the same in this study.[37] Other investigators reported a higher specificity (100%) for ADC in differentiating responders from non-responders than for volume (50%) and diameter measurements (70%). After one cycle of NAC, a significant increase in the ADC was observed between the clinical responders from the non-responders. The mean percentage decrease in volume and diameter was not significantly different between the responders and non-responders.[38] The preliminary results on DWI from these single centers suggest the promise of ADC as a prognostic indicator of treatment response.

SUMMARY

Over the last decade, there have been numerous trials from several countries assessing the role of breast MR imaging in monitoring tumor response to neoadjuvant chemotherapy. Comparison of these published data is difficult because of the different definitions of response, the different chemotherapy agents used, and the chemotherapy regimens. Most of the MR imaging examinations were performed on a 1.5 Tesla (T) magnetic system, with only a few studies performed on a 0.5T and 1.0T systems. The majority of the studies were single center trials with a small set of subjects. The suggested MR imaging response prediction test needs to be evaluated prospectively with patients from multiple institutions. Standardization of the chemotherapeutic agents would minimize the validation concerns of different chemotherapeutic agents having different effects on the performance of the MR imaging test. Besides the timing and dosing regimen standardization, the MR imaging examinations also need to be standardized. Preliminary results of the functional imaging MR techniques are promising. Because the ultimate outcome of a successful chemotherapy regimen is destruction of the tumor, including its neo-vascular system, dynamic contrast-enhanced breast MR imaging coupled with one or more of the functional imaging MR techniques should improve the accuracy and minimize the false negative rate in the assessment of residual disease after NAC.

REFERENCES

1. Fisher B, Bryant J, Wolmark N, et al. Effect of preoperative chemotherapy on the outcome of women with operable breast cancer. J Clin Oncol 1998;16: 2672–85.
2. Fisher ER, Wang J, Bryant J, et al. Pathobiology of preoperative chemotherapy: findings from the National Surgical Adjuvant Breast and Bowel (NSABP) protocol B-18. Cancer 2002;95:681–95.
3. Wolmark N, Wang J, Mamounas E, et al. Preoperative chemotherapy in patients with operable breast cancer: nine-year results from National Surgical Adjuvant Breast and Bowel Project B-18. J Natl Cancer Inst Monogr 2001;30:96–102.
4. Feldman LD, Hortobagyi GN, Budzar AU, et al. Pathologic assessment of response to induction chemotherapy in breast cancer. Breast Cancer Res Treat 1986;46:2578–81.
5. Heys SD, Eremin JM, Sarkar TK, et al. Role of multimodality therapy in the management of locally advanced carcinoma of the breast. J Am Coll Surg 1994;179(4):493–504.
6. Cocconi G, Di Blasio B, Alberti G, et al. Problems in evaluating response of primary breast cancer to systemic therapy. Breast Cancer Res Treat 1984;4: 309–13.

7. Herrada J, Iyer RB, Atkinson EN, et al. Relative value of physical examination, mammography, and breast sonography in evaluating the size of the primary tumor and regional lymph node metastases in women receiving neoadjuvant chemotherapy for locally advanced breast carcinoma. Clin Cancer Res 1997;3:1565–9.

8. Finlayson CA, MacDermott TA. Ultrasound can estimate the pathologic size of infiltrating ductal carcinoma. Arch Surg 2000;135:158–9.

9. Peintinger F, Kuerer HM, Anderson K, et al. Accuracy of the combination of mammography and sonography in predicting tumor response in breast cancer patients after neoadjuvant chemotherapy. Ann Surg Oncol 2006;13(11):1443–9.

10. Gribbestad IS, Nilsen G, Fjosne H, et al. Contrast-enhanced magnetic resonance imaging of the breast. Acta Oncol 1992;31(8):833–42.

11. Segara D, Krop IE, Garber JE, et al. Does MRI predict pathologic tumor response in women with breast cancer undergoing preoperative chemotherapy? J Surg Oncol 2007;96:474–80.

12. Abraham DC, Jones RC, Jones SE, et al. Evaluation of neoadjuvant chemotherapeutic response of locally advanced breast cancer by magnetic resonance imaging. Cancer 1996;78(1):91–100.

13. Akazawa K, Tamaki Y, Taguchi T, et al. Preoperative evaluation of residual tumor extent by three-dimensional magnetic resonance imaging in breast cancer patients treated with neoadjuvant chemotherapy. Breast J 2006;12(2):130–7.

14. Balu-Maestro C, Chapellier C, Bleuse A, et al. Imaging in evaluation of response to neoadjuvant breast cancer treatment benefits of MRI. Breast Cancer Res Treat 2002;72:145–52.

15. Cheung YC, Chen SC, Su MY, et al. Monitoring the size and response of locally advanced breast cancers to neoadjuvant chemotherapy (weekly paclitaxel and epirubicin) with serial enhanced MRI. Breast Cancer Res Treat 2003;78:51–8.

16. Gilles R, Guinebretière JM, Toussaint C, et al. Locally advanced breast cancer: contrast-enhanced subtraction MR imaging of response to preoperative chemotherapy. Radiology 1994;191:633–8.

17. Yeh E, Slanetz P, Kopans DB, et al. Prospective comparison of mammography, sonography, and MRI in patients undergoing neoadjuvant chemotherapy for palpable breast cancer. Am J Roentgenol 2005;184(3):868–77.

18. Rosen EL, Blackwell KL, Baker JA, et al. Accuracy of MRI in the detection of residual breast cancer after neoadjuvant chemotherapy. AJR Am J Roentgenol 2003;181(5):1275–82.

19. Lorenzon M, Zuiani C, Londero V, et al. Assessment of breast cancer response to neoadjuvant chemotherapy: is volumetric MRI a reliable tool? Eur J Radiol 2009;71(1):82–8.

20. Prati PR, Minami CA, Gornbein JA, et al. Accuracy of clinical evaluation of locally advanced breast cancer in patients receiving neoadjuvant chemotherapy. Cancer 2009;115:1194–202.

21. Wasser K, Sinn HP, Fink C, et al. Accuracy of tumor size measurement in breast cancer using MRI is influenced by histological regression induced by neoadjuvant chemotherapy. Eur Radiol 2003;13(6):1213–23.

22. Partridge SC, Gibbs JE, Lu Y, et al. MRI measurements of breast tumor volume predict response to neoadjuvant chemotherapy and recurrence-free survival. AJR Am J Roentgenol 2005;184:1774–81.

23. Martincich L, Montemurro F, De RG, et al. Monitoring response to primary chemotherapy in breast cancer using dynamic contrast enhanced magnetic resonance imaging. Breast Cancer Res Treat 2004;83:67–76.

24. Rieber A, Brambs HJ, Gabelmann A, et al. Breast MRI for monitoring response of primary breast cancer to neoadjuvant chemotherapy. Eur Radiol 2002;12:1711–9.

25. Kim HJ, Im YH, Han BK, et al. Accuracy of MRI for estimating residual tumor size after neoadjuvant chemotherapy in locally advanced breast cancer: Relation to response patterns on MRI. Acta Oncol 2007;46:996–1003.

26. Denis F, Desbiez-Bourcier AV, Chapiron C, et al. Contrast enhanced magnetic resonance imaging underestimates residual disease following neoadjuvant docetaxel based chemotherapy for breast cancer. Eur J Surg Oncol 2004;30:1069–76.

27. Trecate G, Ceglia E, Stabile F, et al. Locally advanced breast tumors. Role of magnetic resonance in the assessment of response to preoperative therapy and of neoplastic residue before the operation. Radiol Med 1998;95(5):449–55.

28. Weatherall PT, Evans GF, Metzger GJ, et al. MRI vs histologic measurement of breast cancer following chemotherapy: comparison with x-ray mammography and palpation. J Magn Reson Imaging 2001;13(6):868–75.

29. Loo CE, Teertstra JH, Rodenhuis S, et al. Dynamic contrast-enhanced MRI for prediction of breast cancer response to neoadjuvant chemotherapy: initial results. Am J Roentgenol 2008;191:1331–8.

30. El Khoury C, Servois V, Thibault F, et al. MR quantification of the washout changes in breast tumors under preoperative chemotherapy: feasibility and preliminary results. Am J Roentgenol 2005;184(5):1499–504.

31. Padhani AR, Hayes C, Assersohn L, et al. Prediction of clinicopathologic response of breast cancer to primary chemotherapy at contrast-enhanced MR imaging: initial clinical results. Radiology 2006;239:361–74.

32. Bartella L, Thakur SB, Morris EA, et al. Enhancing nonmass lesions in the breast: evaluation with

proton (1H) MR spectroscopy1. Radiology 2007; 245:80–7.

33. Jagannathan NR, Kumar M, Seenu V, et al. Evaluation of total choline from in-vivo volume localized proton MR spectroscopy and its response to neoadjuvant chemotherapy in locally advanced breast cancer. Br J Cancer 2001;84:1016–22.

34. Meisamy S, Bolan PJ, Baker EH, et al. Predicting response to neoadjuvant chemotherapy of locally advanced breast cancer with in vivo 1H MRS: a pilot study at 4 Tesla. Radiology 2004;233:424–31.

35. Baek H-M, Chen J-H, Nie K, et al. Predicting pathologic response to neoadjuvant chemotherapy in breast cancer by using MR Imaging and quantitative 1H MR spectroscopy. Radiology 2009;251:653–62.

36. Buijs M, Vossen JA, Hong K, et al. Assessment of metastatic breast cancer response to chemoembolization with contrast agent enhanced and diffusion-weighted MR imaging. Am J Roentgenol 2008; 191(1):285–9.

37. Kuroki Y, Nasu K. Advances in breast MRI: diffusion-weighted imaging of the breast. Breast Cancer 2008;15:212–7.

38. Sharma SU, Danishada KK, Seenub V, et al. Longitudinal study of the assessment by MRI and diffusion-weighted imaging of tumor response in patients with locally advanced breast cancer undergoing neoadjuvant chemotherapy. NMR Biomed 2009;22:104–13.

39. Ah-See ML, Makris A, Taylor NJ, et al. Early changes in functional dynamic magnetic resonance imaging predict for pathologic response to neoadjuvant chemotherapy in primary breast cancer. Clin Cancer Res 2008;14(20):6580–9.

40. Bahri S, Chen JH, Mehta RS, et al. Residual breast cancer diagnosed by MRI in patients receiving neoadjuvant chemotherapy with and without bevacizumab. Ann Surg Oncol 2009;16:1619–28.

41. Chou CP, Wu MT, Chang HT, et al. Monitoring breast cancer response to neoadjuvant systemic chemotherapy using parametric contrast-enhanced MRI: a pilot study. Acad Radiol 2007;14:561–73.

42. Johansen R, Jensen LR, Rydland J, et al. Predicting survival and early clinical response to primary chemotherapy for patients with locally advanced breast cancer using DCE-MRI. J Magn Reson Imaging 2009;29:1300–7.

43. Nicoletto MO, Nitti D, Pescarini L, et al. Correlation between magnetic resonance imaging and histopathological tumor response after neoadjuvant chemotherapy in breast cancer. Tumori 2008;94:481–8.

44. Belli P, Romani M, Costantini M, et al. Role of magnetic resonance imaging in the pre and post-chemotherapy evaluation in locally advanced breast carcinoma. Rays 2002;27(4):279–90.

45. Pickles MD, Lowry M, Manton DJ, et al. Role of dynamic contrast enhanced MRI in monitoring early response of locally advanced breast cancer to neoadjuvant chemotherapy. Breast Cancer Res Treat 2005;91:1–10.

46. Chen JH, Feig B, Agrawal G, et al. MRI evaluation of pathologically complete response and residual tumors in breast cancer after neoadjuvant chemotherapy. Cancer 2008;112(1):17–26.

47. Warren RM, Bobrow LG, Earl HM, et al. Can breast MRI help in the management of women with breast cancer treated by neoadjuvant chemotherapy? Br J Cancer 2004;5(90):1349–60.

48. Bhattacharyya M, Ryan D, Carpenter R, et al. Using MRI to plan breast-conserving surgery following neoadjuvant chemotherapy for early breast cancer. Br J Cancer 2008;98(2):289–93.

49. Choi JH, Lim HI, Lee SK, et al. The role of PET CT to evaluate the response to neoadjuvant chemotherapy in advanced breast cancer: comparison with ultrasonography and magnetic resonance imaging. J Surg Oncol 2009. Available at: http://www3.interscience. wiley.com/journal/122667168/abstract?CRETRY=1 &SRETRY=0. Accessed February 5, 2010.

50. Belli P, Costantini M, Malaspina C, et al. MRI accuracy in residual disease evaluation in breast cancer patients treated with neoadjuvant chemotherapy. Clin Radiol 2006;61(11):946–53.

The Effectiveness of MR Imaging in the Assessment of Invasive Lobular Carcinoma of the Breast

Ritse M. Mann, MD

KEYWORDS

- Breast cancer • Invasive lobular carcinoma
- Breast MR imaging • Preoperative staging

Invasive lobular carcinoma (ILC) is the second most common form of breast cancer, reported in 5% to 20% of patients. The relative frequency of ILC has been increasing in the last decades, probably related to the increased use of complete hormone replacement therapy in perimenopausal women.[1,2] The reduced use of this therapy in recent years may already have resulted in a small decrease of the incidence of ILC.[3] ILC derives its name from the old assumption that the tumor arises from the lobules,[4] whereas the more common form of breast cancer, invasive ductal carcinoma (IDC), arises from the milk ducts. Because most breast cancers, including IDC and ILC, have been shown to arise from the terminal ductal lobular units, these common breast cancers are somewhat awkwardly named.[5,6]

The main difference between IDC and ILC is their growth pattern, with ILC tending to grow more diffusely. The "classic type" lobular carcinoma consists of relatively small, uniform cells that grow in a loosely cohesive fashion, forming lines of cells infiltrating the healthy tissue—so-called Indian files (**Fig. 1**). Formation of webs around healthy ducts, referred to as targetoid growth, is often reported. Furthermore, skip lesions, that is, areas of tumor separated from the index lesion by normal breast tissue, are more common than in IDC.[7,8] Moreover, synchronous and metachronous contralateral carcinomas are more often observed in ILC.[9]

The genetic basis for these differences is probably due to a mutation in the E-cadherin gene (CDH1). E-cadherin is strongly related to cell-cell cohesion, and affects morphology and motility of cells. Hence a lack of E-cadherin expression may

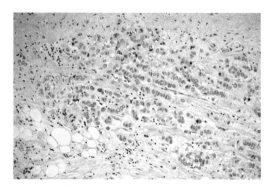

Fig. 1. Ten-times enlarged hematoxylin-eosin stain of an ILC. Note the relative uniformity and the linear arrangement of the small round cancer cells. (*Courtesy of* Peter Bult, MD, PhD, Department of Pathology, Radboud University of Nijmegen Medical Center.)

There are no conflicts of interest to disclose.

Department of Radiology, Radboud University Nijmegen Medical Centre, Huispost 667, Geert Grooteplein 10, P.O. Box 9101, 6500 HB Nijmegen, the Netherlands

E-mail address: r.mann@rad.umcn.nl

Magn Reson Imaging Clin N Am 18 (2010) 259–276

doi:10.1016/j.mric.2010.02.005

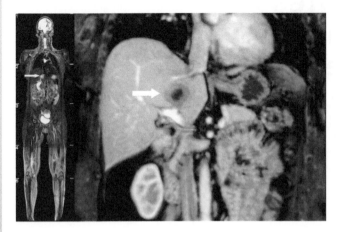

Fig. 2. Images of a 47-year-old woman presenting with a T4 ILC. She underwent whole body MR imaging to screen for distant metastases. The whole body STIR (short time inversion recovery) acquisition (*left*) and the postcontrast (15 mL Gd-DOTA) T1-weighted VIBE (volumetric interpolated breath-hold examination) acquisition (*right*) show a large metastasis central in the liver, with central necrosis (*arrows*). The patient underwent neoadjuvant chemotherapy, to which she responded very well; 6 months later the liver metastasis was no longer visible and the primary tumor was surgically removed.

be the cause for the disjointed growth of ILC.[7,8,10] Apart from the lack of E-cadherin expression, classic ILC biologically resembles low-grade IDC. Similarly, the more aggressive subtype pleomorphic ILC resembles high-grade IDC.

There are only a few other documented differences between IDC and ILC. ILC are generally larger at detection than IDC, and are more often estrogen and progesterone receptor positive. Furthermore, ILC metastasizes to locations that are extremely rare for IDC, such as the gastrointestinal tract, the retroperitoneum, the gynecologic organs, and the leptomeninges.[11,12] However, the most common metastatic sites for ILC are the lungs, the liver, and the bones (**Figs. 2–5**).

Outcomes are not very different, with a 5 year disease-free survival of 85.7% and 83.5% for ILC and IDC, respectively.[9] Some studies suggest even a slightly better outcome for ILC than IDC, regardless of the often larger size of ILC at diagnosis.[13,14] At present, there are no differences in treatment based on the histopathologic differentiation between IDC and ILC.[15]

Despite the relative small differences between IDC and ILC, ILC presents a major diagnostic challenge. The tumors are, due to their diffuse growth pattern, more difficult to detect than IDC. The infiltrative growth pattern is the most likely explanation for why ILC tends to be larger than IDC. Moreover, the diffuse growth pattern of ILC makes mammography and ultrasound unreliable at staging, thus

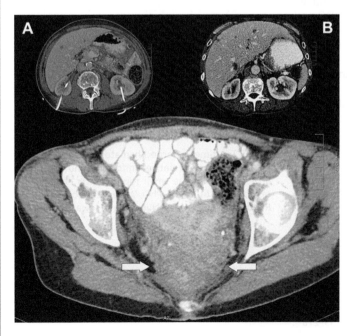

Fig. 3. Postcontrast axial CT images of a 59-year-old woman, 3 years after detection and treatment of a pT3N2a ILC, who presented with bilateral hydronephrosis, caused by a large irregular retroperitoneal mass (*arrows*) obstructing both ureters. Histology was obtained, showing diffuse metastasis of ILC. The hydronephrosis was treated with bilateral nephrostomy (inset *A*). Note also the multiple hypodense liver metastases and sclerotic metastases in the vertebral bodies (insets *A* and *B*).

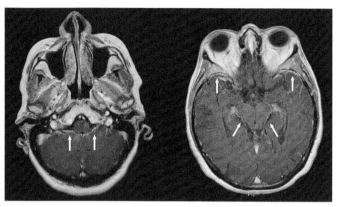

Fig. 4. Axial T1-weighted MR images of the brain after intravenous administration of 15 mL Gd-DOTA in a 62-year-old patient 5 years after detection and treatment of a pT2N3a ILC, who presented with nausea, vomiting, and confusion. Note the diffuse leptomeningeal enhancement (*arrows*), which was later shown to be meningeal carcinomatosis (diffuse ILC metastasis) by lumbar puncture.

causing high rates of tumor reexcision and leading to a common preference by both patients and surgeons to perform mastectomy. Fortunately, studies have shown that mastectomy rates for ILC are decreasing.[16,17]

Because breast MR imaging has been shown to be better at tumor staging, its use may be especially valuable in the preoperative staging of the subgroup of patients with ILC.

CONVENTIONAL IMAGING METHODS IN ILC

In the first evaluation of interval cancers after the initiation of breast cancer screening with

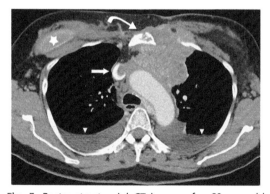

Fig. 5. Postcontrast axial CT image of a 60-year-old woman, 4 years after bilateral mastectomy and reconstruction (*star*) for a pT3N3a ILC in the left breast and a pT1cN0 IDC in the right breast. She presented with thoracic pain and was diagnosed with a large aggressive local recurrence of ILC in the thoracic wall and the superior mediastinum, destroying the sternum (*curved arrow*) and invading the superior vena cava (*straight arrow*). Note also the bilateral pleural effusions (*arrowheads*). She also had multiple lung metastases (not shown).

mammography in the Netherlands, it became clear that ILC was a common pathologic diagnosis in the missed carcinoma group.[18] This finding was attributed to the diffuse infiltrative pattern of the tumors and the poor desmoplastic reaction of the surrounding tissue.[19] In a later, larger study, about one-third of the interval carcinomas were of lobular origin. In a recent evaluation that differentiated between "true" interval carcinomas (fast-growing tumors not present at the time of screening) and false-negative screening mammography, 47% of the latter category were tumors with lobular features.[20,21] This finding may be due to ILC more often being better visualized on craniocaudal (CC) mammographic images than mediolateral oblique (MLO) images, whereas the former are not routinely performed in all screening programs.[22,23] However, even in retrospect 10% to 20% of ILC is not visible at mammography.[23–26]

The hallmark of malignancy on mammography, a spiculated mass, is reported in 28% to 63% of ILC cases (**Figs. 6 and 7**).[23,26–30] Mammographic findings in the remainder of ILC cases are often subtle. There is no association of ILC with microcalcifications, and the tumors are often isodense to fibroglandular tissue.[22,25,27,31,32]

Common descriptors include ill-defined mass (7%–33%),[23,26,29] architectural distortion (10%–24%),[23,26–29] and asymmetry (4%–14%).[23,26] The wide ranges reported probably reflect interreader variability of the descriptive terminology.

Tumor size estimation with mammography is difficult. Reported correlation coefficients range widely from 0.2 to 0.8. Small tumors in fatty breasts are quite accurately assessed, but accuracy decreases rapidly with increasing tumor size and increasing density,[33–35] resulting in structural

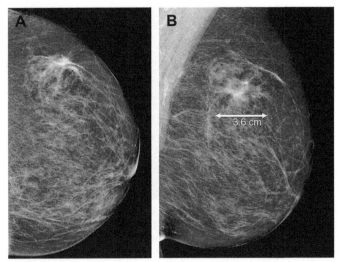

Fig. 6. Mammogram of a 60-year-old woman (*A*: left breast, CC view; *B*: left breast, MLO view) who presented with a palpable mass in the upper outer quadrant of the left breast. There is a hyperdense mass in the upper outer quadrant with an irregular spiculated margin and a maximum diameter of 3.6 cm, which was shown to be a multifocal ILC over an area of 4.2 cm; the largest focus was 2.5 cm.

underestimation of larger tumors. The vague borders commonly seen in ILC make assessment of these tumors particularly difficult, which results in measurements with a stronger negative deviation from pathologic tumor size when compared

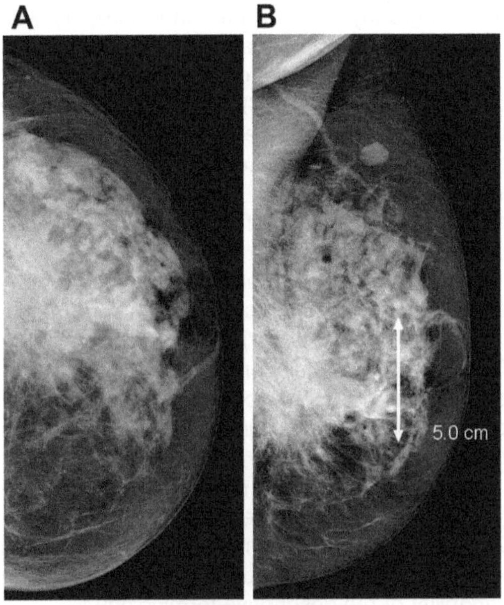

Fig. 7. Mammogram of a 71-year-old woman (*A*: left breast, CC view; *B*: left breast, MLO view) who presented with a palpable lump with skin retraction of the left breast. There is a large architectural distortion in the left breast (at least 5 cm), isointense to the fibroglandular tissue, retracting the whole breast. Histology showed a T4a ILC.

with those seen in IDC.[23,35] Consequently, it has been shown that mammography understages more than one-third of ILC.[36]

Sonography is hardly ever used as a screening modality, hence studies that report on sensitivity of ultrasound in ILC report on lesions that have already been detected by other means (either physical examination or mammography).

Nevertheless, most ILC are visible at sonography, and reported sensitivities range from 78% to 98%.[37–43] In a recent meta-analysis comparing the sensitivity of ultrasound directly with MR imaging, the sensitivity of ultrasound was 83%, with a 95% confidence interval ranging from 71% to 91%.[44]

Although one initial study reported difficulties with the detection of ILC smaller than 1 cm (only 1 out of 4),[45] later studies using more sophisticated equipment reported sensitivities in the normal range.[46,47] Of note, ultrasound sensitivity is also high in lesions that are hardly visible or occult at mammography. Hence ultrasound has complementary value for the detection of ILC in the symptomatic patient.[37] Approximately 60% of ILC lesions exhibit the typical features of malignancy at ultrasound, and present as a hypoechoic heterogeneous mass with ill-defined margins and posterior acoustic shadowing (**Fig. 8**).[37,38,41] Internal hyperechoic patterns are more commonly seen in ILC than in IDC (see **Fig. 8D**),[38,43] and some ILC tumors present as areas of focal shadowing without a discrete mass.[37,41] This latter ultrasound appearance may suggest the classic type of ILC histology.[37]

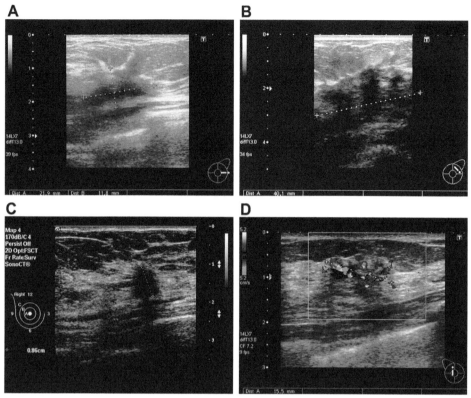

Fig. 8. Ultrasound images of 4 different ILC. The tumors in (*A*), (*B*), and (*C*) exhibit typical malignant features, showing hypoechoic irregular spiculated lesions with posterior acoustic shadowing. The tumor in (*D*) was almost isoechoic to normal fibroglandular breast tissue but showed multiple pathologic Doppler signals, due to extensive neovascularization. The tumor in (*A*) was larger than 5 cm at pathology, in (*B*) larger than 8 cm, in (*C*) 14 mm, and in (*D*) 3.2 cm, showing that ultrasound measurements especially in larger tumors are far from accurate.

Regarding tumor size estimation of ILC, ultrasound performs equally well as mammography, although the spread of reported correlation coefficients is slightly lower, ranging from 0.5 to 0.8.[42,48–50] Similar to mammography, the quality of the tumor size assessment decreases with increasing size of tumor; this holds particularly true for ILC tumors larger than 3 cm, which cannot be accurately assessed with ultrasound.[43,49]

FEATURES OF ILC ON BREAST MR IMAGING

The retrospective sensitivity of breast MR imaging for ILC is high. In a meta-analysis evaluating studies published until April 2006 describing in total 209 patients, the sensitivity was 93.3%, with a 95% confidence interval (CI) ranging from 88% to 96%. Leaving out the results of one very early study that scanned their patients with a far from optimal scan protocol, the sensitivity was even higher, at 96% (95% CI 92%–98%).[44,51–58] Since the publication of this meta-analysis, to the author's knowledge, 3 new studies have appeared in the literature that allowed evaluation of

sensitivity.[59–61] The 2 largest studies both reported a retrospective sensitivity of 100% (in 57 and 69 patients, respectively).[60,61] The third study, which was actually aimed at the evaluation of breast-specific gamma imaging for the detection of ILC, reported 2 false negatives in a series of only 12 patients, resulting in a sensitivity of 83%[59]; this can only be explained by bad luck, as it is far less than the earlier reported confidence intervals.[44]

Almost all available studies are retrospective in design. Only two studies completely report prospective data, and one study is partly prospective.[51,54,60] Francis and colleagues[54] reported a sensitivity of 95% in 22 ILC, Berg and colleagues[51] reported a sensitivity of 97% in 29 ILC, and Caramella and colleagues[60] reported a sensitivity of 100% in 35 ILC. Hence, prospective data are well in line with the results from the retrospective studies.

Nevertheless, all studies evaluated patients that were known to have a carcinoma. Although various investigators report ILC that were incidentally detected in MR imaging examinations performed for other indications, few data are available that report the sensitivity of breast MR imaging for ILC in a screening situation. In general, the sensitivity of breast MR imaging for breast cancer in screening is lower than in preoperative staging, though much better than mammography; reported sensitivities range from 77% to 100%.[62] In the large screening studies too few ILC were detected to produce conclusive results; however, Kriege and colleagues[63] reported a sensitivity of 100% for MR imaging in the detection of 4 ILC, compared with 25% for mammography, suggesting an additional value over mammography of screening for ILC with MR imaging.

For optimal detection of ILC in a screening setting, it is essential to know the appearance of ILC on breast MR imaging. It is commonly stated that ILC appears more often as nonmass-like enhancement and in general enhances less than IDC. At the same time good scientific evidence for these statements is lacking, partly because the interpretation of breast MR imaging, even using the rigorous approach of the BI-RADS lexicon, is subject to considerable interreader variability.[64–66] As a direct consequence, the principal distinction between mass-like and nonmass-like lesions is a very difficult one to make. Different studies report the incidence of nonmass-like enhancement to be between 5% and 69%. Pooling of these data is not possible because of the large heterogeneity in the studies.[44]

In the large group of mass-like lesions, about 85% are described as irregular and spiculated. Therefore, an irregular spiculated mass is in fact the most common appearance of ILC on MR imaging (Fig. 9).[44,60,67] However, round masses with sharp margins have also been described, which subsequently turned out to be ILC.[60,67,68] Nonmass-like enhancement can be either ductal, segmental, regional, or diffuse (Fig. 10).

Evaluation of the enhancement pattern has less often been described. Sittek and colleagues[58] and Trecate and colleagues[69] both noted that peak enhancement was reached relatively late, and washout in the late phase of enhancement was uncommon. Caramella and colleagues[60] noted continuous enhancement in the late phase of enhancement (commonly referred to as a type 1 curve) in 37% of ILC. Two studies that evaluated quantitative enhancement parameters also noted that these values appeared much lower for ILC than in other studies evaluating the same parameters for IDC.[68,70]

In the absence of studies that directly compare morphologic and kinetic descriptors between IDC and ILC, the magnitude of the differences between the appearances of ILC and IDC cannot be adequately assessed. Such direct comparison studies have been performed and reported on, but are so far unpublished.

Newstead and colleagues[71] presented a comparison of 22 ILC with 257 IDC and 83 ductal carcinoma in situ (DCIS) lesions at the 2005 meeting of the Radiological Society of North America. These investigators reported that 55% of ILC presented as a mass, compared with 76% of IDC and only 16% of DCIS lesions. Time to peak enhancement was twice as long for ILC as for IDC (270 ± 112 seconds vs 131 ± 90 seconds) and enhancement after 68 seconds was consequently lower in ILC than in IDC.

Mann and colleagues[72] reported at the 2008 meeting of the International Society for Magnetic Resonance in Medicine a comparison of 33 ILC with 103 IDC, in which 75% of ILC presented as a mass compared with 84% of IDC. Interreader variability was moderate ($\kappa = 0.41$), comparable to literature values, and similar for ILC and IDC. Peak enhancement was not different between ILC and IDC (360% vs 382%), but at visual assessment washout was less common in ILC (48% vs 84%). Using a computer-aided diagnosis (CAD) application, this difference was blotted out; washout was detected in 88% of ILC and 94% of IDC, suggesting that CAD applications may be especially helpful in the assessment of ILC (Fig. 11). This finding is explained by the observation that the fraction of the lesion that shows washout is generally smaller in ILC (<10% of the dominant focus in 64% of ILC vs 30% of IDC). The results of pharmacokinetic analysis also showed that ILC in general enhance slower than IDC, but not less.

Lastly, at the 2009 European Congress of Radiology, Dietzel and colleagues[73] reported on a comparison of 108 ILC with 347 IDC. In their series ILC were more often irregular lesions than IDC (62% vs 55%), though this did not reach statistical significance. An essential finding was, however, that internal necrosis (and hence ring enhancement) was less common in ILC than in IDC (3% vs 15%) and that perifocal edema was less often observed (30% vs 45%). Moreover, they also noted that washout was less frequent in ILC than in IDC (57% vs 73%). Both tumor types were nearly always iso- to hypointense compared with glandular breast tissue on T2-weighted imaging.

In summary, almost all ILC are retrospectively visible. Most ILC still present as an irregular spiculated mass, but the frequency of nonmass-like enhancement (between 20% and 40% approximately) is slightly higher than in IDC. Ring enhancement and surrounding edema are less frequently

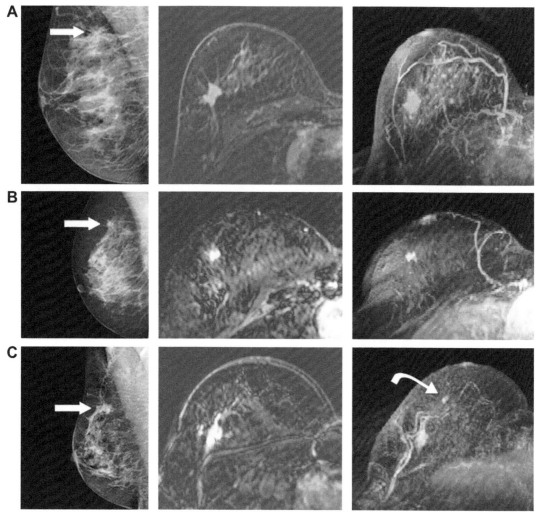

Fig. 9. Three examples (rows *A*, *B*, and *C*) of mass-like ILC in the right breast of 3 different patients at respectively mammography (*first column*), subtraction MR imaging (*second column*), and maximum intensity projection of the MR imaging (*third column*). These masses are all irregular and especially the mass in *A* is heavily spiculated. Note that all masses were also visible at mammography (*straight arrows*); the additional tumor focus in patient *C*, more anteriorly located and in these images only visible on the MIP (*curved arrow*), was only detected at MR imaging.

observed. Contrast enhancement is slower than in IDC, but not necessarily less, which results in a higher proportion of lesions that do not show a typical washout curve. CAD applications may help to adequately assess the most malignant curve shape; however, the morphologic appearance is usually that of a suspicious lesion and should not be misinterpreted in the absence of a washout curve.

AGREEMENT OF MR IMAGING FINDINGS WITH PATHOLOGIC ASSESSMENT OF ILC

Because both mammography and ultrasound findings do not correlate well with the pathologic assessment of ILC, many studies have focused on the correlation of MR findings with pathology.[52,54–57,60,61,74–76] In general, multifocal disease can be correctly predicted in approximately 80% to 90% of patients. Caramella and colleagues[60] showed a kappa coefficient of 0.87 for the detection of multifocal disease compared with pathology, which can be translated as excellent interreader agreement. This result compares with 0.22 for both mammography and ultrasound, which translates into poor to fair agreement. Nevertheless, both overestimation and underestimation of the number of tumor foci occurs. Overestimation has been attributed to enhancing lobular carcinoma in situ.[61] Rodenko and

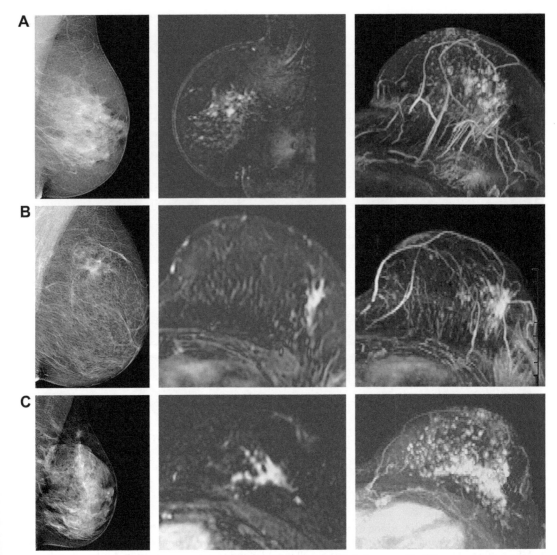

Fig. 10. Three examples (rows *A*, *B*, and *C*) of nonmass-like ILC in the left breast of 3 different patients at respectively mammography (*first column*), subtraction MR imaging (*second column*), and maximum intensity projection of the MR imaging (*third column*). The enhancement was respectively regional (*A*), segmental (*B*), and diffuse (*C*). The tumors in *A* and *C* were palpable but not seen at mammography, while the tumor in *B* was mammographically detected, but its multifocal nature was only depicted at MR imaging.

colleagues[76] noted in a series of 20 patients 2 cases of single quadrant disease that were interpreted as multicentric disease on MR imaging. These 2 cases stress the importance of obtaining histology prior to radical changes to the surgical treatment (**Fig. 12**).

More recently, Onesti and colleagues[75] reported, in a series of 10 ILC, tumor size overestimation of 5 tumors by an average of 1.2 cm. Nonetheless, most studies report good correlation between MR imaging findings and pathology (**Fig. 13**).[52,54–56,60,61,74] Unfortunately, in April 2006 it was not yet possible to perform a meta-analysis due to the large variability among the studies.[44] Nowadays, with the publication of the studies by Caramella and Mann, 7 studies have been published that either calculate Pearson correlation coefficients for tumor size on MR imaging versus pathology, or present sufficient data to calculate this correlation coefficient.[60,61] Because one of the latter studies is an extension to an earlier published study, there are now 6 studies, totaling 220 patients, that can be entered in a meta-analysis as listed in **Table 1**.

Applying simple meta-analytical principles to this data no longer yields significant

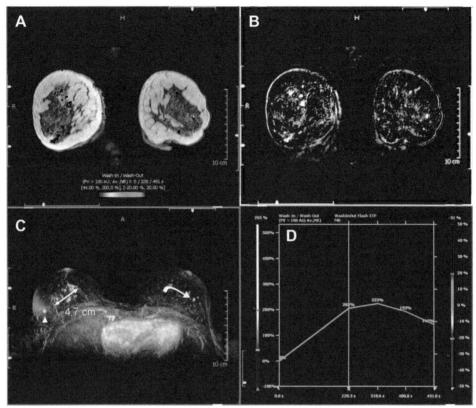

Fig. 11. A 40-year-old woman with strong family history for breast cancer, who presented with nipple discharge. The mammogram showed dense breast tissue with multiple benign calcifications and was thus negative (not shown). Microdochectomy revealed lobular carcinoma in situ. MR imaging was performed, showing a multifocal ILC over an area of 4.7 cm. Although most of the tumor showed continuous enhancement, a small area was detected that showed early washout of the contrast agent. (A) T1w FLASH 3-dimensional acquisition with color-coded overlay of enhancement; the crosshair is placed at the machine detected spot with most suspicious enhancement curve. (B) Subtraction image of pre- and postcontrast MR imaging. (C) Maximum intensity projection; note the tumor area (double-headed arrow), an ipsilateral intramammary lymph node (arrowhead), and the biopsy-proven fibroadenoma in the contralateral breast (curved arrow). (D) Machine-detected most malignant enhancement curve (corresponding to the crosshair in A).

heterogeneity ($Q = 9.75$, [$P = .084$], $I^2 = 49\%$) and consequently data pooling can be performed. The estimated correlation coefficient for MR imaging compared with pathology is 0.89 (95% CI 0.84–0.93), which is much better than what can be achieved by mammography or ultrasound, even in the hands of experienced practitioners.

The bad performance of conventional imaging methods is partly explained because MR imaging detects in many patients tumor foci separate from the index lesion in the ipsilateral breast that were mammographically and sonographically occult. Such additional tumor foci are present in approximately 32% of patients (95% CI 22%–44%), and can be both multifocal as well as multicentric.[44,53,57,77–79]

CONSEQUENCES FOR THE THERAPEUTIC APPROACH OF ILC

The good correlation of MR imaging findings with pathology and the frequent detection of additional tumor foci has a huge impact on the therapeutic approach in patients with ILC. Because the primary treatment of breast cancer, ILC and IDC alike, is usually surgery, the performance of preoperative breast MR imaging and visualization of additional sites in many patients initiates more extensive surgery. The surgical plan changes in approximately 28% of cases (95% CI 20%–39%).[44,53,55,56,76,78] In 12% to 33% of patients, breast-conserving surgery (BCS) followed by radiotherapy is replaced by

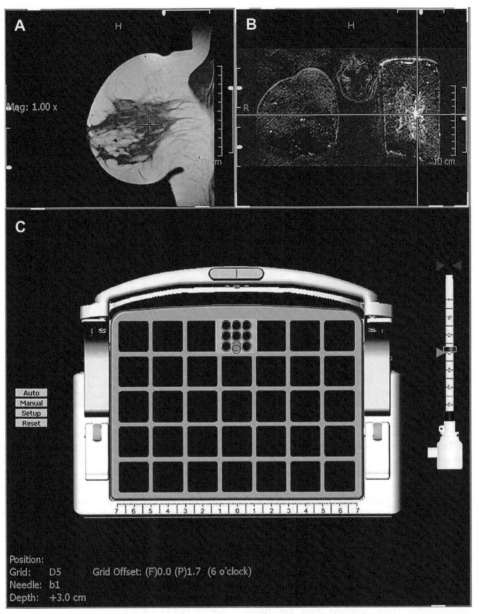

Fig. 12. MR imaging–guided breast biopsy of a multifocal ILC in the left breast, after negative mammography and negative second-look ultrasound. A computer program (DynaCAD; Invivo, Orlando, FL, USA) is used to accurately position the needle. (*A*) A native sagittal T1 image of the left breast; the needle is currently aimed at the crosshair. (*B*) A subtraction image in the coronal plane of both breasts, which is used to locate the lesion. The lesion is in the center of the crosshair. (*C*) The biopsy grid, showing where to position the biopsy block (*purple block with holes*) and in which of the holes to insert the needle (*yellow dot*) to come closest to the optimal position (*red circle*). The necessary depth can be read at the bottom of the screen. Using vacuum-assisted biopsy, the diagnostic yield is approximately 95%.

mastectomy.[53,55,56,60,76,78] Change of therapy in the other direction due to better delineation of the tumor has been reported, but in a substantially smaller percentage of patients (approximately 5%).[60] Consequently, it has been estimated that overall the primary therapy shifts from breast-conserving therapy to mastectomy in 15% to 20% of patients.[80] Furthermore, preoperative MR imaging is able to stratify some patients to neoadjuvant chemotherapy or vice versa, from chemotherapy to direct surgery, due to better tumor evaluation.

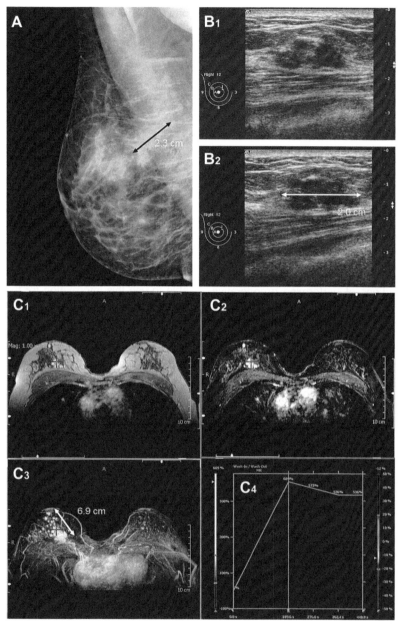

Fig. 13. Images of a 37-year-old woman, known to be a BRCA2 mutation carrier. At mammography (*A*) an isointense spiculated mass was observed with a maximum diameter of 2.3 cm. At sonography (*B*) a hypoechoic mass with minimal posterior acoustic shadowing was observed. The maximum diameter of the tumor appeared to be 2.0 cm (*B2*). The MR imaging, shown in (*C*) (*C1*: native T1 postcontrast acquisition, *C2*: subtraction image, *C3*: maximum intensity projection, *C4*: enhancement versus time curve corresponding with the crosshair in the other images) reveals a multifocal tumor over an area of 6.9 cm. Consequently mastectomy was performed. At pathology, a multicentric ILC was seen over an area of 7.3 cm.

Moreover, MR imaging can also be used to evaluate the effect of neoadjuvant chemotherapy (**Fig. 14**).

About 88% (95% CI 75%–95%) of changes based on MR imaging are subsequently deemed correct by pathologic confirmation of tumor in the specimen.[44]

EFFECT OF PREOPERATIVE BREAST MR IMAGING ON OUTCOME IN PATIENTS WITH ILC

So far there is no evidence that suggests an increase in survival for patients with ILC due to the performance of preoperative MR imaging.

Table 1
Studies evaluating the correlation between MR imaging measured tumor size and pathology

Study	N	Pearson Correlation Coefficient
Munot et al[56]	20	0.97
Kneeshaw et al[55]	21	0.86
Francis et al[54]	22	0.87
Kepple et al[74]	33	0.88
Caramella et al[60]	57	0.88
Mann et al[72]	67	0.85

Reported correlation coefficients of MR imaging measured sizes with sizes of ILC at pathology. N indicates the number of patients included in the study.

The 2 studies that have evaluated recurrence and survival as functions of performing preoperative breast MR imaging have thus far not specifically addressed ILC, nor have they convincingly shown an increased survival for all women with breast cancer.[81,82] The rate of recurrence after BCS followed by radiotherapy is at approximately 0.6% to 1% per year. This rate is acceptably low, and one can hardly expect this to decrease much further by the addition of MR imaging in all

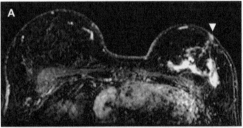

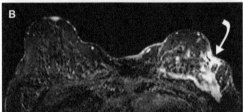

Fig. 14. Two subtraction images of a 47-year-old woman, who presented with a T4 ILC in the left breast. Initial assessment with MR imaging (A) shows a large diffuse-growing tumor within the left breast, with involvement of the skin (arrowhead). She was initially treated with neoadjuvant chemotherapy. The control MR image (B) unfortunately shows that the tumor did not respond well but in fact had grown, while the patient became much thinner. Moreover, the skin involvement worsened (curved arrow). Consequently salvage mastectomy was performed.

patients, further implying that at least some of the additional lesions detected by MR imaging and not surgically excised are adequately treated by radiotherapy and adjuvant chemotherapy. However, reported reexcision rates for ILC in the literature due to failure to radically excise the tumor at the first attempt are unacceptably high, ranging from 29% to 67%.[83–87] Moreover, 16% to 48% of BCS attempts are still converted to mastectomy after initial unsuccessful surgery.[87–92]

These facts are devastating to the mental health of the patient, who already has to deal with the fact that she has breast cancer. Moreover, reexcision is detrimental to the cosmetic outcome.[93]

It may be clear that MR imaging is the best diagnostic imaging modality currently available for ILC. The question is no longer whether the tumor is correctly depicted, but whether surgeons are able to use this information for the benefit of the patient. The high rate of changes induced by preoperative MR imaging should assign patients directly to the correct therapy (either BCS or mastectomy), without unnecessarily assigning patients to mastectomy. The surgeon needs to be able to appreciate breast tumors in 3-dimensional images rather than on flattened mammography images, which requires training and skill. Moreover, it is necessary to transform the MR image mentally from the prone position in which the patient is scanned to the supine position in which the patient is operated, taking into account the movement of the breast tissue in all directions.

A recent retrospective study evaluated the reexcision rate in 267 patients with ILC, of whom 99 underwent preoperative MR imaging.[80] Initially, 145 of these patients underwent BCS, 90 without preoperative MR imaging and 55 with preoperative MR imaging. Reexcision was deemed necessary in 24 patients (27%) without preoperative MR imaging and in 5 patients (9%) with preoperative MR imaging. An odds ratio for reexcision without preoperative MR imaging of 3.64 (95% CI 1.30–10.20) was calculated. In other words, patients who did not undergo preoperative MR imaging had a more than 3.5-times higher chance to need a reexcision and, unfortunately, a 23% chance of ending with a mastectomy, compared with only 7% in the group of patients who underwent preoperative breast MR imaging and were surgically treated by surgeons used to working with breast MR imaging. The final rate of mastectomies appeared even lower in the group of patients who underwent MR imaging (48% vs 59%), though this did not reach statistical significance. Finally, the total treatment time (approximately 42 days) was not dependent on the performance of MR imaging, but was extended by the need for reexcision.

At present, there are only 2 other studies published that evaluate the effect of preoperative MR imaging on margin status,[94,95] none of which specifically addressed ILC. Pengel and colleagues[95] included 52 patients with ILC, of whom half underwent preoperative MR imaging. Excision was extensively incomplete (and thus requiring reexcision) for 3 of 26 patients (12%) with preoperative MR imaging and for 5 of 26 patients (19%) without preoperative MR imaging. In this study, the overall reported reexcision rates (much lower than in the previous mentioned study due to the large fraction of IDC) are more than twice as high in the group of patients who did not undergo preoperative MR imaging (10.6% vs 5%), but the investigators do not report on statistical significance concerning the reexcision rate. The study by Bleicher and colleagues[94] does not provide sufficient data to extract numbers for ILC, but in general did not detect a reduction in the rate of positive margins, nor in the number of patients that finally underwent mastectomy. Apparently, they were thus unable to use the increased knowledge from MR imaging for the benefit of the patients, which underlines the need for training and experience not only of radiologists but also of surgeons.

EVALUATION OF THE CONTRALATERAL BREAST WITH MR IMAGING IN PATIENTS WITH ILC

Apart from staging of the known cancer, breast MR imaging in the preoperative setting serves a second purpose that may be even more important. According to Arpino and colleagues,[9] contralateral carcinoma is present in 20.9% of patients with ILC compared with 11.2% of patients with IDC. Overall, MR imaging is estimated to detect in approximately 4% of patients a synchronous contralateral carcinoma not detected by any other imaging modality.[96] It may not be surprising that the rate of synchronously detected contralateral breast cancers by MR imaging in ILC is almost double that seen in IDC, and is currently estimated at 7% (95% CI 4%–12%) (Fig. 15).[44,51–54,56,74,77,78,96] This result is independent of tumor size and implies the need for preoperative evaluation with MR imaging in all patients with ILC, not only the subset that initially opts for BCS.

It is essential to realize that the specificity of breast MR imaging in the screening of the contralateral breast is only about 50%.[96] Histologic verification of detected contralateral lesions is thus

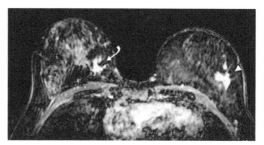

Fig. 15. Subtraction MR image of both breasts of a 48-year-old woman who presented with a palpable lump in the left breast. At mammography and ultrasound (not shown), an ILC of 1.5 cm was detected in the left breast. MR imaging shows a multifocal tumor in the left breast over an area of 3.4 cm (*arrowhead*). A second ILC in the right breast is detected (*curved arrow*), histologically validated using second-look ultrasound.

essential (as well as verification of any lesion in the ipsilateral breast that would largely change the surgical approach). Second-look ultrasound may allow ultrasound-guided breast biopsy in approximately 50% of detected lesions.[97,98] MR imaging–guided breast biopsy is a safe, fast, easy, and conclusive method to assess the remaining 50%, but its easy availability is required (see Fig. 12).[99,100]

The strength, as well as the weakness, of MR imaging in the detection of contralateral carcinomas is that most tumors are identified at an early stage. It is uncertain as to what extent these carcinomas influence prognosis in the setting of an already detected ipsilateral carcinoma, and specific data regarding ILC are completely lacking. Contralateral tumors are different from ipsilateral additional detected tumor foci that receive radiotherapy anyway. Most importantly, contralateral tumors remain untreated if undetected. At the same time, adjuvant systemic therapy if given may prevent these tumors from becoming clinically significant. One would expect that the incidence of metachronous contralateral breast carcinoma decreases in patients who underwent preoperative MR imaging at the time of ipsilateral tumor detection. Unfortunately, the 2 studies that evaluated this issue report conflicting results. Fischer and colleagues[81] reported a reduction in the rate of metachronous contralateral carcinoma from 4% to 1.7% due to preoperative MR imaging, whereas Solin and colleagues[82] reported an incidence of 6% contralateral carcinoma with and without preoperative MR imaging.

Nonetheless, adjuvant therapy alone is generally not considered curative for breast cancer. Because a recent study has shown that early detection of asymptomatic second breast cancer in the ipsilateral breast or the contralateral breast in women with a history of breast cancer increases relative survival by 27% to 47%,[101] one can assume that detection of additional contralateral carcinoma by MR imaging indeed increases survival. The magnitude of this effect remains uncertain.

CURRENT EVIDENCE FOR THE PERFORMANCE OF BREAST MR IMAGING IN ILC, SHORTCOMINGS, AND FUTURE PERSPECTIVES

So far, many studies have shown that MR imaging is able to depict ILC well. MR imaging has also been shown to correlate better with pathology in the assessment of ILC when compared with other commonly available imaging modalities. Moreover, it significantly affects diagnostic thinking and subsequent therapeutic management.

The notion that preoperative MR imaging in ILC affects therapeutic management of these tumors is known as level IV evidence of its value.[102] However, this does not automatically imply that the performance of preoperative MR imaging is also good for the patient (known as level V evidence). At this level of evidence, the rate of re-excisions is the shortest term outcome parameter that can be evaluated, but also reductions in unwanted side effects of therapy, local recurrence, and other metachronous carcinomas can be evaluated. Moreover, the ultimate gain for a patient is increase in survival or even better quality-adjusted life years, which is therefore the principal outcome parameter in many studies.

The first studies evaluating outcome parameters after preoperative MR imaging have only very recently been published,[80–82,94,95] with only one of these studies specifically addressing ILC.[80] The retrospective study discussed earlier shows that in experienced hands preoperative breast MR imaging can reduce the rate of reexcisions in patients with ILC. However, it does not show an effect on tumor recurrence, metachronous contralateral carcinoma, or survival, nor does it evaluate cost-effectiveness. Regarding these issues, only indirect evidence is available. Evidence in favor of preoperative breast MR imaging in patients with ILC at the fifth level is only moderate, and further studies are essential. Moreover, the sixth (and highest) level of evidence, which questions whether the use of preoperative breast MR imaging in ILC is beneficial to society and hence is dependent on a cost-effectiveness analysis from a societal viewpoint, has not been addressed.

The author of this article is, on the other hand, of the opinion that the currently available evidence in favor of preoperative breast MR imaging in patients with ILC is substantial. The inherent benefits of breast MR imaging for patients are large (lowering the chance of incomplete excision and subsequent need for reexcision, and possibly improving survival), whereas the detrimental effects of preoperative MR imaging, if adequately performed, are only minor with the possible additional need for biopsy. Consequently, based on the currently available data, it is strongly recommended that preoperative MR imaging be conducted in all patients with ILC prior to therapy.

REFERENCES

1. Li CI, Anderson BO, Daling JR, et al. Trends in incidence rates of invasive lobular and ductal breast carcinoma. JAMA 2003;289(11):1421–4.
2. Reeves GK, Beral V, Green J, et al. Hormonal therapy for menopause and breast-cancer risk by histological type: a cohort study and meta-analysis. Lancet Oncol 2006;7(11):910–8.
3. Eheman CR, Shaw KM, Ryerson AB, et al. The changing incidence of in situ and invasive ductal and lobular breast carcinomas: United States, 1999–2004. Cancer Epidemiol Biomarkers Prev 2009;18(6):1763–9.
4. Foote FW, Stewart FW. Comparative studies of cancerous versus noncancerous breasts. Ann Surg 1945;121(2):197–222.
5. Wellings SR, Jensen HM, Marcum RG. An atlas of subgross pathology of the human breast with special reference to possible precancerous lesions. J Natl Cancer Inst 1975;55(2):231–73.
6. Wellings SR. Development of human breast cancer. Adv Cancer Res 1980;31:287–314.
7. Hanby AM. Aspects of molecular phenotype and its correlations with breast cancer behaviour and taxonomy. Br J Cancer 2005;92(4):613–7.
8. Hanby AM, Hughes TA. In situ and invasive lobular neoplasia of the breast. Histopathology 2008;52(1):58–66.
9. Arpino G, Bardou VJ, Clark GM, et al. Infiltrating lobular carcinoma of the breast: tumor characteristics and clinical outcome. Breast Cancer Res 2004;6(3):R149–56.
10. Yoder BJ, Wilkinson EJ, Massoll NA. Molecular and morphologic distinctions between infiltrating ductal and lobular carcinoma of the breast. Breast J 2007;13(2):172–9.
11. Doyle DJ, Relihan N, Redmond HP, et al. Metastatic manifestations of invasive lobular breast carcinoma. Clin Radiol 2005;60(2):271–4.
12. Winston CB, Hadar O, Teitcher JB, et al. Metastatic lobular carcinoma of the breast: patterns of spread

in the chest, abdomen, and pelvis on CT. AJR Am J Roentgenol 2000;175(3):795–800.

13. Bharat A, Gao F, Margenthaler JA. Tumor characteristics and patient outcomes are similar between invasive lobular and mixed invasive ductal/lobular breast cancers but differ from pure invasive ductal breast cancers. Am J Surg 2009;198(4):516–9.

14. Li CI, Moe RE, Daling JR. Risk of mortality by histologic type of breast cancer among women aged 50 to 79 years. Arch Intern Med 2003; 163(18):2149–53.

15. National Breast Cancer Organization Netherlands. Guideline for treatment of patients with breast cancer. Kwaliteitsinstituut voor de gezondheidszorg CBO, Available at: http://www.oncoline.nl; 2008. Accessed November 27, 2009.

16. Biglia N, Mariani L, Sgro L, et al. Increased incidence of lobular breast cancer in women treated with hormone replacement therapy: implications for diagnosis, surgical and medical treatment. Endocr Relat Cancer 2007;14(3):549–67.

17. Singletary SE, Patel-Parekh L, Bland KI. Treatment trends in early-stage invasive lobular carcinoma: a report from the National Cancer Data Base. Ann Surg 2005;242(2):281–9.

18. Holland R, Mravunac M, Hendriks JH, et al. So-called interval cancers of the breast. Pathologic and radiologic analysis of sixty-four cases. Cancer 1982;49(12):2527–33.

19. Holland R, Hendriks JH, Mravunac M. Mammographically occult breast cancer. A pathologic and radiologic study. Cancer 1983;52(10):1810–9.

20. Peeters PH, Verbeek AL, Hendriks JH, et al. The occurrence of interval cancers in the Nijmegen screening programme. Br J Cancer 1989;59(6): 929–32.

21. Porter GJ, Evans AJ, Burrell HC, et al. Interval breast cancers: prognostic features and survival by subtype and time since screening. J Med Screen 2006;13(3):115–22.

22. Garnett S, Wallis M, Morgan G. Do screen-detected lobular and ductal carcinoma present with different mammographic features? Br J Radiol 2009;82(973):20–7.

23. Hilleren DJ, Andersson IT, Lindholm K, et al. Invasive lobular carcinoma: mammographic findings in a 10-year experience. Radiology 1991;178(1): 149–54.

24. Adler OB, Engel A. Invasive lobular carcinoma. Mammographic pattern. Rofo 1990;152(4):460–2.

25. Krecke KN, Gisvold JJ. Invasive lobular carcinoma of the breast: mammographic findings and extent of disease at diagnosis in 184 patients. AJR Am J Roentgenol 1993;161(5):957–60.

26. Le Gal M, Ollivier L, Asselain B, et al. Mammographic features of 455 invasive lobular carcinomas. Radiology 1992;185(3):705–8.

27. Evans WP, Warren Burhenne LJ, Laurie L, et al. Invasive lobular carcinoma of the breast: mammographic characteristics and computer-aided detection. Radiology 2002;225(1):182–9.

28. Helvie MA, Paramagul C, Oberman HA, et al. Invasive lobular carcinoma. Imaging features and clinical detection. Invest Radiol 1993;28(3):202–7.

29. Tan SM, Behranwala KA, Trott PA, et al. A retrospective study comparing the individual modalities of triple assessment in the pre-operative diagnosis of invasive lobular breast carcinoma. Eur J Surg Oncol 2002;28(3):203–8.

30. Uchiyama N, Miyakawa K, Moriyama N, et al. Radiographic features of invasive lobular carcinoma of the breast. Radiat Med 2001;19(1):19–25.

31. Mendelson EB, Harris KM, Doshi N, et al. Infiltrating lobular carcinoma: mammographic patterns with pathologic correlation. AJR Am J Roentgenol 1989;153(2):265–71.

32. Newstead GM, Baute PB, Toth HK. Invasive lobular and ductal carcinoma: mammographic findings and stage at diagnosis. Radiology 1992;184(3): 623–7.

33. Dummin LJ, Cox M, Plant L. Prediction of breast tumor size by mammography and sonography—A breast screen experience. Breast 2007;16(1):38–46.

34. Fasching PA, Heusinger K, Loehberg CR, et al. Influence of mammographic density on the diagnostic accuracy of tumor size assessment and association with breast cancer tumor characteristics. Eur J Radiol 2006;60(3):398–404.

35. Heusinger K, Lohberg C, Lux MP, et al. Assessment of breast cancer tumor size depends on method, histopathology and tumor size itself. Breast Cancer Res Treat 2005;94(1):17–23.

36. Veltman J, Boetes C, van Die L, et al. Mammographic detection and staging of invasive lobular carcinoma. Clin Imaging 2006;30(2):94–8.

37. Butler RS, Venta LA, Wiley EL, et al. Sonographic evaluation of infiltrating lobular carcinoma. AJR Am J Roentgenol 1999;172(2):325–30.

38. Cawson JN, Law EM, Kavanagh AM. Invasive lobular carcinoma: sonographic features of cancers detected in a BreastScreen Program. Australas Radiol 2001;45(1):25–30.

39. Chapellier C, Balu-Maestro C, Bleuse A, et al. Ultrasonography of invasive lobular carcinoma of the breast: sonographic patterns and diagnostic value: report of 102 cases. Clin Imaging 2000;24(6):333–6.

40. Rissanen T, Tikkakoski T, Autio AL, et al. Ultrasonography of invasive lobular breast carcinoma. Acta Radiol 1998;39(3):285–91.

41. Selinko VL, Middleton LP, Dempsey PJ. Role of sonography in diagnosing and staging invasive lobular carcinoma. J Clin Ultrasound 2004;32(7): 323–32.

42. Skaane P, Skjorten F. Ultrasonographic evaluation of invasive lobular carcinoma. Acta Radiol 1999; 40(4):369–75.

43. Watermann DO, Tempfer C, Hefler LA, et al. Ultrasound morphology of invasive lobular breast cancer is different compared with other types of breast cancer. Ultrasound Med Biol 2005;31(2): 167–74.

44. Mann RM, Hoogeveen YL, Blickman JG, et al. MRI compared to conventional diagnostic work-up in the detection and evaluation of invasive lobular carcinoma of the breast: a review of existing literature. Breast Cancer Res Treat 2008;107(1):1–14.

45. Paramagul CP, Helvie MA, Adler DD. Invasive lobular carcinoma: sonographic appearance and role of sonography in improving diagnostic sensitivity. Radiology 1995;195(1):231–4.

46. Evans N, Lyons K. The use of ultrasound in the diagnosis of invasive lobular carcinoma of the breast less than 10 mm in size. Clin Radiol 2000; 55(4):261–3.

47. Mesurolle B, Mignon F, riche-Cohen M, et al. [Invasive infra centimetric breast lobular carcinoma: ultrasonographic features]. J Radiol 2003;84(2 Pt 1):147–51 [in French].

48. Golshan M, Fung BB, Wiley E, et al. Prediction of breast cancer size by ultrasound, mammography and core biopsy. Breast 2004;13(4):265–71.

49. Pritt B, Ashikaga T, Oppenheimer RG, et al. Influence of breast cancer histology on the relationship between ultrasound and pathology tumor size measurements. Mod Pathol 2004;17(8):905–10.

50. Tresserra F, Feu J, Grases PJ, et al. Assessment of breast cancer size: sonographic and pathologic correlation. J Clin Ultrasound 1999;27(9):485–91.

51. Berg WA, Gutierrez L, NessAiver MS, et al. Diagnostic accuracy of mammography, clinical examination, US, and MR imaging in preoperative assessment of breast cancer. Radiology 2004; 233(3):830–49.

52. Boetes C, Veltman J, van Die L, et al. The role of MRI in invasive lobular carcinoma. Breast Cancer Res Treat 2004;86(1):31–7.

53. Fabre DN, Boulet P, Prat X, et al. [Breast MRI in invasive lobular carcinoma: diagnosis and staging]. J Radiol 2005;86(9 Pt 1):1027–34 [in French].

54. Francis A, England DW, Rowlands DC, et al. The diagnosis of invasive lobular breast carcinoma. Does MRI have a role? Breast 2001;10(1):38–40.

55. Kneeshaw PJ, Turnbull LW, Smith A, et al. Dynamic contrast enhanced magnetic resonance imaging aids the surgical management of invasive lobular breast cancer. Eur J Surg Oncol 2003;29(1):32–7.

56. Munot K, Dall B, Achuthan R, et al. Role of magnetic resonance imaging in the diagnosis and single-stage surgical resection of invasive lobular carcinoma of the breast. Br J Surg 2002; 89(10):1296–301.

57. Schelfout K, Van GM, Kersschot E, et al. Preoperative breast MRI in patients with invasive lobular breast cancer. Eur Radiol 2004;14(7):1209–16.

58. Sittek H, Perlet C, Untch M, et al. [Dynamic MR-mammography in invasive lobular breast cancer]. Rontgenpraxis 1998;51(7):235–42 [in German].

59. Brem RF, Ioffe M, Rapelyea JA, et al. Invasive lobular carcinoma: detection with mammography, sonography, MRI, and breast-specific gamma imaging. AJR Am J Roentgenol 2009;192(2): 379–83.

60. Caramella T, Chapellier C, Ettore F, et al. Value of MRI in the surgical planning of invasive lobular breast carcinoma: a prospective and a retrospective study of 57 cases: comparison with physical examination, conventional imaging, and histology. Clin Imaging 2007;31(3):155–61.

61. Mann RM, Veltman J, Barentsz JO, et al. The value of MRI compared to mammography in the assessment of tumour extent in invasive lobular carcinoma of the breast. Eur J Surg Oncol 2008;34(2):135–42.

62. Saslow D, Boetes C, Burke W, et al. American Cancer Society guidelines for breast screening with MRI as an adjunct to mammography. CA Cancer J Clin 2007;57(2):75–89.

63. Kriege M, Brekelmans CT, Peterse H, et al. Tumor characteristics and detection method in the MRISC screening program for the early detection of hereditary breast cancer. Breast Cancer Res Treat 2007; 102(3):357–63.

64. Ikeda DM, Hylton NM, Kinkel K, et al. Development, standardization, and testing of a lexicon for reporting contrast-enhanced breast magnetic resonance imaging studies. J Magn Reson Imaging 2001; 13(6):889–95.

65. Kim SJ, Morris EA, Liberman L, et al. Observer variability and applicability of BI-RADS terminology for breast MR imaging: invasive carcinomas as focal masses. AJR Am J Roentgenol 2001;177(3):551–7.

66. Stoutjesdijk MJ, Futterer JJ, Boetes C, et al. Variability in the description of morphologic and contrast enhancement characteristics of breast lesions on magnetic resonance imaging. Invest Radiol 2005;40(6):355–62.

67. Levrini G, Mori CA, Vacondio R, et al. MRI patterns of invasive lobular cancer: T1 and T2 features. Radiol Med 2008;113(8):1110–25.

68. Yeh ED, Slanetz PJ, Edmister WB, et al. Invasive lobular carcinoma: spectrum of enhancement and morphology on magnetic resonance imaging. Breast J 2003;9(1):13–8.

69. Trecate G, Tess JD, Vergnaghi D, et al. Lobular breast cancer: how useful is breast magnetic resonance imaging? Tumori 2001;87(4):232–8.

70. Qayyum A, Birdwell RL, Daniel BL, et al. MR imaging features of infiltrating lobular carcinoma of the breast: histopathologic correlation. AJR Am J Roentgenol 2002;178(5):1227–32.

71. Newstead GM, Arkani S, Abe H, et al. Dynamic breast MR imaging: comparison of kinetic and morphologic characteristics of malignant lesions by tumor type and grade. In: Proceedings of the RSNA. 2005 [abstract no. SSM01-05]. Available at: http://rsna2005.rsna.org/rsna2005/V2005/conference/event_display.cfm?em_id=4417024. Accessed February 5, 2010.

72. Mann RM, Huisman H, Veltman J, et al. Morphologic and dynamic differences between invasive ductal and invasive lobular carcinomas of the breast. Proc Intl Soc Mag Reson Med 2008;16:3769.

73. Dietzel M, Baltzer PA, Herzog A, et al. MRI of invasive lobular carcinoma - prospective study comparing invasive lobular and ductal carcinomas vs. benign lesions in 891 cases. Eur Radiol 2009;19(Suppl 1): S283 [abstract no. B-613].

74. Kepple J, Layeeque R, Klimberg VS, et al. Correlation of magnetic resonance imaging and pathologic size of infiltrating lobular carcinoma of the breast. Am J Surg 2005;190(4):623–7.

75. Onesti JK, Mangus BE, Helmer SD, et al. Breast cancer tumor size: correlation between magnetic resonance imaging and pathology measurements. Am J Surg 2008;196(6):844–8.

76. Rodenko GN, Harms SE, Pruneda JM, et al. MR imaging in the management before surgery of lobular carcinoma of the breast: correlation with pathology. AJR Am J Roentgenol 1996;167(6): 1415–9.

77. Diekmann F, Diekmann S, Beljavskaja M, et al. [Preoperative MRT of the breast in invasive lobular carcinoma in comparison with invasive ductal carcinoma]. Rofo 2004;176(4):544–9 [in German].

78. Quan ML, Sclafani L, Heerdt AS, et al. Magnetic resonance imaging detects unsuspected disease in patients with invasive lobular cancer. Ann Surg Oncol 2003;10(9):1048–53.

79. Weinstein SP, Orel SG, Heller R, et al. MR imaging of the breast in patients with invasive lobular carcinoma. AJR Am J Roentgenol 2001; 176(2):399–406.

80. Mann RM, Loo CE, Wobbes T, et al. The impact of preoperative breast MRI on the re-excision rate in invasive lobular carcinoma of the breast. Breast Cancer Res Treat 2010;119(2):415–22.

81. Fischer U, Zachariae O, Baum F, et al. The influence of preoperative MRI of the breasts on recurrence rate in patients with breast cancer. Eur Radiol 2004;14(10):1725–31.

82. Solin LJ, Orel SG, Hwang WT, et al. Relationship of breast magnetic resonance imaging to outcome after breast-conservation treatment with radiation for women with early-stage invasive breast carcinoma or ductal carcinoma in situ. J Clin Oncol 2008;26(3):386–91.

83. Keskek M, Kothari M, Ardehali B, et al. Factors predisposing to cavity margin positivity following conservation surgery for breast cancer. Eur J Surg Oncol 2004;30(10):1058–64.

84. O'Sullivan MJ, Li T, Freedman G, et al. The effect of multiple reexcisions on the risk of local recurrence after breast conserving surgery. Ann Surg Oncol 2007;14(11):3133–40.

85. Smitt MC, Horst K. Association of clinical and pathologic variables with lumpectomy surgical margin status after preoperative diagnosis or excisional biopsy of invasive breast cancer. Ann Surg Oncol 2007;14(3):1040–4.

86. van den Broek N, van der Sangen MJ, van de Poll-Franse LV, et al. Margin status and the risk of local recurrence after breast-conserving treatment of lobular breast cancer. Breast Cancer Res Treat 2007;105(1):63–8.

87. Waljee JF, Hu ES, Newman LA, et al. Predictors of re-excision among women undergoing breast-conserving surgery for cancer. Ann Surg Oncol 2008;15(5):1297–303.

88. Dillon MF, Hill AD, Fleming FJ, et al. Identifying patients at risk of compromised margins following breast conservation for lobular carcinoma. Am J Surg 2006;191(2):201–5.

89. Hussien M, Lioe TF, Finnegan J, et al. Surgical treatment for invasive lobular carcinoma of the breast. Breast 2003;12(1):23–35.

90. Molland JG, Donnellan M, Janu NC, et al. Infiltrating lobular carcinoma—a comparison of diagnosis, management and outcome with infiltrating duct carcinoma. Breast 2004;13(5):389–96.

91. Morrow M, Keeney K, Scholtens D, et al. Selecting patients for breast-conserving therapy: the importance of lobular histology. Cancer 2006;106(12): 2563–8.

92. Yeatman TJ, Cantor AB, Smith TJ, et al. Tumor biology of infiltrating lobular carcinoma. Implications for management. Ann Surg 1995;222(4): 549–59.

93. Al-Ghazal SK, Blamey RW, Stewart J, et al. The cosmetic outcome in early breast cancer treated with breast conservation. Eur J Surg Oncol 1999; 25(6):566–70.

94. Bleicher RJ, Ciocca RM, Egleston BL, et al. Association of routine pretreatment magnetic resonance imaging with time to surgery, mastectomy rate, and margin status. J Am Coll Surg 2009;209(2): 180–7.

95. Pengel KE, Loo CE, Teertstra HJ, et al. The impact of preoperative MRI on breast-conserving surgery of invasive cancer: a comparative cohort study. Breast Cancer Res Treat 2009;116(1):161–9.

96. Brennan ME, Houssami N, Lord S, et al. Magnetic resonance imaging screening of the contralateral breast in women with newly diagnosed breast cancer: systematic review and meta-analysis of incremental cancer detection and impact on surgical management. J Clin Oncol 2009;27(33):5640–9.

97. LaTrenta LR, Menell JH, Morris EA, et al. Breast lesions detected with MR imaging: utility and histopathologic importance of identification with US. Radiology 2003;227(3):856–61.

98. Linda A, Zuiani C, Londero V, et al. Outcome of initially only magnetic resonance mammography-detected findings with and without correlate at second-look sonography: distribution according to patient history of breast cancer and lesion size. Breast 2008;17(1):51–7.

99. Floery D, Helbich TH. MRI-Guided percutaneous biopsy of breast lesions: materials, techniques, success rates, and management in patients with suspected radiologic-pathologic mismatch. Magn Reson Imaging Clin N Am 2006;14(3):411–25, viii.

100. Veltman J, Boetes C, Wobbes T, et al. Magnetic resonance-guided biopsies and localizations of the breast: initial experiences using an open breast coil and compatible intervention device. Invest Radiol 2005;40(6):379–84.

101. Houssami N, Ciatto S, Martinelli F, et al. Early detection of second breast cancers improves prognosis in breast cancer survivors. Ann Oncol 2009;20(9):1505–10.

102. Sardanelli F, Hunink MG, Gilbert FJ, et al. Evidence-based radiology: why and how? Eur Radiol 2010;20(1):1–15.

A Clinical Oncologic Perspective on Breast Magnetic Resonance Imaging

Sara Bloom, MD[a], Monica Morrow, MD[a,b],*

KEYWORDS
• Magnetic resonance imaging
• Breast-conserving therapy • Local recurrence
• Occult cancer • Neoadjuvant therapy

Breast cancer mortality in the United States, as well as in other parts of the world, has decreased in recent years, a finding attributable in part to the use of screening mammography and in part to improved treatment, particularly the use of adjuvant endocrine therapy and chemotherapy.[1] It is now recognized that breast cancer survival and local control are a function of the interaction between the fundamental biology of the cancer, the disease burden, and the availability of effective therapy. Traditionally, disease burden has been the major consideration in selecting local therapy. In patients treated with breast-conserving therapy (BCT) consisting of excision of the tumor and whole-breast irradiation, randomized trials have shown that failure to reduce the tumor burden in the breast to a subclinical level is associated with an increased risk of local recurrence.[2,3] This has resulted in multicentric cancer and margins that cannot be cleared of cancer cells being accepted as indications for mastectomy.[4,5] As experience with BCT has been gained, local recurrence rates have steadily decreased[6,7] as a result of the routine inking of specimen margins, more extensive pathologic evaluation of margin surfaces, standardization of radiation doses, and the widespread use of adjuvant endocrine therapy and chemotherapy.

Magnetic resonance (MR) imaging is a technology capable of detecting small foci of cancer in the breast that were previously only evident on detailed pathology evaluation. Although it seems intuitively obvious that an improved ability to detect cancer would be beneficial, evidence of improved patient outcomes is lacking. This article considers the available data on the effect of MR imaging on short- and long-term outcomes of surgical treatment of operable breast cancer based on what is known today about patient selection for BCT and the incidence, detection, and management of local recurrence. Other relevant clinical areas, including the effect of MR imaging on selection of patients for partial breast irradiation, and its role in the multidisciplinary care of the patient receiving neoadjuvant therapy, are also addressed. When considering therapy from a clinical perspective, oncologic end points of relevance to the patient, such as disease-free survival or quality of life, and not the rate of cancer detection, must be considered. The authors have attempted to address these end points in the context of current thinking regarding the role of local control in improving survival and what is known about the biologic diversity of breast cancer.

[a] Breast Service, Department of Surgery, Memorial Sloan-Kettering Cancer Center, Evelyn H. Lauder Breast Center, 300 East 66th Street, New York, NY 10065, USA
[b] Department of Surgery, Weill Medical College of Cornell University, 425 East 61st Street, New York, NY 10065, USA
* Corresponding author. Breast Service, Department of Surgery, Memorial Sloan-Kettering Cancer Center, Evelyn H. Lauder Breast Center, 300 East 66th Street, New York, NY 10065.
E-mail address: morrowm@mskcc.org

Magn Reson Imaging Clin N Am 18 (2010) 277–294
doi:10.1016/j.mric.2010.02.007

MR IMAGING FOR TREATMENT SELECTION

Clinically and radiographically, breast cancer is usually a unicentric lesion, with multicentric carcinoma identified by physical examination or mammography in fewer than 10% of cases.[8] However, pathology studies using serial subgross sectioning of mastectomy specimens have documented that additional tumor foci are frequently present in the same quadrant (multifocal) or other quadrants (multicentric) of a breast with what seems to be clinically unicentric tumor.

In one such study, Holland and colleagues[9] evaluated mastectomy specimens of 282 patients with unicentric cancers 5 cm or less in size and found additional tumor foci in 63%. In 20% of cases, the additional tumor was identified within 2 cm of the index tumor, and in the remaining 43% at a greater distance from the primary site, although usually within 4 cm. The likelihood of identifying additional tumor foci was not related to the size of the primary tumor.

Studies examining the incidence of pathologic multifocality or multicentricity in clinically localized tumors are summarized in **Table 1**.[9–15] In spite of variable inclusion criteria, additional tumor foci were identified in 21% to 63% of cases, including a 44% incidence in patients with mammographically detected lesions. Such studies were initially used to argue that the treatment of breast cancer with approaches that did not remove the entire breast was inappropriate and would result in high rates of local recurrence. Extensive clinical experience, including multiple prospective randomized trials, has since demonstrated that survival after BCT, consisting of excision of the tumor to negative margins and whole-breast irradiation, is equal to survival after mastectomy. In the current era of the routine use of adjuvant systemic therapy in breast cancer, 10-year rates of local recurrence after BCT are less than 10%,[16,17] considerably lower than the incidence of multifocality/multicentricity seen in the pathology studies included in **Table 1**. These findings indicate that although subclinical tumor foci are present in significant numbers of women with clinically localized breast cancer, most of these subclinical tumor foci are controlled with radiotherapy (XRT), and it is this paradox that lies at the heart of the debate over the benefit of MR imaging for cancer staging and treatment selection.

It is clear that, in women with breast cancer, MR imaging identifies additional cancer foci that are not evident on clinical examination, mammogram, or ultrasound. In a meta-analysis of 19 studies, including 2610 patients with breast cancer, Houssami and colleagues[18] reported that additional cancer was identified by MR imaging in 16% of patients, with a range of 6% to 34% in individual studies. In studies restricted to patients with infiltrating lobular carcinoma, the detection of additional disease is even more frequent.

In a meta-analysis of MR imaging in lobular carcinoma reported by Mann and colleagues,[19] which included 18 studies and 450 cancers, additional disease was detected with MR imaging in 32% of cases (95% confidence interval [CI] 22%–44%). The usefulness of MR imaging in ductal carcinoma in situ (DCIS) is unclear.

Some studies have reported that MR imaging is less effective at detecting DCIS than invasive carcinoma. Sardanelli and colleagues[20] observed a sensitivity of only 40% for the detection of DCIS by MR imaging when the results of serial subgross sectioning were used as the standard. In contrast, Kuhl and colleagues[21] reported that MR imaging was significantly more sensitive than mammography for the detection of DCIS when

Table 1
Pathologic studies of breast cancer multifocality/multicentricity

Study	No. of Cases	Population	Multifocal/ Multicentric (%)
Qualheim and Gall[13]	157	Not stated	54
Rosen et al[14]	203	Invasive carcinoma	33
Lagios[12]	85	Not stated	21
Egan[11]	118	Not stated	60
Schwartz et al[15]	43	Nonpalpable cancer	44
Anastassiades et al[10]	366	Invasive ≤7 cm, noninvasive	49
Holland et al[9]	282	Clinically unicentric invasive cancer <5 cm	63

conventional pathologic evaluation was used. Of 167 women with DCIS who had undergone mammography and MR imaging preoperatively, DCIS was diagnosed by mammography in 56% of cases, and by MR imaging in 98%, with the superior performance of MR imaging particularly evident in high-grade DCIS.

Although it is possible that some of the enhancement patterns seen with DCIS were not well recognized as abnormal in early studies of MR imaging, resulting in a lower sensitivity, the clinical questions regarding the significance of the low-volume disease detected by MR imaging, whether DCIS or invasive carcinoma, are similar.

It is reasonable to ask whether the tumor foci identified by MR imaging are the same tumor foci identified by pathologists using serial subgross sectioning. This question was most directly addressed by Sardanelli and colleagues,[20] who performed MR imaging on 90 patients before mastectomy, then processed the mastectomy specimens with serial subgross sectioning and correlated the pathologic tumor location with the findings of the preoperative MR imaging. The overall sensitivity of MR imaging for the detection of tumor was 81%; 89% for invasive carcinoma and 40% for DCIS. In the 90 breasts studied, MR imaging failed to identify microscopic multifocal or multicentric disease in 19, and incorrectly indicated additional disease in 30, and correctly identifying the extent of tumor in 50. The mean diameter of malignant lesions not seen by MR imaging was 5 mm and ranged from 0.5 mm to 15 mm. These findings strongly suggest that MR imaging is capable of finding some, but not all, of the tumor foci identified with detailed pathologic sectioning.

Indirect evidence also suggests that the same tumor is identified with both techniques. Berg and colleagues[22] observed that in 40 of 46 breasts with additional tumor foci detected with MR imaging, the tumor foci were within 4 cm of the index lesion. Liberman and colleagues[23] also noted that most of the additional tumors detected were in the same quadrant as the index lesion. These findings correspond well to the observations of Holland and colleagues[9] that 96% of pathologically detected tumor foci were within 4 cm of the index tumor, and provide further support for the concept that MR imaging is a technology capable of detecting some, but not all, of the tumors seen on serial subgross sectioning.

Until relatively recently, it has been assumed that the finding of additional cancer on MR imaging was clearly of benefit to the patient. In the meta-analyses of Houssami and colleagues,[18] the results of the MR imaging examination changed surgical therapy in 7.8% to 33.3% of cases in individual studies, and virtually always in the direction of more extensive surgery, such as a wider excision or a mastectomy that would not otherwise have been performed. In a study of 5405 patients treated at the Mayo Clinic, Rochester, MN, the use of MR imaging increased from 10% of newly diagnosed breast cancers in 2003 to 26% in 2006. A significant increase in the mastectomy rate was also observed during this period, and after adjustment for age, stage, and the presence of contralateral carcinoma, women who had MR imaging were 1.7 times more likely to undergo mastectomy than their counterparts who did not have the examination, although the mastectomy rate was also noted to increase in this group over time.[24] If the more extensive surgery that occurs as a result of MR imaging findings is truly beneficial to patients, it should result in improvement in either short-term outcomes of surgery, such as the improved ability to identify patients requiring a mastectomy preoperatively, or an increased likelihood of achieving negative margins with a single operative procedure. Alternatively, the benefit of MR imaging may be to improve long-term outcomes by decreasing the incidence of local recurrence after BCT or allowing the synchronous detection of contralateral breast cancer.

THE EFFECT OF MR IMAGING ON SHORT-TERM SURGICAL OUTCOMES

The identification of patients who are appropriate candidates for BCT is not a major problem at the present time. Standard guidelines for the use of BCT have been developed,[5] and contraindications to the procedure are reliably identified with a history, physical examination, and diagnostic mammography. Morrow and colleagues[25] reported that of 263 consecutive patients selected for BCT between 1989 and 1993 using a history, physical examination, and diagnostic mammography, conversion to mastectomy was necessary in only 2.9%. In a population-based sample of 800 women from the Los Angeles and Detroit Surveillance Epidemiology and End Results (SEER) sites attempting BCT between June 2005 and May 2006, 12% required conversion to mastectomy, although in 8%, mastectomy occurred after a single attempt at BCT.[26] Two retrospective studies[27,28] and 1 prospective randomized trial[29] have examined whether the use of MR imaging reduces the need for mastectomy in patients attempting BCT. Bleicher and colleagues[27] retrospectively reviewed 290 patients attempting BCT who had a multidisciplinary preoperative evaluation between July

2004 and December 2006, and found no significant difference in the likelihood of requiring conversion from BCT to mastectomy based on a preoperative MR imaging. Pengel and colleagues[28] compared outcomes among 355 women treated at a single institution. Those who had an MR imaging were part of a study evaluating the procedure, and the control group consisted of patients who declined to enter the study. Again, no significant differences in the rate of unanticipated conversion to mastectomy were noted (**Table 2**).[27–29]

The most robust data addressing this question came from the COMICE trial, a prospective randomized study involving 107 participating surgeons in the United Kingdom that was designed to address the question of the role of MR imaging in improving outcomes in patients undergoing BCT.[29] The sample included 1623 women believed to be candidates for BCT who were stratified by age, breast density, and treating surgeon, and randomized to receive an MR imaging scan or not. In the MR imaging group, 58 patients (7.1%) underwent an immediate mastectomy as a result of the MR imaging findings, and 10 patients in the no MR imaging group (1.2%) changed their treatment decision after randomization and opted for a mastectomy. Of the remainder who attempted BCT, conversion to mastectomy was required in 5.9% of the MR imaging group and 7.6% of the no MR imaging group ($P = $ NS, see **Table 2**).[29] The overall result was a 13% mastectomy rate in the MR imaging group and an 8.8% rate in the no MR imaging group. In the study of Pengel and colleagues,[28] the mastectomy rate was doubled in the MR imaging group (11.6% vs 5.1%), and in the report of Bleicher and colleagues,[27] the use of MR imaging increased the mastectomy rate from 25% to 38%, an odds ratio of 1.80 after adjustment for tumor size and patient age ($P = .024$). These studies provide no suggestion that MR imaging decreases the likelihood of unplanned mastectomy, but do show a consistent pattern of an increased mastectomy rate in patients undergoing MR imaging.

In contrast to patient selection for BCT, which is not a major clinical problem, the need for reexcision because of margins involved with tumor after the initial lumpectomy is a common clinical occurrence. Morrow and colleagues[26] observed that 22% of 800 women undergoing successful BCT in a population-based sample derived from the SEER registry required at least 1 reexcision to complete surgical therapy. Reexcision is traumatic to patients, costly to the health care system, and delays the initiation of adjuvant therapy. Strategies to reduce the need for reexcision would address a substantial problem in breast cancer surgery. **Table 3** summarizes 4 retrospective studies and 1 prospective study that have addressed the question of the effect of MR imaging on the need for reexcision.[27–31] In spite of the inclusion of almost 2500 patients in total, none of the individual studies show a significant reduction in the need for reexcision in patients undergoing MR imaging. One study limited to patients with infiltrating lobular carcinoma has shown a benefit for MR imaging. Mann and colleagues[32] studied 90 patients who did not have MR imaging and 55 who did in whom BCT was attempted and reported a 27% rate of reexcision in the no MR imaging group compared with 9% in the MR imaging group ($P = .01$), as well as a significantly higher mastectomy rate in the no MR imaging group (23% vs 7%; $P = .013$). Patients included in this study were treated between 1993 and 2005, and it is not clear if those undergoing MR imaging were more commonly treated later in the study period and if criteria for reexcision were uniform over time. Other studies have not confirmed a difference in the need for reexcision in patients with infiltrating lobular and infiltrating ductal histology. In a study of 318 patients with infiltrating lobular cancer who were matched by stage, year of diagnosis, and menopausal status to 2 controls with infiltrating ductal cancer (n =

Table 2
Effect of MR imaging on the need for unplanned mastectomy

| Author | No. of Patients | Mastectomy (%) | | P Value |
		No MR Imaging	MR Imaging	
Bleicher et al[27]	290	5.9	9.8	NS
Pengel et al[28]	355	5.1	2.5	NS
Turnbull et al[29]	1623	7.6	5.9	NS

Abbreviation: NS, not significant.

Table 3
Effect of MR imaging on the likelihood of positive margins after initial surgical excision

Author	No. of Patients	% Positive Margins		P Value
		No MR Imaging	MR Imaging	
Bleicher et al[27]	290	14	22	NS
Pengel et al[28]	355	19	14	NS
Schiller et al[31]	730	18	14	NS
Hwang et al[30]	472	14	12	NS
Turnbull et al[29]	1623	11	10	NS

Abbreviation: NS, not significant.

636), 25% of patients with lobular cancer required reexcision compared with 21% of those with ductal cancer, a difference that was not statistically significant after adjusting for tumor size and patient age.[33] One potential explanation for the inability of MR imaging to reduce the need for reexcision has to do with its accuracy in determining tumor size. Although multiple studies have shown that MR imaging is more accurate than mammography in determining tumor size,[34–36] the degree of precision of measurement, and the ability to translate the imaging findings to the amount of tissue removed in the operating room, may be insufficient to see a reduction in margin positivity. For example, Grimsby and colleagues[37] compared tumor size as determined by MR imaging for 190 invasive breast cancers with pathologic size measurements and found that MR imaging estimated size within 5 mm of the pathologic measurement in only about half of cases, overestimating the size in one-third of cases, and underestimating in 15%. As previously discussed, when serial subgross sectioning was used as the standard, MR imaging underestimated disease extent for 19% of invasive foci and a far higher percentage of DCIS foci. Because margin specimens are often subjected to detailed pathologic scrutiny, some of this disease will be identified as positive margins.

The available data on the use of MR imaging in the setting of newly diagnosed breast cancer do not provide evidence of patient benefit in short-term surgical outcomes, and raise some concerns. In addition to the increased mastectomy rate seen in patients undergoing MR imaging (discussed earlier), there are also concerns about false-positive findings and the need for additional radiologic workup to evaluate these findings, leading to increased health care costs and delays in therapy. In the meta-analysis of Houssami and colleagues,[18] the false-positive rate of MR imaging was 5.5% (95% CI 3.1%–9.5%), and it is likely that

false-positive rates outside of the centers of expertise included in this meta-analysis are higher. Petit and colleagues[38] reported that 36 of 410 patients believed to be candidates for BCT were converted to mastectomy because of additional MR imaging lesions. In 23 cases, biopsy confirmation of malignancy in the additional lesion was not performed, and no additional cancer was found in more than half of these patients. Although it is clear that the problem of inappropriate surgery because of false-positive MR imaging results can be minimized with biopsy confirmation of malignancy, there are some practical difficulties associated with this approach.

The current algorithm for evaluating an MR imaging abnormality involves a targeted ultrasound to try and identify the lesion to allow an ultrasound-guided biopsy. If the lesion cannot be visualized by ultrasound and the patient is seeking treatment at a different institution than the 1 in which the MR imaging was obtained, then the MR imaging is often repeated to verify the presence of a target before the time of biopsy. In the study of Bleicher and colleagues,[27] there was a 22.4-day delay in the time from histologic diagnosis to initial surgery in patients who had MR imaging compared with those who did not (P = .01). The need for additional biopsies, particularly at multiple sites, is traumatic for patients, and Berg and colleagues[22] found that 12% of patients underwent a medically unnecessary mastectomy rather than undergo further workup of abnormal MR imaging findings. The risk of unnecessary surgery is present in the ipsilateral and the contralateral breast. King and colleagues[39] compared presenting characteristics of 2558 women who underwent unilateral mastectomy with 407 who had a contralateral prophylactic mastectomy (CPM) between 1997 and 2005 at Memorial Sloan-Kettering Cancer Center. Patients having preoperative MR imaging were significantly more likely to undergo CPM (43% vs 16%; P = .0001), and this was particularly true if the unaffected breast required a biopsy for a benign finding.

EFFECT OF MR IMAGING ON LONG-TERM CANCER OUTCOMES
Local Recurrence

A potential major benefit to patients of preoperative MR imaging would be a reduction in the incidence of local recurrence after BCT. Since the publication of the initial trials that established the suitability of BCT as a breast cancer treatment modality, rates of local recurrence have steadily declined. This decrease can be attributed to improvements in mammography, the routine inking of surgical margins and more detailed evaluation of margin specimens, and particularly to the increased use of adjuvant systemic therapy. Pass and colleagues[7] examined the effect of changes in the processes of care between 1981 and 1996 on local recurrence rates in a group of 607 patients treated at a single institution. Between 1981 and 1985, the 5-year rate of ipsilateral breast tumor recurrence (IBTR) was 8%, decreasing to 1% between 1991 and 1996. In this period, the proportion of patients with negative margins increased from 48% to 76%, and the mean number of pathology slides examined to determine margin status increased from 11 to 21 per patient. The use of tamoxifen increased from 10% to 61% of cases. In a similar study, Ernst and colleagues[6] observed 8-year rates of locoregional recurrence after BCT to decrease from 20.1% between 1985 and 1992, to 5.4% from 1993 to 1999. In contrast, rates of locoregional recurrence after mastectomy did not change between the 2 time periods. In the National Surgical Adjuvant Breast and Bowel Project (NSABP) trials conducted since the 1990s, rates of IBTR at 10 years were less than 8% in node-positive and node-negative women receiving systemic therapy.[16,17] These findings emphasize that local recurrence may be caused by 2 mechanisms:

> The first mechanism, an excessive tumor burden in the breast that cannot be controlled with XRT, is the type of local recurrence that is potentially amenable to reduction through the use of MR imaging for patient selection.
> The second mechanism, local recurrence that occurs because of biologically aggressive disease, is actually a first site of metastases and will only be affected by improvements in systemic therapy.

The proportion of local recurrences caused by each of these mechanisms is unknown; however, the observation from the Early Breast Cancer Trialists overview analysis[40] that local recurrence is seen on the chest wall after mastectomy and XRT in 3% of node-negative cases and 7% of node-positive cases (figures similar to current rates of IBTR after BCT) strongly suggests that most recurrences after BCT in the current era are caused by aggressive biology, not a heavy residual disease burden in the breast.

Three studies have retrospectively examined the effect of patient selection with MR imaging on IBTR. Fischer and colleagues[41] retrospectively compared 121 patients who had preoperative MR imaging to 225 who did not. After a mean follow-up of approximately 40 months, IBTR occurred in 1.2% of the MR imaging group and 6.8% of the no MR imaging group (P<.001). The 6.8% incidence of IBTR at less than 5 years follow-up is unusually high by current standards, making the outcome of this study difficult to interpret. In addition, although patients in the MR imaging group were more likely to have T1 tumors (64% vs 48%), more likely to be node-negative (61% vs 54%), and less likely to have high-grade lesions (13% vs 28%), no adjustments for differences in tumor characteristics between the groups were made. In spite of the more favorable profile of the MR imaging patients, chemotherapy was administered to 95% of patients in this group with indications for treatment, compared with 82% in the no MR imaging group, and no adjustment was made for this difference. The combination of an unusually high rate of IBTR in the no MR imaging group compared with other large datasets of patients treated without MR imaging in the same time period,[16,17] and the lack of adjustment for major differences in tumor and treatment variables which affect the incidence of IBTR, make it difficult to draw reliable conclusions from this study. Solin and colleagues[42] also examined the effect of MR imaging on IBTR in 215 patients who had the examination and 541 who did not. Appropriate statistical adjustments were made for differences between patient groups. At 8 years, the rate of IBTR in the MR imaging group was 3% and was 4% in the non-IBTR group. Hwang and colleagues[30] also examined the effect of MR imaging on IBTR with adjustment for differences between groups. After a median follow-up of 54 months, the 8-year actuarial rates of local recurrence were 1.8% in the MR imaging group and 2.5% in the no MR imaging group, a nonsignificant difference.

What is noteworthy about this study and the study of Solin and colleagues[42] is that based on the results of the Houssami and colleagues[18] meta-analysis showing a 6% to 11% conversion rate from BCT to mastectomy based on the findings of MR imaging, between 21 and 38 of the patients in the study by Hwang and colleagues[30] and 32 to 60 patients in the study by Solin and colleagues[42] who were treated without MR imaging had inappropriate BCT; yet the actual number of patients who recurred was 9 and 13, respectively. The COMICE trial will provide additional data on MR imaging and IBTR when further follow-up is available. However, the information available now suggests that the use of MR imaging may not have an effect on breast cancer-specific survival.

The Early Breast Cancer Trialists overview[40] showed that, to observe a survival difference at 15 years, differences in local failure rates of 10% or greater between treatments must be present at 5 years of follow-up. Differences of this magnitude are seen in patients treated with BCT with or without XRT, whether node-positive or node-negative, and in node-positive women undergoing mastectomy treated with and without XRT. The rate of IBTR after BCT in patients selected for the procedure without MR imaging is less than 10% at 10 years, so a difference of the magnitude needed to show a survival gain cannot be anticipated with the addition of MR imaging. Even if the group that seems to be at the highest risk for IBTR after BCT (women with estrogen receptor [ER], progesterone receptor [PR], and human epidermal growth factor receptor 2 [HER2]-negative disease[43]) were to be studied, it is unlikely that MR imaging would result in a survival benefit because these patients also have the highest risk for local recurrence after mastectomy,[44] strongly suggesting that these recurrences are a reflection of aggressive tumor biology rather than a heavy tumor burden in the breast.

Contralateral Cancer

The other long-term outcome with the potential to be affected by MR imaging is the synchronous versus metachronous diagnosis of contralateral breast cancer. Women with unilateral breast carcinoma are recognized as being at increased risk for the development of second cancers, but the absolute magnitude of this risk is relatively low in women who do not have BRCA gene mutations. In 134,501 women diagnosed with unilateral DCIS, stage 1 and stage 2 breast carcinoma between 1973 and 1996 and reported to SEER, the 10-year actuarial risk of a contralateral cancer was 6.1%, and the 20-year risk was 12%.[45] For those less than 45 years of age at initial diagnosis,

these figures were 3.1% and 6.2%, respectively. A diagnosis of DCIS was associated with a 6.0% risk of a second cancer at 10 years, and a diagnosis of infiltrating lobular carcinoma was associated with a 6.4% risk at 10 years. Based on these low incidence rates, it is difficult to argue that more intensive surveillance of the contralateral breast added to an annual mammogram is a cost-effective strategy for the general population of women with breast cancer. However, Lehman and colleagues[46] examined the role of MR imaging for evaluation of the contralateral breast in 969 women with unilateral breast cancer. Cancer was detected by MR imaging in 30 women (3.1%) with clinically and mammographically normal breasts within 12 months of the initial breast cancer diagnosis. The mean patient age was 53.3 years, and only 19.6% had 1 or more first-degree relatives with breast cancer. Of the cancers detected, 18 were invasive carcinoma and 12 were DCIS. An additional 3 cases of DCIS not detected by MR imaging were identified in prophylactic mastectomy specimens. The investigators concluded that MR imaging of the contralateral breast at the time of a unilateral breast cancer diagnosis was useful to allow the detection of early-stage carcinoma, and synchronous rather than metachronous treatment of second primary tumors. The same arguments have been used to support the use of mirror image, contralateral breast biopsy, a procedure with similar results. Cody[47] identified contralateral cancer with mirror image biopsy in 3% of 871 women with unilateral cancer and a normal examination and mammogram treated between 1979 and 1993, and half of the cancers were invasive; Pressman[48] reported a 6.2% identification rate with contralateral biopsy in an earlier time period. To reconcile the findings of Lehman and colleagues[46] and the contralateral biopsy studies[47,48] with the low rates of cancer observed at 5 and 10 years in the SEER study of Gao and colleagues,[45] one must make the assumption that virtually all contralateral cancer that occurs in the first 5 years after diagnosis is present at the time of diagnosis, and that it is all detectable by MR imaging. This seems unlikely and also ignores clinical data that indicate that the use of endocrine therapy reduces the clinical incidence of contralateral breast cancer by 50%.[49] Even the use of conventional chemotherapy reduces contralateral cancer by 20%,[49] raising the distinct possibility that MR imaging of the contralateral breast identifies some cancers that would never become clinically evident, resulting in unnecessary treatment. In a meta-analysis of MR imaging of the contralateral breast, Brennan and colleagues[50] reported a 9.3% incidence of abnormalities detected by MR imaging in the contralateral breast (true-positive plus false-positive), with a positive predictive value (PPV) of 47.9%. In the already anxious woman with a new diagnosis of breast cancer, this relatively low PPV may have significant clinical consequences. In a large study examining factors associated with CPM, King and colleagues[39] found that undergoing a preoperative MR imaging increased the risk of contralateral prophylactic mastectomy by a factor of 3.2 in multivariate analysis. Similarly, Sorbero and colleagues[51] examined the use of CPM in 3606 stage 1 to 3 patients with breast cancer between 1998 and 2005 and found that in multivariate analysis, the use of preoperative MR imaging was associated with an increased use of contralateral prophylactic mastectomy (odds ratio 2.04; $P = .001$) in women with stage 1 and 2 disease, although the overall rates of contralateral prophylactic mastectomy were significantly lower than those reported by King and colleagues.[39]

In addition, the 1-year follow-up in the study of Lehman and colleagues[46] is insufficient to judge the effect of MR imaging on the incidence of contralateral cancer, and limited clinical data are available that address this question. Solin and colleagues[42] reported a 6% incidence of cancer at 8 years of follow-up in women who did and did not have preoperative MR imaging, indicating that more data are needed before concluding that MR imaging is routinely indicated in women with unilateral cancer for the purpose of screening the contralateral breast.

MR IMAGING FOR OCCULT BREAST CANCER

Fewer than 1% of breast cancers present as axillary nodal metastases with an occult primary tumor that cannot be detected by physical examination, mammography, or ultrasound. Traditionally, these cases have been treated with mastectomy to ensure removal of the primary tumor, but in approximately one-third of the breast specimens, cancer is not identified by pathologic evaluation.[52] Although mastectomy was a reasonable approach to this problem in earlier years where the tumor burden that was undetected clinically could be quite large, in more recent studies,[53,54] the identification of cancer in the breast specimen has been infrequent, and those cancers that were found were often quite small. Although breast conservation has been successfully performed in patients with occult tumors using whole-breast irradiation without surgical excision, this deprives the patient of the benefit of a boost dose of radiation to the primary tumor site. The use of MR imaging to identify the primary tumor, allowing surgical excision and the use of a radiation boost, is a clinically valuable tool in this uncommon circumstance.

Studies evaluating the use of MR imaging in cases of occult breast cancer have been small and retrospective, but typically demonstrate detection of tumor in more than two-thirds of these cases with low false-negative rates (as summarized in **Table 4**).[55–61] A meta-analysis by de Bresser and colleagues[62] summarized the results of 220 patients in 8 of these studies. MR imaging identified a suspicious lesion in 72% of cases with a sensitivity of 90% and a specificity of 31% (range 22%–50%). The mean size of tumors identified on pathologic examination ranged from 5 mm to 16 mm, and more than 90% (pooled mean, 96%) were invasive carcinomas.

The largest study included in the meta-analysis by Buchanan and colleagues[55] examined 55 patients with axillary lymphadenopathy and occult primary without evidence of distant disease. MR imaging revealed suspicious lesions in 76%, of which 62% (26 of 42) proved pathologically to be the primary tumor, resulting in 15 of these patients

Table 4
MR imaging in occult breast cancer presenting as axillary adenopathy: identification and false-negative rates

Study	No. of Patients	MR Imaging-Detected Cancer (%)	False-Negatives
Buchanan et al[55]	55	26/55 (47)	2/13
McMahon et al[58]	18	12/18 (67)	NA
Olson et al[60]	40	28/40 (70	1/5
Orel et al[61]	22	17/20 (85)	2/3
Henry-Tillman et al[56]	10	8/8 (100)	0/2
Morris et al[59]	12	9/12 (75)	0/2
Ko et al[57]	12	10/12 (83)	NA

Abbreviations: NA, not applicable.

being considered candidates for BCT. Conversely, MR imaging failed to identify the primary tumor in 25 patients (12 false-positive MR imaging scans and 13 negative MR imaging scans). Twelve of these patients underwent mastectomy, yielding cancer in only 4 cases (33%).

In an earlier investigation from the same institution (and an overlapping study period), Olson and colleagues[60] looked at the effect of MR imaging on breast conservation in 40 women with occult breast cancer. Of the 28 patients whose primary tumors were identified by MR imaging, 11 elected lumpectomy/axillary lymph node dissection (ALND). Two of the lumpectomy patients ultimately required mastectomy because of positive margins. Of the 12 patients with negative MR imaging scans, 5 underwent mastectomy, yielding cancer in only 1 patient. A negative MR imaging in this group of patients was predictive of low tumor yield, and potentially identified a subset of patients that could be adequately treated with whole-breast irradiation instead of mastectomy. This course of treatment was selected in 7 patients with negative MR imaging who underwent ALND and whole-breast irradiation. With a median follow-up of 19 months, no local recurrences were observed in either the patients treated with lumpectomy/ALND/XRT or those treated with ALND/XRT. Ultimately, the breasts were conserved in 16 (47%) patients in this study. Varadarajan and colleagues[63] looked at the outcomes of 10 patients, most of whom had negative MR imaging scans and received XRT to the breast. In this select group of patients with occult breast cancer, there have been no IBTR with a median follow-up of 57 months.

In summary, MR imaging is proving to be useful in patients with occult breast cancer, resulting in identification of the primary tumor in approximately 60% of cases. Patients with small unifocal tumors are candidates for conventional BCT.

Negative MR imaging provides reassurance that a large tumor burden is unlikely and that the patient may be adequately treated locally with axillary dissection and whole-breast irradiation. Despite this, as illustrated in **Table 5**,[55,57–61] mastectomy remains the most common form of local therapy in this situation even when MR imaging is used.

MR IMAGING TO SELECT PATIENTS FOR ACCELERATED PARTIAL BREAST IRRADIATION

The use of a short course of radiation therapy (RT) limited to the region of the tumor bed, known as accelerated partial breast irradiation (APBI), is currently a subject of great interest. APBI is not believed to be a more effective method of radiotherapy than conventional whole-breast RT, but is intended to increase the convenience of RT by reducing the 6.0- to 6.5-week treatment time of standard RT to 5 days or less. In addition to convenience, APBI offers the theoretic advantage of decreasing the radiation dose delivered to areas of the breast not involved with carcinoma, decreasing the radiation dose to adjacent organs, and improving cosmetic outcome.[64] It is anticipated that the availability of a more convenient form of RT would decrease the number of women who are candidates for BCT but choose to undergo mastectomy to avoid RT,[65,66] at the same time preserving the survival advantage that is seen when BCT without RT is compared with BCT with whole-breast RT.[40]

A major part of the rationale for APBI is the clinical observation that in women treated with whole-breast RT, most local recurrences occur in proximity to the primary tumor. Thus, a requirement for APBI to be successful is that tumor not be present outside the quadrant of the known primary tumor. Several studies have been conducted on APBI using clinical selection criteria,

Table 5
Selected treatments for patients with occult breast cancer with preoperative MR imaging evaluation

Study	No. of Patients	Mastectomy/ ALND (%)	Lumpectomy/ ALND/XRT (%)	ALND/XRT (%)	Other
Buchanan et al[55]	55	29 (53)	9 (16)	13 (24)	4
McMahon et al[58]	18	8 (44)	3 (17)	0	7
Olson et al[60]	40	18 (45)	9 (23)	7 (18)	6
Orel et al[61]	22	14 (67)	7 (32)	0	1
Morris et al[59]	12	8 (67)	4 (33)	0	0
Ko et al[57]	12	2 (17)	6 (50)	2 (17)	2

Abbreviations: ALND, axillary lymph node dissection; XRT, radiotherapy.

and although individual selection criteria varied slightly between studies, eligibility was generally limited to patients with T1 and T2 tumors, clear margins, no extensive intraductal component, and fewer than 4 positive nodes. With relatively short periods of follow-up, local recurrences have been infrequent, occurring in fewer than 4% of women at 4 years of follow-up.[67–70] The potential of MR imaging to improve on these outcomes is uncertain. Several studies have examined the frequency with which MR imaging findings would theoretically render a patient ineligible for APBI when the eligibility criteria for the ongoing NSABP/Radiation Therapy Oncology Group (RTOG) trial of APBI are used. These include

- Unifocal tumor with a size 3 cm or less
- Involvement of fewer than 4 axillary nodes
- Negative surgical margins.

In a study of 260 patients with a median age of 57 years, MR imaging identified additional cancer foci in the ipsilateral breast in 4.2%.[71] In contrast, Al-Hallaq and colleagues[72] reported the identification of additional cancer with MR imaging in 8.1% of 110 patients meeting clinical eligibility criteria for the protocol. In 4.5% of cases (95% CI 2.0%–10.2%) the disease was multicentric, and in 3.6% (95% CI 1.4%–9.0%) it was multifocal, leading them to conclude that MR imaging should be used to assess eligibility for APBI. In the work of Godinez and colleagues,[73] MR imaging identified additional foci of tumor in 38% of cases believed to be eligible for APBI, with multicentric disease present in 10%. These findings parallel the results of studies of patient selection for BCT with whole-breast RT using MR imaging; namely that MR imaging identifies significantly more disease than is manifest as local recurrence.

In the case of patients receiving whole-breast RT, it is relatively easy to assume that the disease identified by MR imaging is controlled with RT. In patients with disease outside the quadrant of the known primary tumor who are treated with APBI without the use of MR imaging to identify eligibility, the low rates of local recurrence observed to date might be explained as a function of the limited follow-up periods available or because the additional disease identified with MR imaging is biologically indolent disease that is unlikely to become clinically evident during the patient's lifetime. This situation should be clarified as further follow-up becomes available, but at present, the consensus panel on APBI for the American Society for Radiation Oncology (ASTRO) concluded that "there are insufficient data to justify the routine use of MRI."[74] APBI is not the standard approach to irradiation in BCT, but one that is reserved for women with favorable tumors at relatively low risk for local recurrence, so the possibility of APBI does not provide a rationale for the use of MR imaging in all women with newly diagnosed breast cancer.

MR IMAGING–NEOADJUVANT CHEMOTHERAPY

Neoadjuvant chemotherapy is used to downstage breast cancer to allow inoperable tumors to be resected, and to allow patients requiring mastectomy if surgery is the initial therapy to become candidates for breast conservation. Approximately 80% of patients will respond with a 50% or greater reduction in tumor diameter after neoadjuvant therapy, with 6% to 19% showing a pathologic complete response (CR) in initial studies.[75] With newer combinations of anthracyclines and taxanes, pathologic CR is seen in approximately 25% of patients,[76,77] and the combination of chemotherapy and trastuzumab is associated with pathologic CR in 55% to 65% of cases.[77]

Determination of posttreatment extent of disease is critical to determining subsequent surgical intervention, and difficulty with this process remains a major impediment to increased rates of BCT after neoadjuvant therapy. This is well illustrated in the NSABP B-27 trial in which patients received either 4 cycles of doxorubicin and cyclophosphamide (AC) or 4 cycles of AC followed by 4 cycles of docetaxel (T) before surgery.[76] Although the pathologic CR rate was increased from 14% to 26% (P<.001) with the addition of T, the rates of BCT were 62% in the AC arm and 64% in the ACT arm (p = NS). Physical examination, mammography, and ultrasound play an important role before the initiation of neoadjuvant chemotherapy in identifying patients who are not candidates for down staging to a breast-conserving approach. These include patients with multicentric carcinoma and those with extensive indeterminate or suspicious microcalcifications throughout the breast. However, none of these modalities are particularly accurate in evaluating the response of the tumor to chemotherapy. In 1 study of 189 patients treated with neoadjuvant therapy, the correlation coefficients for residual tumor size as estimated by physical examination, ultrasound, and mammography were 0.42, 0.42, and 0.41, respectively. More importantly, from the perspective of clinical decision making, tumor size as estimated by each of these modalities was within 1 cm of the actual pathologic size in only 66% to 75% of cases.[78]

Similar results were reported by Peintinger and colleagues,[79] who observed that the accuracy of mammography and sonography in predicting pathologic CR was 89%, and that pathologic tumor size was within 0.5 cm of the predicted size in 69% of patients. Some of the inaccuracy of physical examination, mammography, and ultrasonography in predicting the extent of residual tumor results from the inability of these modalities to distinguish the fibrosis and tumor cell death that occurs in response to treatment from viable residual tumor.

The clinical observation, discussed previously, that high rates of response to chemotherapy are frequent, yet a relatively small proportion of women treated with neoadjuvant therapy undergo breast conservation, indicates that improved methods of evaluating the extent of residual tumor would be clinically beneficial. An increasing body of literature suggests that MR imaging is more accurate than ultrasound, physical examination, or mammography in predicting the extent of disease after neoadjuvant therapy (**Table 6**).[80–84] Ultrasound and physical examinations were compared with MR imaging in a study of 68 patients by Segara and colleagues,[84] in which MR imaging was found to be a significantly better predictor of pathologic size. The correlation coefficient was 0.75 for MR imaging, compared with 0.61 for ultrasound and 0.44 for physical examination. In this study, MR imaging was also able to correctly predict complete pathologic responses in 8 of 11 patients. A study by Rosen and colleagues[83] also showed a correlation coefficient of 0.75 for MR imaging, and found that the extent of disease on MR imaging was within 1 cm of the pathologic extent of disease in 12 of 21 (57%) patients. MR imaging overestimated the extent of disease in 7 (33%) patients, and underestimated tumor extent in 2 (10%) patients, including 1 false-negative examination.

MR imaging is also more accurate than mammography at predicting residual tumor.[85–87] In a prospective study of 31 patients, Yeh and colleagues[88] compared clinical evaluation, mammography, ultrasound, and MR imaging to pathology findings. Agreement with the pathologic extent of response occurred in 19%, 26%, 35%, and 71% of cases, respectively. In this study, MR imaging was noted to overestimate the extent of residual disease in 6% of cases and underestimate the extent in 29% (95% CI 14%–48%). Abraham and colleagues[85] looked at 39 patients with stage II, III, or IV disease and compared the accuracy of physical examination, mammography, and MR imaging in predicting response to neoadjuvant therapy. This study showed a high correlation (97%) between MR imaging and pathologic findings. Of 12 patients who failed to show a mammographic response, 8 were found to have marked reduction in tumor by MR imaging evaluation. Similarly, Julius and colleagues[87] found MR imaging correctly identified tumor size in 24/29 (83%) cases, but mammography correlated in only 10/26 (38%). The accuracy of MR imaging in predicting response seems to vary based on the characteristics of the tumor[89] and the degree of response. In general, there is agreement that MR imaging is most accurate in patients who are nonresponders and those with partial responses to treatment.[90,91] Although the decrease or loss of enhancement is evidence of response, it is not a guarantee that no residual tumor is present. Multiple small nests of tumor may persist even in the absence of enhancement, and although the pathogenesis of this is uncertain, decreased vascular permeability and chemotherapy-induced loss of neovascularization are believed to play a role.

Although there is much information correlating tumor size and MR imaging findings, there is a relative paucity of data on the effect of MR imaging on the selection of the appropriate surgical procedure in the neoadjuvant setting. A study by Julius and colleagues[87] looked at changes in surgical

Table 6
Correlation of imaging studies to pathologic extent of disease after neoadjuvant therapy

| Study | No. of Patients | Correlation Coefficient | | | |
		MR Imaging	Mammogram	Ultrasound	Physical Examination
Belli et al[80]	45	0.96			
Segara et al[84]	68	0.75		0.61	0.44
Rosen et al[83]	21	0.75			0.61
Bhattacharyya et al[81]	32	0.71	Not measureable	0.65	
Prati et al[82]	45	0.36	0.15		0.66

management based on MR imaging evaluation. Thirty-four patients were assessed before neoadjuvant therapy as requiring mastectomy (n = 22) or as being inoperable (n = 12). After chemotherapy, only 2 patients were still considered inoperable. Eighteen patients were felt to be candidates for BCT based on a decrease in tumor size, but 2 of these patients eventually required mastectomy because of persistent positive margins. Chen and colleagues[92] showed 2 experienced breast surgeons pre- and post-chemotherapy MR imaging scans and asked them to state which surgical procedure they believed was appropriate. They were then provided with the final pathology reports and asked if their recommendation would differ. Of 21 patients believed to require a mastectomy based on imaging findings, 7 to 10 were felt to be appropriate candidates for BCT based on minimal residual disease at pathology, indicating a significant amount of overestimation of disease by MR imaging. In contrast, of 22 patients believed to be candidates for lumpectomy, only 2 had extensive residual disease at pathology that was believed to necessitate mastectomy.

A pathologic CR to neoadjuvant chemotherapy is predictive of greater disease-free and overall survival, and the ability to predict which tumors are responding before the administration of several cycles of chemotherapy has the potential to save patients who are resistant to particular drugs from unnecessary treatment toxicity. The study of MR imaging characteristics that are predictive of treatment response is a subject of great research interest. Loo and colleagues[93] performed MR imaging pretreatment and after 2 cycles of chemotherapy. They found that a change in largest late enhancement diameter was the single most predictive MR imaging characteristic of tumor response. A less than 25% decrease in diameter indicated residual tumor. Pickles and colleagues[94] looked at pretreatment MR imaging of 54 patients to identify predictive parameters. They found patients who showed high levels of pretreatment perfusion and vessel permeability had a lower disease-free and overall survival. Similarly, a low preoperative mean diffusivity has been suggested by Iacconi and colleagues[95] to be predictive of greater tumor response in terms of percentage of volume reduction. Others have suggested that the morphology of the tumor on MR imaging is predictive of the likelihood of pathologic response,[96] and not surprisingly, unicentric tumors with well-defined boundaries were more likely to be suitable for breast conservation after neoadjuvant chemotherapy.

Ongoing studies should clarify the role of MR imaging in predicting tumor biology. At present, clinical examination, mammography, and MR imaging are all useful in evaluating the extent of disease after neoadjuvant therapy. In addition to providing the most accurate estimate of lesion size, MR imaging also allows visualization of the pattern of residual tumor (**Fig. 1**), which may indicate that the patient is not a candidate for breast conservation. In cases where the findings do not clearly indicate that mastectomy is necessary, breast conservation should be attempted if that is the patient's preferred treatment because it is clear that imaging modalities may overestimate the extent of viable residual tumor. In the circumstance of breast conservation after neoadjuvant therapy, patients should be counseled regarding the potential need for additional surgery, either re-excision or mastectomy, because even MR imaging is known to underestimate residual disease growing as microscopic tumor nests.

MR IMAGING FOR DETECTION OF LOCAL RECURRENCE

The current recommendations for detection of local recurrence after BCT are monthly breast self-examination by the patient; physician examination every 3 to 6 months for 5 years, then annually; and a mammogram 6 to 12 months after the completion of RT, and then yearly.[5] With this approach, one-half to one-third of recurrences are identified as nonpalpable lesions detected by mammography alone, and 85% to 90% of patients have operable disease when a local recurrence is detected.[97,98] Evidence suggests that current methods of surveillance are highly successful; the inoperable recurrences are primarily inflammatory type skin recurrences, an aggressive subtype of recurrence whose biology is unlikely to be affected by detection method,[99] and the average size of recurrent tumors is 1 to 2 cm.[100,101] It is not clear if there is any benefit to detecting local recurrence at a smaller size.

Mastectomy is the standard treatment of local recurrence, regardless of size, in patients who have received previous whole-breast irradiation, so the choice of therapy is not related to tumor size. Attempts to reconserve the breast with wide excision alone, even for small tumors with favorable histologic characteristics, have resulted in further local recurrence in 19% to 48% of cases,[98,100,102–104] an unacceptable rate given what is understood about the effect of failure to maintain local control on long-term survival.[40]

Perhaps most importantly, there is no evidence that earlier identification of local recurrence

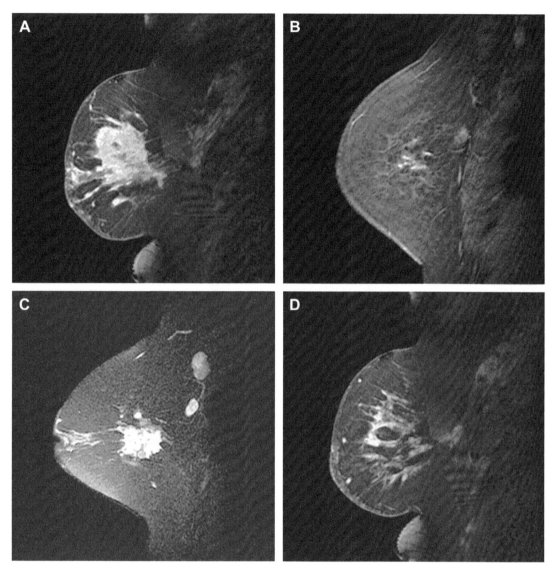

Fig. 1. Different patterns of response to neoadjuvant chemotherapy demonstrated by MR imaging. (*A, B*) Pre- and posttreatment studies with concentric shrinkage of the tumor, which is now suitable for breast-conserving surgery. (*C, D*) Although there is tumor shrinkage on the posttreatment view, it is discontinuous, and tumor is still scattered over a large area of the breast, necessitating mastectomy.

improves patient outcomes. Most studies indicate that tumors with aggressive biology recur locally and distantly in a shorter time interval. In a study by Millar and colleagues,[105] the 10-year rate of IBTR for Luminal A cancers (ER and/or PR positive, HER2-negative) was 3.6%, and the median time to recurrence was 80.5 months. For Basal cancers (ER, PR, HER2-negative) there was a 9.6% incidence of IBTR at 10 years, with a median time to recurrence of 20 months. In spite of the shorter time to the detection of IBTR in the Basal group, the incidence of breast cancer death at a median follow-up of 96 months was 13.5% compared with 7.4% in the Luminal A group.

Veronesi and colleagues[101] reported that the risk of distant metastases after a local recurrence detected within 1 year of initial treatment was 6.6 times the risk seen in patients with local recurrence detected more than 3 years after surgery (*P* = .004). Other studies have confirmed the association between a short interval to the detection of local recurrence and poor survival.[102,106,107] Thus, the extrapolation from trials of screening mammography in which detection of a tumor at a smaller size, and presumably earlier in its natural history, results in a survival advantage does not seem relevant to the problem of local recurrence. In addition, given current rates of local recurrence of less than 1% per year[16,17] and the relatively prolonged period of risk for local recurrence, which occurs at a median interval of 5 to 6 years after treatment,[101,102,105] the cost-effectiveness of follow-up with MR imaging in these cases may be called into question.

SUMMARY

MR imaging is a technology that is able to visualize small tumor deposits that previously could only be identified on pathologic examination. Although this presents new opportunities, it also presents problems when this information results in more aggressive therapy in clinical situations where outcomes are well documented and known to be good. At present, the clinical value of MR imaging is most evident in areas where patient management has been problematic. These include determining tumor response after neoadjuvant therapy and identification of the primary tumor site in patients presenting with axillary adenopathy. The role of MR imaging for treatment selection in the patient with newly diagnosed breast cancer remains extremely controversial. Success rates for patients selected for BCT without MR imaging are high, and rates of IBTR are low. An expanding body of evidence indicates that tumor biology, as well as tumor burden, is a major factor in the outcome of local and systemic therapy. Future efforts to improve the local therapy for breast cancer must acknowledge the heterogeneity of the disease and tailor approaches to the biology of individual subsets, as has been done in newer trials of systemic therapy. This can only be accomplished through a multidisciplinary approach to studies that examine the applications of newer diagnostic modalities such as MR imaging.

REFERENCES

1. Berry DA, Cronin KA, Plevritis SK, et al. Effect of screening and adjuvant therapy on mortality from breast cancer. N Engl J Med 2005;353(17):1784–92.
2. Poggi MM, Danforth DN, Sciuto LC, et al. Eighteen-year results in the treatment of early breast carcinoma with mastectomy versus breast conservation therapy: the National Cancer Institute Randomized Trial. Cancer 2003;98(4):697–702.
3. van Dongen JA, Voogd AC, Fentiman IS, et al. Long-term results of a randomized trial comparing breast-conserving therapy with mastectomy: European Organization for Research and Treatment of Cancer 10801 trial. J Natl Cancer Inst 2000; 92(14):1143–50.
4. Kaufmann M, Morrow M, von Minckwitz G, et al. The Biedenkopf Expert Panel Members. Local-regional treatment of primary breast cancer: consensus recommendations from an international expert panel. Cancer 2010;116(5):1184–91.
5. Morrow M, Harris JR. Practice guideline for breast conservation therapy in the management of invasive breast cancer. J Am Coll Surg 2007;205:362–76.
6. Ernst MF, Voogd AC, Coebergh JW, et al. Using loco-regional recurrence as an indicator of the quality of breast cancer treatment. Eur J Cancer 2004;40(4):487–93.
7. Pass H, Vicini FA, Kestin LL, et al. Changes in management techniques and patterns of disease recurrence over time in patients with breast carcinoma treated with breast-conserving therapy at a single institution. Cancer 2004;101(4):713–20.
8. Morrow M, Bucci C, Rademaker A. Medical contraindications are not a major factor in the underutilization of breast conserving therapy. J Am Coll Surg 1998;186(3):269–74.
9. Holland R, Veling SH, Mravunac M, et al. Histologic multifocality of Tis, T1-2 breast carcinomas. Implications for clinical trials of breast-conserving surgery. Cancer 1985;56(5):979–90.
10. Anastassiades O, Iakovou E, Stavridou N, et al. Multicentricity in breast cancer. A study of 366 cases. Am J Clin Pathol 1993;99(3):238–43.
11. Egan RL. Multicentric breast carcinomas: clinical-radiographic-pathologic whole organ studies and 10-year survival. Cancer 1982;49(6):1123–30.
12. Lagios MD. Multicentricity of breast carcinoma demonstrated by routine correlated serial subgross and radiographic examination. Cancer 1977;40(4): 1726–34.
13. Qualheim RE, Gall EA. Breast carcinoma with multiple sites of origin. Cancer 1957;10(3):460–8.
14. Rosen PP, Fracchia AA, Urban JA, et al. "Residual" mammary carcinoma following simulated partial mastectomy. Cancer 1975;35(3):739–47.
15. Schwartz GF, Patchesfsky AS, Feig SA, et al. Multicentricity of non-palpable breast cancer. Cancer 1980;45(12):2913–6.
16. Anderson SJ, Wapnir I, Dignam JJ, et al. Prognosis after ipsilateral breast tumor recurrence and locoregional recurrences in patients treated by breast-conserving therapy in five National Surgical Adjuvant Breast and Bowel Project protocols of node-negative breast cancer. J Clin Oncol 2009; 27(15):2466–73.
17. Wapnir IL, Anderson SJ, Mamounas EP, et al. Prognosis after ipsilateral breast tumor recurrence and locoregional recurrences in five National Surgical Adjuvant Breast and Bowel Project node-positive adjuvant breast cancer trials. J Clin Oncol 2006; 24(13):2028–37.

18. Houssami N, Ciatto S, Macaskill P, et al. Accuracy and surgical impact of magnetic resonance imaging in breast cancer staging: systematic review and meta-analysis in detection of multifocal and multicentric cancer. J Clin Oncol 2008;26(19): 3248–58.

19. Mann RM, Hoogeveen YL, Blickman JG, et al. MRI compared to conventional diagnostic work-up in the detection and evaluation of invasive lobular carcinoma of the breast: a review of existing literature. Breast Cancer Res Treat 2008; 107(1):1–14.

20. Sardanelli F, Giuseppetti GM, Panizza P, et al. Sensitivity of MRI versus mammography for detecting foci of multifocal, multicentric breast cancer in fatty and dense breasts using the whole-breast pathologic examination as a gold standard. AJR Am J Roentgenol 2004;183(4):1149–57.

21. Kuhl CK, Schrading S, Bieling HB, et al. MRI for diagnosis of pure ductal carcinoma in situ: a prospective observational study. Lancet 2007; 370(9586):485–92.

22. Berg WA, Gutierrez L, NessAiver MS, et al. Diagnostic accuracy of mammography, clinical examination, US, and MR imaging in preoperative assessment of breast cancer. Radiology 2004; 233(3):830–49.

23. Liberman L, Morris EA, Dershaw DD, et al. MR imaging of the ipsilateral breast in women with percutaneously proven breast cancer. AJR Am J Roentgenol 2003;180(4):901–10.

24. Katipamula R, Degnim AC, Hoskin T, et al. Trends in mastectomy rates at the Mayo Clinic Rochester: effect of surgical year and preoperative magnetic resonance imaging. J Clin Oncol 2009;27(25): 4082–8.

25. Morrow M, Schmidt R, Hassett C. Patient selection for breast conservation therapy with magnification mammography. Surgery 1995;118(4):621–6.

26. Morrow M, Jagsi R, Alderman AK, et al. Surgeon recommendations and receipt of mastectomy for treatment of breast cancer. JAMA 2009;302(14): 1551–6.

27. Bleicher RJ, Ciocca RM, Egleston BL, et al. Association of routine pretreatment magnetic resonance imaging with time to surgery, mastectomy rate, and margin status. J Am Coll Surg 2009;209(2): 180–7 [quiz: 294–5].

28. Pengel KE, Loo CE, Teertstra HJ, et al. The impact of preoperative MRI on breast-conserving surgery of invasive cancer: a comparative cohort study. Breast Cancer Res Treat 2009;116(1):161–9.

29. Turnbull LW, Brown SR, Olivier C, et al. Multicentre randomized controlled trial examining the cost-effectiveness of contrast enhanced high field magnetic resonance imaging in women with primary breast cancer scheduled for wide local excision (COMICE). Health Technology Assessment 2010;14(1):1–155.

30. Hwang N, Schiller DE, Crystal P, et al. Magnetic resonance imaging in the planning of initial lumpectomy for invasive breast carcinoma: its effect on ipsilateral breast tumor recurrence after breast-conservation therapy. Ann Surg Oncol 2009;16(11):3000–9.

31. Schiller DE, Le LW, Cho BC, et al. Factors associated with negative margins of lumpectomy specimen: potential use in selecting patients for intraoperative radiotherapy. Ann Surg Oncol 2008;15(3):833–42.

32. Mann RM, Loo CE, Wobbes T, et al. The impact of preoperative breast MRI on the re-excision rate in invasive lobular carcinoma of the breast. Breast Cancer Res Treat 2010;119(2):415–22.

33. Morrow M, Keeney K, Scholtens D, et al. Selecting patients for breast-conserving therapy: the importance of lobular histology. Cancer 2006;106(12): 2563–8.

34. Schouten van der Velden AP, Boetes C, Bult P, et al. Magnetic resonance imaging in size assessment of invasive breast carcinoma with an extensive intraductal component. BMC Med Imaging 2009;9:5.

35. Van Goethem M, Schelfout K, Kersschot E, et al. MR mammography is useful in the preoperative locoregional staging of breast carcinomas with extensive intraductal component. Eur J Radiol 2007;62(2):273–82.

36. Wasif N, Garreau J, Terando A, et al. MRI versus ultrasonography and mammography for preoperative assessment of breast cancer. Am Surg 2009; 75(10):970–5.

37. Grimsby GM, Gray R, Dueck A, et al. Is there concordance of invasive breast cancer pathologic tumor size with magnetic resonance imaging? Am J Surg 2009;198(4):500–4.

38. Pettit K, Swatske ME, Gao F, et al. The impact of breast MRI on surgical decision-making: are patients at risk for mastectomy? J Surg Oncol 2009;100(7):553–8.

39. King TA, Sakr R, Gurevich I, et al. Clinical management factors contribute to the decision for contralateral prophylactic mastectomy. Cancer Res 2009;69(Suppl 24):494s #38.

40. Clarke M, Collins R, Darby S, et al. Effects of radiotherapy and of differences in the extent of surgery for early breast cancer on local recurrence and 15-year survival: an overview of the randomised trials. Lancet 2005;366(9503):2087–106.

41. Fischer U, Zachariae O, Baum F, et al. The influence of preoperative MRI of the breasts on recurrence rate in patients with breast cancer. Eur Radiol 2004;14(10):1725–31.

42. Solin LJ, Orel SG, Hwang WT, et al. Relationship of breast magnetic resonance imaging to outcome

after breast-conservation treatment with radiation for women with early-stage invasive breast carcinoma or ductal carcinoma in situ. J Clin Oncol 2008;26(3):386–91.

43. Nguyen PL, Taghian AG, Katz MS, et al. Breast cancer subtype approximated by estrogen receptor, progesterone receptor, and HER-2 is associated with local and distant recurrence after breast-conserving therapy. J Clin Oncol 2008; 26(14):2373–8.

44. Kyndi M, Sorensen FB, Knudsen H, et al. Estrogen receptor, progesterone receptor, HER-2, and response to postmastectomy radiotherapy in high-risk breast cancer: the Danish Breast Cancer Cooperative Group. J Clin Oncol 2008; 26(9):1419–26.

45. Gao X, Fisher SG, Emami B. Risk of second primary cancer in the contralateral breast in women treated for early-stage breast cancer: a population-based study. Int J Radiat Oncol Biol Phys 2003; 56(4):1038–45.

46. Lehman CD, Gatsonis C, Kuhl CK, et al. MRI evaluation of the contralateral breast in women with recently diagnosed breast cancer. N Engl J Med 2007;356(13):1295–303.

47. Cody HS 3rd. Routine contralateral breast biopsy: helpful or irrelevant? Experience in 871 patients, 1979–1993. Ann Surg 1997;225(4):370–6.

48. Pressman PI. Selective biopsy of the opposite breast. Cancer 1986;57(3):577–80.

49. Early Breast Cancer Trialists' Collaborative Group (EBCTCG). Effects of chemotherapy and hormonal therapy for early breast cancer on recurrence and 15-year survival: an overview of the randomised trials. Lancet 2005;365(9472):1687–717.

50. Brennan ME, Houssami N, Lord S, et al. Magnetic resonance imaging screening of the contralateral breast in women with newly diagnosed breast cancer: systematic review and meta-analysis of incremental cancer detection and impact on surgical management. J Clin Oncol 2009;27(33):5640–9.

51. Sorbero ME, Dick AW, Beckjord EB, et al. Diagnostic breast magnetic resonance imaging and contralateral prophylactic mastectomy. Ann Surg Oncol 2009;16(6):1597–605.

52. Fourquet A, Kirova YM, Campana F. Occult primary cancer with axillary metastases. In: Harris JR, Lippman ME, Morrow M, et al, editors. Diseases of the breast. 4th edition. Philadelphia: Lippincott Williams & Wilkins; 2010. p. 817–21.

53. Ellerbroek N, Holmes F, Singletary E, et al. Treatment of patients with isolated axillary nodal stases from an occult primary carcinoma consistent with breast origin. Cancer 1990;66(7):1461–7.

54. Kemeny MM, Rivera DE, Terz JJ, et al. Occult primary adenocarcinoma with axillary metastases. Am J Surg 1986;152(1):43–7.

55. Buchanan CL, Morris EA, Dorn PL, et al. Utility of breast magnetic resonance imaging in patients with occult primary breast cancer. Ann Surg Oncol 2005;12(12):1045–53.

56. Henry-Tillman RS, Harms SE, Westbrook KC, et al. Role of breast magnetic resonance imaging in determining breast as a source of unknown metastatic lymphadenopathy. Am J Surg 1999;178(6): 496–500.

57. Ko EY, Han BK, Shin JH, et al. Breast MRI for evaluating patients with metastatic axillary lymph node and initially negative mammography and sonography. Korean J Radiol 2007;8(5):382–9.

58. McMahon K, Medoro L, Kennedy D. Breast magnetic resonance imaging: an essential role in malignant axillary lymphadenopathy of unknown origin. Australas Radiol 2005;49(5):382–9.

59. Morris EA, Schwartz LH, Dershaw DD, et al. MR imaging of the breast in patients with occult primary breast carcinoma. Radiology 1997; 205(2):437–40.

60. Olson JA Jr, Morris EA, Van Zee KJ, et al. Magnetic resonance imaging facilitates breast conservation for occult breast cancer. Ann Surg Oncol 2000; 7(6):411–5.

61. Orel SG, Weinstein SP, Schnall MD, et al. Breast MR imaging in patients with axillary node stases and unknown primary malignancy. Radiology 1999;212(2):543–9.

62. de Bresser J, de Vos B, van der Ent F, et al. Breast MRI in clinically and mammographically occult breast cancer presenting with an axillary metastasis: a systematic review. Eur J Surg Oncol 2010;36(2):114–9.

63. Varadarajan R, Edge SB, Yu J, et al. Prognosis of occult breast carcinoma presenting as isolated axillary nodal metastasis. Oncology 2006;71(5–6): 456–9.

64. Smith BD, Smith GL, Roberts KB, et al. Baseline utilization of breast radiotherapy before institution of the Medicare practice quality reporting initiative. Int J Radiat Oncol Biol Phys 2009;74(5): 1506–12.

65. Katz SJ, Lantz PM, Janz NK, et al. Patient involvement in surgery treatment decisions for breast cancer. J Clin Oncol 2005;23(24):5526–33.

66. Katz SJ, Lantz PM, Janz NK, et al. Patterns and correlates of local therapy for women with ductal carcinoma-in-situ. J Clin Oncol 2005;23(13): 3001–7.

67. Arthur DW, Koo D, Zwicker RD, et al. Partial breast brachytherapy after lumpectomy: low-dose-rate and high-dose-rate experience. Int J Radiat Oncol Biol Phys 2003;56(3):681–9.

68. Chen PY, Wallace M, Mitchell C, et al. Four-year efficacy, cosmesis, and toxicity using three-dimensional conformal external beam radiation therapy to

deliver accelerated partial breast irradiation. Int J Radiat Oncol Biol Phys 2009. [Epub ahead of print].

69. Kuske RR, Winter K, Arthur DW. A phase II trial of brachytherapy alone following lumpectomy for stage I or II breast cancer: initial outcomes of RTOG 9517. (A565). J Clin Oncol 2004;22(Suppl 14):18s.

70. Wazer DE, Berle L, Graham R, et al. Preliminary results of a phase I/II study of HDR brachytherapy alone for T1/T2 breast cancer. Int J Radiat Oncol Biol Phys 2002;53(4):889–97.

71. Tendulkar RD, Chellman-Jeffers M, Rybicki LA, et al. Preoperative breast magnetic resonance imaging in early breast cancer: implications for partial breast irradiation. Cancer 2009;115(8): 1621–30.

72. Al-Hallaq HA, Mell LK, Bradley JA, et al. Magnetic resonance imaging identifies multifocal and multicentric disease in breast cancer patients who are eligible for partial breast irradiation. Cancer 2008; 113(9):2408–14.

73. Godinez J, Gombos EC, Chikarmane SA, et al. Breast MRI in the evaluation of eligibility for accelerated partial breast irradiation. AJR Am J Roentgenol 2008;191(1):272–7.

74. Smith BD, Arthur DW, Buchholz TA, et al. Accelerated partial breast irradiation consensus statement from the American Society for Radiation Oncology (ASTRO). Int J Radiat Oncol Biol Phys 2009; 74(4):987–1001.

75. Kaufmann M, von Minckwitz G, Smith R, et al. International expert panel on the use of primary (preoperative) systemic treatment of operable breast cancer: review and recommendations. J Clin Oncol 2003;21(13):2600–8.

76. Bear HD, Anderson S, Brown A, et al. The effect on tumor response of adding sequential preoperative docetaxel to preoperative doxorubicin and cyclophosphamide: preliminary results from National Surgical Adjuvant Breast and Bowel Project Protocol B-27. J Clin Oncol 2003;21(22):4165–74.

77. Buzdar AU, Valero V, Ibrahim NK, et al. Neoadjuvant therapy with paclitaxel followed by 5-fluorouracil, epirubicin, and cyclophosphamide chemotherapy and concurrent trastuzumab in human epidermal growth factor receptor 2-positive operable breast cancer: an update of the initial randomized study population and data of additional patients treated with the same regimen. Clin Cancer Res 2007;13(1):228–33.

78. Chagpar AB, Middleton LP, Sahin AA, et al. Accuracy of physical examination, ultrasonography, and mammography in predicting residual pathologic tumor size in patients treated with neoadjuvant chemotherapy. Ann Surg 2006;243(2):257–64.

79. Peintinger F, Kuerer HM, Anderson K, et al. Accuracy of the combination of mammography and sonography in predicting tumor response in breast cancer patients after neoadjuvant chemotherapy. Ann Surg Oncol 2006;13(11):1443–9.

80. Belli P, Costantini M, Malaspina C, et al. MRI accuracy in residual disease evaluation in breast cancer patients treated with neoadjuvant chemotherapy. Clin Radiol 2006;61(11):946–53.

81. Bhattacharyya M, Ryan D, Carpenter R, et al. Using MRI to plan breast-conserving surgery following neoadjuvant chemotherapy for early breast cancer. Br J Cancer 2008;98(2):289–93.

82. Prati R, Minami CA, Gornbein JA, et al. Accuracy of clinical evaluation of locally advanced breast cancer in patients receiving neoadjuvant chemotherapy. Cancer 2009;115(6):1194–202.

83. Rosen EL, Blackwell KL, Baker JA, et al. Accuracy of MRI in the detection of residual breast cancer after neoadjuvant chemotherapy. AJR Am J Roentgenol 2003;181(5):1275–82.

84. Segara D, Krop IE, Garber JE, et al. Does MRI predict pathologic tumor response in women with breast cancer undergoing preoperative chemotherapy? J Surg Oncol 2007;96(6): 474–80.

85. Abraham DC, Jones RC, Jones SE, et al. Evaluation of neoadjuvant chemotherapeutic response of locally advanced breast cancer by magnetic resonance imaging. Cancer 1996;78(1):91–100.

86. Gilles R, Guinebretiere JM, Toussaint C, et al. Locally advanced breast cancer: contrast-enhanced subtraction MR imaging of response to preoperative chemotherapy. Radiology 1994; 191(3):633–8.

87. Julius T, Kemp SE, Kneeshaw PJ, et al. MRI and conservative treatment of locally advanced breast cancer. Eur J Surg Oncol 2005;31(10):1129–34.

88. Yeh E, Slanetz P, Kopans DB, et al. Prospective comparison of mammography, sonography, and MRI in patients undergoing neoadjuvant chemotherapy for palpable breast cancer. AJR Am J Roentgenol 2005;184(3):868–77.

89. Chen JH, Feig B, Agrawal G, et al. MRI evaluation of pathological complete response and residual tumors in breast cancer after neoadjuvant chemotherapy. Cancer 2008;112(1):17–26.

90. Partridge SC, Gibbs JE, Lu Y, et al. Accuracy of MR imaging for revealing residual breast cancer in patients who have undergone neoadjuvant chemotherapy. AJR Am J Roentgenol 2002; 179(5):1193–9.

91. Rieber A, Brambs HJ, Gabelmann A, et al. Breast MRI for monitoring response of primary breast cancer to neo-adjuvant chemotherapy. Eur Radiol 2002;12(7):1711–9.

92. Chen JH, Feig BA, Hsiang DJ, et al. Impact of MRI-evaluated neoadjuvant chemotherapy response on change of surgical recommendation in breast cancer. Ann Surg 2009;249(3):448–54.

93. Loo CE, Teertstra HJ, Rodenhuis S, et al. Dynamic contrast-enhanced MRI for prediction of breast cancer response to neoadjuvant chemotherapy: initial results. AJR Am J Roentgenol 2008;191(5):1331–8.

94. Pickles MD, Manton DJ, Lowry M, et al. Prognostic value of pre-treatment DCE-MRI parameters in predicting disease free and overall survival for breast cancer patients undergoing neoadjuvant chemotherapy. Eur J Radiol 2009;71(3):498–505.

95. Iacconi C, Giannelli M, Marini C, et al. The role of mean diffusivity (MD) as a predictive index of the response to chemotherapy in locally advanced breast cancer: a preliminary study. Eur Radiol 2010;20(2):303–8.

96. Esserman L, Kaplan E, Partridge S, et al. MRI phenotype is associated with response to doxorubicin and cyclophosphamide neoadjuvant chemotherapy in stage III breast cancer. Ann Surg Oncol 2001;8(6):549–59.

97. van Tienhoven G, Voogd AC, Peterse JL, et al. Prognosis after treatment for loco-regional recurrence after mastectomy or breast conserving therapy in two randomised trials (EORTC 10801 and DBCG-82TM). EORTC Breast Cancer Cooperative Group and the Danish Breast Cancer Cooperative Group. Eur J Cancer 1999;35(1):32–8.

98. Voogd AC, van Tienhoven G, Peterse HL, et al. Local recurrence after breast conservation therapy for early stage breast carcinoma: detection, treatment, and outcome in 266 patients. Dutch Study Group on Local Recurrence after Breast Conservation (BORST). Cancer 1999;85(2):437–46.

99. Gage I, Schnitt SJ, Recht A, et al. Skin recurrences after breast-conserving therapy for early-stage breast cancer. J Clin Oncol 1998; 16(2):480–6.

100. Fisher ER, Anderson S, Redmond C, et al. Ipsilateral breast tumor recurrence and survival following lumpectomy and irradiation: pathological findings from NSABP protocol B-06. Semin Surg Oncol 1992;8(3):161–6.

101. Veronesi U, Marubini E, Del Vecchio M, et al. Local recurrences and distant metastases after conservative breast cancer treatments: partly independent events. J Natl Cancer Inst 1995; 87(1):19–27.

102. Galper S, Blood E, Gelman R, et al. Prognosis after local recurrence after conservative surgery and radiation for early-stage breast cancer. Int J Radiat Oncol Biol Phys 2005;61(2):348–57.

103. Kurtz JM, Jacquemier J, Amalric R, et al. Is breast conservation after local recurrence feasible? Eur J Cancer 1991;27(3):240–4.

104. Salvadori B, Veronesi U. Conservative methods for breast cancer of small size: the experience of the National Cancer Institute, Milan (1973–1998). Breast 1999;8(6):311–4.

105. Millar EK, Graham PH, O'Toole SA, et al. Prediction of local recurrence, distant metastases, and death after breast-conserving therapy in early-stage invasive breast cancer using a five-biomarker panel. J Clin Oncol 2009;27(28):4701–8.

106. Fortin A, Larochelle M, Laverdiere J, et al. Local failure is responsible for the decrease in survival for patients with breast cancer treated with conservative surgery and postoperative radiotherapy. J Clin Oncol 1999;17(1):101–9.

107. Fourquet A, Campana F, Zafrani B, et al. Prognostic factors of breast recurrence in the conservative management of early breast cancer: a 25-year follow-up. Int J Radiat Oncol Biol Phys 1989; 17(4):719–25.

MR Imaging in the Evaluation of Equivocal Clinical and Imaging Findings of the Breast

Jessica W.T. Leung, MD

KEYWORDS

- Breast • Breast cancer • Mammography
- MR imaging • Magnetic resonance

Mammography, sonography, and magnetic resonance (MR) imaging are established imaging modalities for detecting breast cancer. While MR imaging is known to be a sensitive method for depicting breast cancer, its precise range of clinical applications remains controversial, especially in the era of cost containment. The costs of MR imaging include not only the scan itself but also the downstream costs of evaluating incidental lesions and false-positive results, leading to financial costs, patient anxiety, and potential morbidity from biopsy and intravenous gadolinium administration. A meta-analysis of 44 studies supported the commonly accepted notion that breast MR imaging is associated with a high sensitivity but relatively limited specificity.[1] Nevertheless, MR imaging tends to have a higher negative predictive value than conventional breast imaging studies, such as mammography and ultrasound.[2]

It is important to define the appropriate applications of MR imaging in breast imaging to optimize its clinical use. In 2008, the American College of Radiology published guidelines for clinical applications of breast MR imaging.[3] These guidelines include:

1. Screening of high-risk patients, the contralateral breast in patients with recent diagnosis of breast cancer, and patients with augmented or reconstructed breasts.

2. Defining extent of disease after diagnosis of invasive carcinoma and/or ductal carcinoma in situ (DCIS), including relationship of disease to the fascia, pectoralis major, serratus anterior, and/or intercostals muscles, residual disease in patients after lumpectomy with positive margins, and monitoring of neoadjuvant chemotherapy patients.

3. Additional evaluation of clinical or imaging findings, including tumor recurrence at lumpectomy site, metastatic axillary lymphadenopathy of unknown primary, lesion characterization when mammography, ultrasound, and physical examination findings are equivocal and biopsy is not possible, and suspected tumor in reconstructed breast.

A similar consensus document was published in Europe in 2007.[4] This group specifically contended that MR imaging should not be used as a diagnostic tool in the setting of equivocal findings at conventional imaging if biopsy (especially percutaneous core biopsy) could be performed for tissue diagnosis.

This review focuses on the use of MR imaging in the additional evaluation of clinical or imaging findings. In the setting of a worrisome or suspicious clinical or imaging finding where biopsy is possible, it is well accepted that MR imaging cannot negate the need for biopsy.[3–9] However,

Breast Health Center, California Pacific Medical Center, 3698 California Street, 2nd Floor, San Francisco, CA 94118, USA
E-mail address: leungjw@sutterhealth.org

Magn Reson Imaging Clin N Am 18 (2010) 295–308
doi:10.1016/j.mric.2010.02.012

MR imaging may be useful in solving remaining questions after thorough assessment using mammography and sonography, especially when biopsy is not technically possible. Such use falls into 2 categories:

1. Clinical problems that cannot be sufficiently addressed with conventional imaging methods such as mammography and ultrasound.
2. Imaging findings that are indeterminate despite thorough evaluation.

A high negative predictive value is the underlying premise for this use of MR imaging.[6,10–12] In other words, even when MR imaging does not provide a specific answer, it may be used to exclude malignancy in many circumstances. To realize the high negative predictive value of MR imaging, radiologists must optimize all MR imaging parameters, including imaging equipment and technique, interpretation criteria, and correlation with mammography and ultrasound.[13]

CLINICAL SYMPTOMS

At this time, MR imaging has a limited role in the evaluation of clinical symptoms in the absence of suspicious imaging findings, with the exception of assessing patients who present with nipple discharge.

Palpable Lump

A palpable lump is a very common clinical complaint. Although most palpable lumps do not represent breast cancer, it is the most common clinical symptom of breast cancer. Therefore, it is important to properly evaluate palpable lumps, both to diagnose breast cancer in a timely fashion and to accomplish this goal in a cost-effective manner. In the setting of a clinically significant palpable lump, diagnostic mammography and ultrasound should be performed as the initial examinations.[10,14] The combination of properly performed diagnostic mammography and ultrasound carries a very high negative predictive value (nearly 100%).[15–17] In the setting of a suspicious imaging finding or persistent clinical suspicion (despite lack of an imaging correlate), tissue diagnosis via percutaneous core biopsy is often performed.[14,18] Although MR imaging may depict the palpable lump in question, diagnostic mammography and ultrasound are more efficacious and cost-effective methods for evaluation. The American College of Radiology (ACR) Appropriateness Criteria rated MR imaging as very low in appropriateness in the initial evaluation of palpable breast masses.[14] On a scale of 1 to 9

(1 = least appropriate; 9 = most appropriate), MR imaging was given a rating of 1, whereas diagnostic mammography and ultrasound were each given a rating of 9.

Breast Pain

Although pain (both focal and diffuse) is the most common breast complaint, there are no data to support the use of MR imaging for evaluation of this symptom, especially in the absence of a palpable lump or other clinical findings of breast cancer. Unilateral, focal, noncyclical pain is of greater clinical concern than bilateral, diffuse, cyclical pain that waxes and wanes with the menstrual cycle, which is almost always benign. A study of 110 targeted ultrasound examinations in 99 patients who presented with focal breast pain (in the absence of an associated palpable finding) did not reveal any cancers.[19] It was concluded that ultrasound (and perhaps other imaging studies) is most useful for patient reassurance in this setting, rather than for diagnosis of breast cancer. Similarly, MR imaging has no particular role in evaluating patients with breast pain, particularly given its high costs and relatively limited specificity.

Nipple Discharge

Of all clinical symptoms in the breast, pathologic nipple discharge is the symptom with the best documented diagnostic role for MR imaging. Investigators have advocated this use of MR imaging because of its high diagnostic performance, even when conventional imaging modalities are negative.[6,9,20–24] At the Consensus Conference of the Congress "Attualita in Senologia" in 2007, the Italian scientific societies supported this use of MR imaging when mammography, ultrasound, and galactography results are negative or ambiguous.[4]

Nipple discharge is most significant when it is bloody (serosanguinous) or spontaneous.[25–27] In the majority of cases, even if bloody and spontaneous, nipple discharge stems from a benign cause. Most (80%–90%) cases of nipple discharge result from ductal ectasia and/or papillomas.[28] Although invasive, surgical duct exploration remains the definitive method of evaluation.[25] Imaging studies are primarily performed to establish or exclude the presence of lesions (both benign and malignant). Exact diagnosis at imaging is often not possible because many lesions have overlapping, nonspecific imaging findings.

The optimal imaging workup protocol for nipple discharge remains controversial. Galactography has traditionally been performed. However, this requires duct cannulation and may be both techni-cally challenging, with up to 10% failure rates even when performed by experienced practitioners,[29] and uncomfortable for the patient. Furthermore, the diagnostic information that this study yields may be limiting. The reported sensitivities of galac-tography for cancer ranged between 0% and 55%.[30–32] Although preoperative wire localization is possible,[33] it remains technically challenging. In up to 20% of cases where galactography re-vealed a lesion, subsequent surgical excision was unsuccessful.[34,35]

In a study of 23 patients with nipple discharge who had undergone MR imaging evaluation, Orel and colleagues[24] found that 73% of the MR imaging findings correlated with pathology and concluded that MR imaging may serve as a nonin-vasive method of duct evaluation (instead of gal-actography). Similarly, Ballesio and colleagues[36] examined 44 patients and reported that MR imaging was able to show the galactographic find-ings. Nakahara and colleagues[23] compared ultra-sound, galactography, and MR imaging in 55 patients and found that MR imaging showed the location and distribution of lesions best, especially in cases of DCIS. Although galactography is sensi-tive in depicting papillomas, MR imaging was found to be better in demonstrating the location and distribution of lesions, particularly important in processes (such as DCIS or papillomatosis) that may extend over a large region (**Fig. 1**).[10,37]

The use of MR imaging in evaluating patients with nipple discharge and negative conventional imaging has also been investigated.[22–24] Speci-ficity remains limited, and differentiation between benign papilloma and malignancy (either invasive or in situ) is usually not possible.[6]

MR imaging galactography is a novel imaging test consisting of indirect and direct MR galactog-raphy. In the former setting, heavily T2-weighted sequences are used,[38] with no contrast agent. Similar to conventional galactography, dilated ducts are seen as tubular structures with high signal intensity. Lesions may be seen as defects in intraductal signal, duct wall irregularity, or ductal obstruction.

Direct MR galactography (also known as MR contrast galactography) requires cannulation of the ducts and injection of contrast agent. In a pilot study of 16 patients,[39] gadopentate dimeglumine (0.1 mL) was mixed with nonionic contrast material (0.9 mL), and the resultant 1-mL solution was in-jected using a 30-gauge needle, on cannulation of the secreting ducts. Three-dimensional gradient-echo fat-saturated turboflash sequences were used for imaging. These same patients also under-went conventional galactography. When

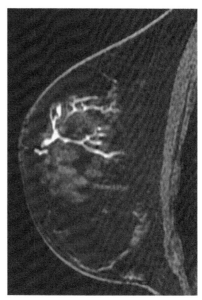

Fig. 1. Three-dimensional, nonenhanced, gradient-echo with fat saturation MR image in the sagittal plane, showing intrinsically hyperintense, branching, tubular structures in a segmental distribution (upper inner quadrant). These findings are consistent with blood with the ducts and may be seen in patients with bloody nipple discharge. MR may be used to reveal or exclude underlying malignancy and demon-strate disease extent. After contrast administration, no abnormal enhancement is seen in this case to suggest malignancy (image not shown). (*Courtesy of* M. Allen Fry, MD, San Francisco, CA.)

compared with surgical and histopathologic results, MR contrast galactography was found to be just as sensitive, but with fewer false positives than conventional galactography.

Schwab and colleagues[40] compared direct MR galactography (using gadopentetate dimeglu-mine), indirect MR galactography, and conven-tional galactography in 23 patients with pathologic nipple discharge. At conventional gal-actography, 57 lesions were identified. Direct MR galactography was more sensitive than indirect galactography when using conventional galactog-raphy results as the gold standard.

Similar to conventional galactography, visuali-zation of the extent of disease is limited with MR galactography (both indirect and direct). There-fore, fusion of MR ductography and MR images of the breasts has been proposed to identify the relationship between the intraductal abnormality and extent of disease.[20]

EQUIVOCAL IMAGING FINDINGS

MR imaging has long been used for additional assessment of indeterminate imaging findings.[41–44]

Nevertheless, this clinical application has been relatively limited, as percutaneous imaging-guided core biopsy is both safe and efficacious,[45] and provides a definitive histologic diagnosis in most cases. However, tissue diagnosis is sometimes not indicated or technically possible. One of the biggest challenges in mammography is the distinction between superimposition of fibroglandular structures (summation artifact) from a true lesion (**Fig. 2**). In other words, one must first determine whether a potential lesion is even real before proceeding farther in the workup. This determination is a prerequisite in biopsy evaluation because biopsy of summation artifact is not indicated. Even when a true lesion is suspected, ideally it should be identified with certainty in 2 projections, preferably orthogonal, before performance of ultrasound or biopsy. Absence of a sonographic correlate or lesion identification in 2 mammographic projections diminishes the likelihood of success of core biopsy and sometimes renders core biopsy technically impossible. Surgical excision is also limited when preoperative wire localization cannot be performed with confidence in 2 mammographic projections.[46]

The question arises as to whether or not MR imaging has a sufficiently high negative predictive value to exclude malignancy when biopsy is not possible. Given the high sensitivity of this modality, high negative predictive values of approximately 98% have been reported.[47,48] These numbers are higher than those reported for other adjunctive breast imaging tests, including nuclear medicine studies of the breasts (positron emission tomography, positron emission mammography, and scintimammography).[49–53] It remains to be demonstrated whether these high negative predictive values reported in single-institution studies from academic centers can be replicated and generalized in the community. An overall negative predictive value of 85.4% was reported in a multi-institutional trial.[8] This number is lower than the traditionally reported negative predictive value of breast MR imaging (usually more than 90%) and likely too low for MR imaging to be used to obviate biopsy. In addition to optimal technique and radiologist interpretation, it appears that case selection is a very important variable in ensuring that MR imaging is of clinical benefit in evaluating equivocal imaging findings.

MR imaging should only be used as a problem-solving tool after full and detailed mammographic assessment.[7] In one of the largest studies to date on the use of MR imaging in evaluating

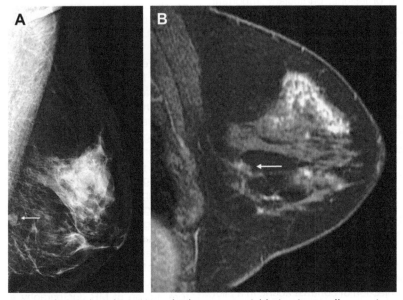

Fig. 2. MR imaging may be used to determine whether a potential lesion is actually superimposition of fibroglandular structures. (*A*) Mammogram in the mediolateral oblique projection showing a round asymmetry in the posterior breast (*arrow*). Despite thorough mammographic assessment, including mammography in the exaggerated craniocaudal lateral and medial projections (not shown), the asymmetry is not identifiable in 2 views. Because lesion location is unknown, the application of ultrasound is limited. (*B*) Three-dimensional, contrast-enhanced gradient-echo with fat saturation MR image in the sagittal plane, showing nonenhancing tissue that correlates to the mammographic one-view asymmetry (*arrow*). (Nonmass enhancement with kinetic features suggesting benignity is seen elsewhere.) Despite its round morphology, the mammographic finding in *A* represents superimposition of fibroglandular structures.

equivocal mammographic findings, Moy and colleagues[11] was careful in the study design to include only cases that had been thoroughly evaluated with supplemental mammographic views (especially when attempting to localize potential lesions in 2 mammographic projections), including true lateral, spot-compression, magnification, rolled or exaggerated craniocaudal, step-oblique views, or a combination of these views.[54,55]

Most lesions and most cancers can be identified in 2 mammographic projections. However, there is a small subset of cancers that are seen only or primarily in one view.[56] The challenge in evaluating one-view-only imaging findings is that malignancy is highly unlikely, but possible. Sickles reviewed 61,273 screening mammography examinations and identified 2023 (3.3%) studies in which findings were prospectively identified in only one standard mammographic projection (mediolateral oblique or craniocaudal). The majority (82.7%) of the cases was considered to represent summation artifact, with this assessment made at either the time of initial screening interpretation (53.7%) or subsequently after recall imaging (29.0%). Of the remaining cases, 36 cancers were identified. Invasive lobular carcinoma was disproportionately represented in this series, constituting 33% of cancers presenting in one view versus 10% of all cancers from the same institution.[56] This trend has also been noted by other investigators.[57]

Diagnostic mammography results in identification of the majority of true lesions (and cancers) in 2 projections. However, there remains a small subset of true lesions (and cancers) that cannot be well visualized in 2 projections despite tailored diagnostic views. Before application of MR imaging in such cases, ultrasound should be part of the initial imaging evaluation. Ultrasound is a very helpful tool in assessing mammographic lesions, particularly in patients with dense breasts.[58–60] However, ultrasound can be limited if the lesion in question has not been identified with certainty in 2 projections.[55,61] In the study by Moy and colleagues,[11] ultrasound was performed as part of the initial imaging evaluation in 72.8% of the study cohort with dense breasts (heterogeneously dense or extremely dense) and 17.6% of those with less dense breasts (scattered fibroglandular densities). In the series of 86 lesions by Lee and colleagues,[12] ultrasound was performed in 47 (55%) of cases. Ultrasound was not performed in the remaining 45% of cases because of the vagueness of the mammographic finding, lack of accuracy in localization, and inability of ultrasound to distinguish between scar and tumor.

Lesion Type

Cancer may be depicted at mammography as mass, calcifications, architectural distortion, or asymmetry. Because case selection is of utmost importance in ensuring the efficacious use of MR imaging in the evaluation of equivocal imaging findings, MR imaging should only be performed in this context for specific lesion types. In general, it is not indicated as a problem-solving modality after identification of mass or calcifications.

Mass

A mass differs from an asymmetry because a mass is a finding that is seen in 2 (or more) projections, characterized by convex outward margins and associated with central density.[62] In many cases, there is a sonographic correlate to the mammographic mass. Biopsy may then be performed using core biopsy (using stereotaxis or ultrasound guidance) or surgical excision (preoperative wire localization may be performed using mammographic or ultrasound guidance) as indicated. Although MR imaging may reveal a correlate to the mammographic mass, it is not indicated because it cannot be used in lieu of a biopsy in most cases. Indeed, the ACR Appropriateness Criteria rated MR imaging as very low in appropriateness in the evaluation of nonpalpable breast masses.[63]

Calcifications

Calcifications may form in breast cancers as a result of dystrophic reaction associated with cell turnover. At the same time, many benign forms of calcifications occur in the breasts. Although linear branching pleomorphic calcifications are characteristic of malignancy, many calcifications are indeterminate,[64] with positive predictive value of malignancy at biopsy of only 21.7% reported in one series.[65] MR imaging has been used in some clinical situations to preclude the need for biopsy, particularly in cases of low-suspicion calcifications, such as amorphous calcifications. However, even in cases of amorphous calcifications the probability of malignancy is 20%.[66]

MR imaging is limited in the additional evaluation of calcifications beyond mammography (using fine-detailed magnification views) because magnetic resonance does not depict calcifications as well as mammography. Furthermore, malignant calcifications are mostly associated with the diagnosis of DCIS rather than invasive cancer,[67] and the sensitivity of MR imaging for DCIS is lower than its sensitivity for invasive cancer, particularly in cases of low-grade DCIS. Therefore, the negative predictive value of MR imaging in the setting of suspicious calcifications at mammography is only approximately 85%, making it insufficient to exclude malignancy.[6] In a multi-institutional Italian trial consisting of 112 cases of calcifications for which biopsy was recommended (assessed as Breast Imaging Reporting and Data System[68] BI-RADS 4, suspicious or BI-RADS 5, highly suggestive of malignancy), the negative predictive value of MR imaging was only 71%.[69] Similarly, in a single-institution study of 55 women with BI-RADS 3 (probably benign), BI-RADS 4 (suspicious), or BI-RADS 5 (highly suggestive of malignancy) calcifications, the reported negative predictive value was 76%.[70]

Therefore, MR imaging cannot be performed as an alternative to biopsy in the setting of suspicious calcifications at mammography. The ACR Appropriateness Criteria rated MR imaging as very low in appropriateness in the evaluation of breast calcifications.[71] After a diagnosis of in-situ cancer is made in the setting of mammographically detected calcifications, MR imaging may play a role in identifying any invasive component and to delineate the extent of disease, especially if DCIS is high grade.[6,72,73]

Architectural distortion

Architectural distortion represents distortion of tissue and may be seen as white lines emanating from a center without a central mass. The most common cause is surgical scarring, but it may result from the desmoplastic reaction that some cancers exert on adjacent tissues. In the absence of a sonographic correlate, management of the finding of architectural distortion may be challenging. Stereotactic-guided core biopsy would be technically challenging, as architectural distortion lacks a central density and may not be identifiable without sufficient compression. Wire-localization surgical excision, besides being invasive, would require confident identification of the finding in 2 (preferably orthogonal) mammographic views.

Benign causes for architectural distortion at mammography include radial scar (complex sclerosing lesion) and sclerosing adenosis.[74] However, in the absence of clinical history that suggests scarring (such as history of surgery), architectural distortion is considered a suspicious finding that requires biopsy (**Fig. 3**). The challenge occurs when it is only identified in one view and when there is no sonographic correlate; biopsy (either core or surgical excision) would not be technically feasible. MR imaging may have a role in such cases, but there are insufficient data currently to support or negate this potential role.

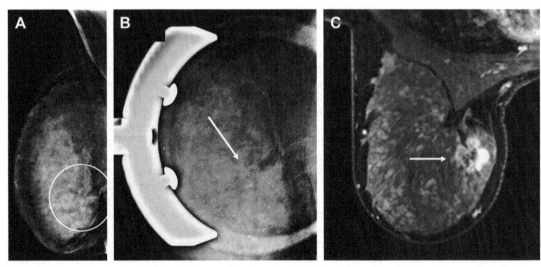

Fig. 3. MR imaging may be used for further evaluation of architectural distortion. MR imaging confirms the presence of a true lesion and reveals its location, allowing for biopsy and diagnosis of invasive ductal carcinoma. (*A*) Mammogram in the mediolateral oblique projection showing an area of architectural distortion (*circle*) in a patient with no history of surgical biopsy or breast trauma. (*B*) Spot-compression magnification mammography in the mediolateral projection showing persistence of architectural distortion (*arrow*). However, this finding could not be localized at mammography in the craniocaudal projection (not shown). Benign-appearing scattered calcifications (unrelated to the finding of architectural distortion) are also present, most of which represent milk-of-calcium. (*C*) Three-dimensional, contrast-enhanced gradient-echo with fat saturation MR image in the axial plane, showing an irregular heterogeneous enhancing mass (*arrow*) in the inner breast. Benign-appearing enhancing foci are seen scattered in the breast. Subsequent core biopsy of the enhancing mass reveals invasive ductal carcinoma. Postbiopsy and clip-placement mammograms confirm that the enhancing mass at MR imaging correlate with the architectural distortion at mammography.

Perfetto and colleagues[74] examined the MR imaging results in 20 patients with focal architectural distortion at mammography. Their study investigated whether or not MR imaging can be used to determine which patients need to proceed to surgical excision (vs imaging follow-up). Twenty-four mammographic lesions were present in these 20 patients. It is unknown whether these mammographic lesions were identified in 1 or 2 views. At mammography, 8 of these 24 mammographic lesions were assessed as BI-RADS 3 (probably benign), 8 as BI-RADS 4 (suspicious), and 8 as BI-RADS 5 (highly suggestive of malignancy). At MR imaging, 24 lesions were identified, 7 of which were cancers. The investigators reported a high negative predictive value (100%) in that no cancers were missed without MR imaging showing malignant features. Although this was a small study, one may infer from its results that MR imaging may play a role in excluding cancer in cases of architectural distortion where biopsy is not technically feasible.

Asymmetry

Mammographic asymmetry differs from a mass in that it is characterized by concave (rather than convex) outward margins and may be interspersed with fat.[61,62,75,76] According to the most current edition of Breast Imaging Reporting and Data System, there are 3 types of asymmetries[65]:

1. Asymmetry (see **Fig. 2**)
2. Global asymmetry
3. Focal asymmetry.

An asymmetry is a finding seen primarily in one view, whereas a focal asymmetry is seen in 2 views. Global asymmetry is diffuse increase in breast tissue in one breast when compared with the other breast. In addition to these 3 types of asymmetries, the term developing asymmetry has been defined as a focal asymmetry that is new or increasing in size or conspicuity when compared with a prior mammographic examination (**Figs. 4 and 5**).[75,76] Of all mammographic lesions, MR imaging has demonstrated the greatest clinical utility in assessing asymmetries (vs mass, calcifications, or architectural distortion).

The probability of malignancy ranges from 12.8% for developing asymmetry[75] to 1.8% for one-view asymmetry[56] to 0% for nonpalpable global asymmetry.[77] The role of MR imaging has only been studied peripherally in studies of asymmetries because these lesions occur infrequently, so an exact role for MR imaging has yet to be established.[75,76] In a study of 311 cases of developing asymmetries obtained from a cohort of 180,801 consecutive screening and 27,330 consecutive diagnostic mammography examinations, MR imaging was performed in only 2 cases.[75] In one case, MR imaging showed non-mass enhancement with plateau kinetics as the correlate to the developing asymmetry, and biopsy revealed pseudoangiomatous stromal hyperplasia. In the second case, MR imaging was negative (with no correlate), and the patient was cancer-free at follow-up.

Empirical Data

To date, there are only a small number of well-controlled studies on the use of MR imaging in resolving equivocal imaging findings, partly because biopsy, rather than MR imaging, is performed in many circumstances.[6] Comparison of the major studies is limited given that each study was designed in a slightly different way and focused on different parameters. Given that the equivocal imaging findings that may benefit from MR imaging occur only infrequently, multi-institutional trials may be necessary with large enough sample sizes to produce results that can be generalized to different centers.

In the 1990s, Orel and colleagues[9] reported the use of MR imaging in assessing one-view mammographic findings or equivocal changes in sites of prior biopsy. Sardanelli and colleagues[78] studied 19 cancers with inconclusive mammographic findings that had been imaged with MR imaging, reported 1 false-negative and 2 false-positive MR imaging examinations, and concluded that MR imaging was helpful.

Lee and colleagues[12] retrospectively identified 86 lesions that were evaluated by MR imaging because of equivocal findings at mammography. Inclusion criteria for this use included:

1. Definite mammographic finding identified but its significance was unclear (n = 26)
2. Inconclusive mammographic finding (with or without addition of ultrasound) as to whether a true lesion existed (n = 20)
3. Suspicious finding identified but its true location was uncertain (n = 16)
4. Possible mammographic change representing tumor recurrence versus posttreatment change in patients who had undergone breast conservation therapy (n = 15)
5. Increased density or distortion at site of prior benign biopsy (n = 9).

Of these 86 lesions, 58 (67%) were breast asymmetries, and 28 (33%) were cases of architectural distortion.

Contrast-enhanced MR imaging using 1.5-Tesla magnet was performed. The earlier examinations

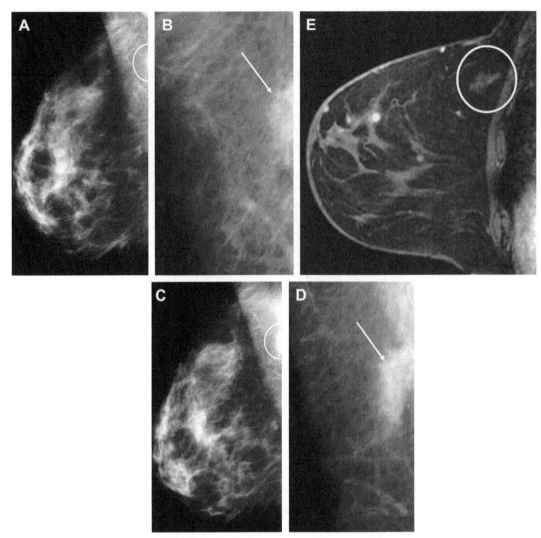

Fig. 4. MR imaging may be used for further evaluation of developing asymmetry. In most cases, MR imaging is used to exclude malignancy and not necessarily to reveal etiology of the mammographic finding. In this case, MR imaging reveals a direct correlate (focus of fibroglandular tissue) that correlates with the mammographic finding. It is benign because it does not enhance. (*A*) Baseline mammogram in the mediolateral oblique projection showing an asymmetry in the upper posterior breast at edge of the image (*circle*). (*B*) Photographic enlargement of the asymmetry in **Fig. 3A** showing an irregular margin. (*C*) One year later, mammogram in the mediolateral oblique projection showing that the same asymmetry is more prominent, suggesting the presence of a developing asymmetry (*circle*). (*D*) Photographic enlargement of the asymmetry in **Fig. 3C** showing the increase in size and margin irregularity since baseline mammogram (*arrow*). (*E*) Three-dimensional, contrast-enhanced gradient-echo with fat saturation MR image in the sagittal plane, showing nonenhancing tissue in the upper posterior breast adjacent to the pectoralis muscle (*circle*) corresponding to the mammographic finding.

during the study period were performed using a 2-dimensional spin echo sequence; the later examinations were performed using a 3-dimensional fast spoiled gradient sequence with fat suppression. MR imaging was considered positive if focal enhancement (either mass or nonmass) was identified. MR imaging was considered negative if there was no enhancement, or if enhancement was either diffuse and uniform or similar to that of background parenchyma. The MR imaging finding was considered a correlate if it accounted for the mammographic finding based on location; otherwise, it was considered an incidental finding. Twenty-six (30%) correlates were identified at MR imaging, along with 12 incidental lesions. All 26 correlates were biopsied, and 9 cancers were diagnosed. No cancer was identified in the remaining 60 mammographic lesions that had no

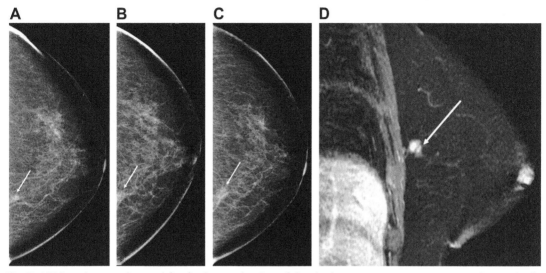

Fig. 5. MR imaging may be used for further evaluation of developing asymmetry. An asymmetry is seen in the medial posterior breast. The asymmetry appears to increase over the course of 2 years, but it is uncertain that the apparent increase is real (vs inclusion of additional tissues). Absence of identification of this finding in the second mammographic projection limits the utility of ultrasound. MR imaging reveals an enhancing correlate, and biopsy shows invasive ductal carcinoma. (A) Baseline mammogram in the craniocaudal projection showing an asymmetry in the inner posterior breast at edge of the image (arrow). (B) One year later, mammogram in the craniocaudal oblique projection showing that the same asymmetry is more prominent, suggesting the presence of a developing asymmetry (arrow). (C) Two years later, mammogram in the craniocaudal oblique projection showing that the same asymmetry is even more prominent, confirming the presence of a developing asymmetry (arrow). (D) Three-dimensional, contrast-enhanced gradient-echo with fat saturation MR image in the sagittal plane, showing a round homogeneous enhancing mass with dark septations (arrow) in the posterior breast, corresponding to the developing asymmetry at mammography. Although dark septations may be present in fibroadenoma, subsequent core biopsy of the enhancing mass reveals invasive ductal carcinoma. Postbiopsy and clip-placement mammograms confirm that the enhancing mass at MR imaging correlate with the developing asymmetry at mammography.

correlate at MR imaging, 6 of which were excised with benign results, and 54 of which were stable at mammographic follow-up (mean, 19 months).

The largest series on the use of MR imaging in evaluating equivocal imaging findings was published in 2009.[11] Moy and colleagues[11] retrospectively reviewed 115 MR imaging examinations that were performed after inconclusive mammographic findings: asymmetries without associated microcalcifications (n = 98, 85.2%), architectural distortion (n = 12, 10.4%), and change at prior benign biopsy site (n = 5, 4.3%). MR imaging was performed using T1-weighted fat-suppressed 3-dimensional fast spoiled recalled echo sequence. No suspicious MR imaging correlate was present in 100 (87%) of 115 cases. These negative cases were stable at imaging (either mammography or MR imaging) follow-up, with mean follow-up interval of 34 months. In 15 (13%) of the 115 cases, enhancing masses were identified that corresponded to the mammographic finding. At biopsy, 6 of the 15 masses were malignant. Of these 6 cancers, 4 were seen in one mammographic

view only. Although none were identified at initial ultrasound, 2 of the 6 cancers were identified at second-look ultrasound. When compared with mammography, MR imaging had a higher specificity (91.7% vs 80.7%, P = .029), positive predictive value (40% vs 8.7%, P = .032), and accuracy (92.2% vs 78.3%, P = .0052). Because MR imaging identified all 6 cancers, its sensitivity in this series was 100%.

In contrast to the study by Lee and colleagues,[12] Moy and colleagues[11] excluded cases of mammographic changes at the lumpectomy site because the utility of MR imaging for differentiating tumor recurrence versus surgical scar had already been proven by other published studies. Also excluded were suspicious lesions amenable to mammographic or sonographic localization for biopsy, suspicious calcifications, and questionable findings correlating with palpable lumps. In other words, the study by Moy and colleagues[11] sought to address the utility of MR imaging in evaluating equivocal imaging questions in a cohort in which biopsy was not possible.

Surgical Scar

Surgical scars are often associated with spiculation and tissue distortion at mammography, making it difficult to distinguish from tumor, either recurrent after lumpectomy, or new in a site of prior benign surgical biopsy. Ultrasound is often challenging as well, as scars are often associated with significant posterior acoustic shadowing and variable echogenicity and may mimic cancers.[12] Clinical examination is also of limited utility because scarring and tumor may not be discernible when the clinical presentation is induration and palpable thickening.

On the other hand, MR imaging is particularly useful for distinguishing scar tissue from recurrent tumor (**Fig. 6**).[43,79–83] This is one area, among the various equivocal imaging findings, where MR imaging has been proven to be of significant clinical use. If performed and interpreted properly, MR imaging is both sensitive and specific in distinguishing recurrent tumor from surgical scar.[6,9,84,85] Optimal technique is required for this distinction, as kinetic evaluation plays

a significant role. In a study of 20 women with suspected tumor recurrence after breast conservation surgery, Kerslake and colleagues[80] found that benign scars enhance slowly and less strongly, whereas tumor recurrence demonstrated rapid, early, and avid enhancement.

Of note, MR imaging is limited in specificity in the early time period after treatment, defined as within 6 months of surgery and 9 months of radiation therapy in one series,[81] as enhancement related to treatment may result in false-positive results.[79] Using a greater than 75% increase in signal intensity within the first minute after injection of contrast as a cutoff point in 67 lumpectomy patients, Muuller and colleagues[82] found that MR imaging demonstrated tumor recurrence with sensitivity of nearly 100% and specificity of greater than 90% when patients are imaged more than 12 months after completion of therapy. Although specificities are decreased within the first year after therapy, these investigators nevertheless found MR imaging to be a helpful clinical tool. Others contend that if performed using optimal technique and interpreted by

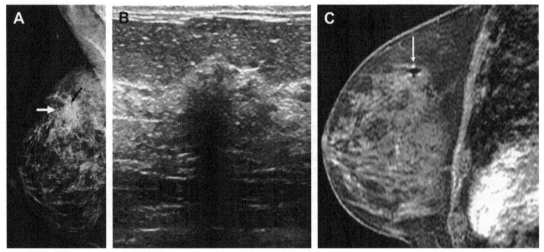

Fig. 6. MR imaging may be used to distinguish between surgical scar and tumor recurrence in breast conservation therapy patients with mammographic changes at the site of surgery. (*A*) Mammogram in the mediolateral oblique projection showing an irregular asymmetry in the upper breast (*white arrow*) in a patient with history of breast conservation surgery. The asymmetry appears larger and more irregular than at prior mammograms (not shown). A surgical clip (*black arrow*) is present in the asymmetry. Differential includes surgical scar versus tumor recurrence. (*B*) Sonogram of the corresponding region shows an irregular hypoechoic mass with posterior acoustic shadowing. Differential remains surgical scar versus tumor recurrence. Ultrasound-guided core biopsy may be performed. However, if pathology shows surgical scar only, the possibility of sampling error and imaging-histologic discordance persists. (*C*) Three-dimensional, contrast-enhanced gradient-echo with fat saturation MR image in the sagittal plane, showing a signal void (*arrow*) that corresponds to the surgical clip seen at mammography. When compared with the corresponding nonenhanced MR image (not shown), no enhancement is identified to represent tumor recurrence. The heart shows robust enhancement, compatible with intravenous contrast administration. Given the high sensitivity of MR imaging, the lack of enhancement is strong evidence in the exclusion of tumor recurrence.

experienced radiologists, MR imaging may be performed even early after surgery or radiation therapy without compromise in diagnostic performance.[85]

LIMITATIONS

MR imaging may be useful in the evaluation of equivocal imaging findings because of its high sensitivity and negative predictive value. However, it is relatively low in specificity. The resultant false-positive results associated with MR imaging must be considered, as they increase the costs of MR imaging and thereby limit its clinical utility. Although this limitation is present in breast MR imaging in general, it is particularly significant when MR imaging is used to evaluate equivocal imaging findings because of the low likelihood of malignancy in the setting of such findings.[56,76] Stringent and prudent case selection is vital to ensure that MR imaging is properly used as an adjunctive diagnostic imaging modality when conventional imaging is inconclusive.

Incidental enhancing lesions are fairly common at MR imaging of the breast, with reported rates of 25% to 29%.[86,87] The likelihood of cancer is higher if there is a malignancy elsewhere in the breast.[87] In the study of 86 equivocal mammographic lesions by Lee and colleagues,[12] 12 (14%) incidental enhancing lesions were identified, 1 of which was malignant (18-mm invasive ductal carcinoma) at biopsy. However, a developing asymmetry that corresponded to this incidental enhancing MR lesion was visible on retrospective review of the mammograms. In the study of 115 equivocal mammographic lesions by Moy and colleagues,[11] 18 (16%) incidental enhancing lesions were identified. These 18 lesions were further evaluated with mammography and ultrasound, after which 14 lesions were biopsied (10 benign, 4 atypia) and 4 were followed with imaging for 2 years, all without evidence of malignancy.

Another limitation is the relatively subjective nature of MR imaging interpretation and the occasional challenge in correlating the equivocal mammographic lesion with MR imaging enhancement. Proper use of MR imaging in the context of resolving equivocal mammographic findings requires the ability to interpret both mammography and MR imaging, coupled with experience in breast imaging.[11,12] It is important to review the mammography finding at the time of MR imaging interpretation.[12]

Finally, it must be borne in mind that the high negative predictive value of MR imaging can only be achieved with stringent technical standards.

Despite the high sensitivity of MR imaging, false negatives have been reported for DCIS and invasive carcinoma (both ductal and lobular subtypes).[88,89]

SUMMARY

MR imaging of the breast has become increasingly available in recent years but remains an expensive test. In addition to the financial expense of MR imaging, the downstream costs of incidental lesions and false positives, patient anxiety, and potential morbidity need to be considered. MR imaging has no particular role in assessing patients with palpable lump or breast pain while it may contribute to the clinical management of patients with nipple discharge. MR imaging should only be performed after a thorough workup with mammography and ultrasound has been performed. MR imaging is not indicated in assessing mass or calcifications but is primarily reserved for asymmetries and architectural distortion, especially if they are seen in only one mammographic projection and biopsy is not technically feasible. The high negative predictive value of MR imaging in these settings can only be achieved with strict technical standards and proper image interpretation. Appropriate case selection is of utmost importance in the successful clinical implementation of breast MR imaging in the evaluation of equivocal clinical and imaging findings.

REFERENCES

1. Peters NH, Borel Rinkes IH, Zuithoff NP, et al. Meta-analysis of MR imaging in the diagnosis of breast lesions. Radiology 2008;246(1):116–24.

2. Vassiou K, Kanavou T, Vlychou M, et al. Characterization of breast lesions with CE-MR multimodal morphological and kinetic analysis: comparison with conventional mammography and high-resolution ultrasound. Eur J Radiol 2009;70(1):69–76.

3. ACR practice guideline for the performance of contrast-enhanced magnetic resonance imaging (MRI) of the breast. Available at: http://www.acr.org/SecondaryMainMenuCategories/quality_safety/guidelines/breast/mri_breast.aspx. Accessed February 5, 2010.

4. Sardanelli F, Giuseppetti GM, Canavese G, et al. Indications for breast magnetic resonance imaging. Consensus document "Attualita in senologia" Florence 2007. Radiol Med 2008;113(8):1085–95.

5. DeMartini W, Lehman C. A review of current evidence-based clinical applications for breast magnetic resonance imaging. Top Magn Reson Imaging 2008;19(3):143–50.

6. Kuhl CK. Current status of breast MR imaging. Part 2: clinical applications. Radiology 2007;244(3): 672–91.

7. Lee CH. Problem solving MR imaging of the breast. Radiol Clin North Am 2004;42(5):919–34.

8. Bluemke DA, Gatsonis CA, Chen MH, et al. Magnetic resonance imaging of the breast prior to biopsy. JAMA 2004;292(22):2735–42.

9. Orel SG, Hochman MG, Schnall MD, et al. High-resolution MR imaging of the breast: clinical context. Radiographics 1996;16(6):1385–401.

10. Van Goethem M, Verslegers I, Biltjes I, et al. Role of MRI of the breast in the evaluation of the symptomatic patient. Curr Opin Obstet Gynecol 2009;21(1): 74–9.

11. Moy L, Elias K, Patel V, et al. Is breast MRI helpful in the evaluation of inconclusive mammographic findings? AJR Am J Roentgenol 2009; 193(4):986–93.

12. Lee CH, Smith RC, Levine JA, et al. Clinical usefulness of MR imaging of the breast in the evaluation of the problematic mammogram. AJR Am J Roentgenol 1999;173(5):1323–9.

13. Schnall M, Orel S. Breast MR imaging in the diagnostic setting. Magn Reson Imaging Clin N Am 2006;14(3):329–37.

14. American College of Radiology ACR Appropriateness criteria—palpable breast masses. Available at: http://www.acr.org/SecondaryMainMenuCategories/quality_safety/app_criteria/pdf/ExpertPanelonWomensImaging BreastWorkGroup/PalpableBreastMassesDoc3.aspx. Accessed February 5, 2010.

15. Soo MS, Rosen EL, Baker JA, et al. Negative predictive value of sonography with mammography in patients with palpable breast lesions. AJR Am J Roentgenol 2001;177(5):1167–70.

16. Shetty MK, Shah YP, Sharman RS. Prospective evaluation of the value of combined mammographic and sonographic assessment in patients with palpable abnormalities of the breast. J Ultrasound Med 2003;22(3):263–8.

17. Moy L, Slanetz PJ, Moore R, et al. Specificity of mammography and US in the evaluation of a palpable abnormality: retrospective review. Radiology 2002;225(1):176–81.

18. Hazard HW, Hansen NM. Image-guided procedures for breast masses. Adv Surg 2007;41(41):257–72.

19. Leung JW, Kornguth PJ, Gotway MB. Utility of targeted sonography in the evaluation of focal breast pain. J Ultrasound Med 2002;21(5):521–6.

20. Hirose M, Otsuki N, Hayano D, et al. Multi-volume fusion imaging of MR ductography and MR mammography for patients with nipple discharge. Magn Reson Med Sci 2006;5(2):105–12.

21. Ishikawa T, Momiyama N, Hamaguchi Y, et al. Evaluation of dynamic studies of MR mammography for the diagnosis of intraductal lesions with nipple discharge. Breast Cancer 2004;11(3):288–94.

22. Daniel BL, Gardner RW, Birdwell RL, et al. MRI of intraductal papilloma of the breast. Magn Reson Imaging 2003;21(8):887–92.

23. Nakahara H, Namba K, Watanabe R, et al. A comparison of MR imaging, galactography and ultrasonography in patients with nipple discharge. Breast Cancer 2003;10(4):320–9 (16).

24. Orel SG, Dougherty CS, Reynolds C, et al. MR imaging in patients with nipple discharge: initial experience. Radiology 2000;216(1):248–54.

25. Morrogh M, Park A, Elkin EB, et al. Lessons learned from 416 cases of nipple discharge of the breast. Am J Surg 2010. [Epub ahead of print].

26. Sharma R, Dietz J, Wright H, et al. Comparative analysis of minimally invasive microductectomy versus major duct excision in patients with pathologic nipple discharge. Surgery 2005;138(4): 591–6.

27. Markopoulos C, Mantas D, Kouskos E, et al. Surgical management of nipple discharge. Eur J Gynaecol Oncol 2006;27(3):275–8.

28. Cabioglu N, Hunt KK, Singletary SE, et al. Surgical decision making and factors determining a diagnosis of breast carcinoma in women presenting with nipple discharge. J Am Coll Surg 2003; 196(3):354–64.

29. Slawson SH, Johnson BA. Ductography: how to and what if? Radiographics 2001;21(1):133–50.

30. Simmons R, Adamovich T, Brennan M, et al. Nonsurgical evaluation of pathologic nipple discharge. Ann Surg Oncol 2003;10(2):113–6.

31. Dinkel HP, Trusen A, Gassel AM, et al. Predictive value of galactographic patterns for benign and malignant neoplasm of the breast in patients with nipple discharge. Br J Radiol 2000;73(871): 706–14.

32. Dawes LG, Bowen C, Venta LA, et al. Ductography for nipple discharge: no replacement for ductal excision. Surgery 1998;124(4):685–91.

33. Chow JS, Smith DN, Kaelin CM, et al. Case report: galactography-guided wire localization of an intraductal papilloma. Clin Radiol 2001;56(1):72–3.

34. Koskela A, Berg M, Pietilainen T, et al. Breast lesions causing nipple discharge: preoperative galactography-aided stereotactic wire localization. AJR Am J Roentgenol 2005;184(6):1795–8.

35. Baker KS, Davey DD, Stelling CB. Ductal abnormalities detected with galactography: frequency of adequate excisional biopsy. AJR Am J Roentgenol 1994;162(4):821–4.

36. Ballesio L, Maggi C, Savelli S, et al. Role of breast magnetic resonance imaging (MRI) in patients with unilateral nipple discharge: preliminary study. Radiol Med 2008;113(2):249–64.

37. Morrogh M, Morris EA, Liberman L, et al. The positive predictive value of ductography and magnetic resonance imaging in the management of nipple discharge. Ann Surg Oncol 2007;14(12):3369–77.

38. Hirose M, Nobusawa H, Gokan T. MR ductography: comparison with conventional ductography as a diagnostic method in patients with nipple discharge. Radiographics 2007;27(Suppl 1):S183–96.

39. Yucesoy C, Ozturk E, Ozer Y, et al. Conventional galactography and MR contrast galactography for diagnosing nipple discharge: preliminary results. Korean J Radiol 2008;9(5):426–31.

40. Schwab SA, Uder M, Schulz-Wendtland R, et al. Direct MR galactography: feasibility study. Radiology 2008;249(1):54–61.

41. Kelcz F, Santyr G. Gadolinium-enhanced breast MRI. Crit Rev Diagn Imaging 1995;36(4):287–338.

42. Heywang-Kobrunner SH, Schlegel A, Beck R, et al. Contrast-enhanced MRI of the breast after limited surgery and radiation therapy. J Comput Assist Tomogr 1993;17(6):891–900.

43. Gilles R, Guinebretiere JM, Shapeero LG, et al. Assessment of breast cancer recurrence with contrast-enhanced subtraction MR imaging: preliminary results in 26 patients. Radiology 1993;188(2):473–8.

44. Kaiser WA, Zeitler E. MR imaging of the breast: fast imaging sequences with and without Gd-DTPA—preliminary observations. Radiology 1989;170:681–6.

45. Liberman L. Percutaneous image-guided core breast biopsy. Radiol Clin North Am 2002;40(3):483–500.

46. Meyer JE, Sonnenfeld MR, Greenes RA, et al. Cancellation of preoperative breast localization procedures: analysis of 53 cases. Radiology 1988;169(3):629–30.

47. Fischer U, Kopka L, Grabbe E. Breast carcinoma: effect of preoperative contrast-enhanced MR imaging on the therapeutic approach. Radiology 1999;213(3):881–8.

48. Kuhl CK, Schmutzler RK, Leutner CC, et al. Breast MR imaging screening in 192 women proved or suspected to be carriers of a breast cancer susceptibility gene: preliminary results. Radiology 2000;215:267–79.

49. Smyczek-Gargya B, Fersis N, Dittmann H, et al. PET with [^{18}F]fluorothymidine for imaging of primary breast cancer: a pilot study. Eur J Nucl Med Mol Imaging 2004;31:720–4.

50. Samson DJ, Flamm CR, Pisano ED, et al. Should FDG PET be used to decide whether a patient with an abnormal mammogram or breast finding at physical examination undergo biopsy? Acad Radiol 2002;9(7):773–83.

51. Avril N, Rose CA, Schelling M, et al. Breast imaging with positron emission tomography and fluorine-18 fluorodeoxyglucose: use and limitations. J Clin Oncol 2000;18(20):3495–502.

52. Berg WA, Weinberg IN, Narayanan D, et al. High-resolution fluorodeoxyglucose positron emission tomography with compression ("positron emission tomography") is highly accurate in depicting primary breast cancer. Breast J 2006;12(4):309–23.

53. De Cicco C, Trifiro G, Baio S, et al. Clinical utility of 99mTc-Sestamibi scintimammography in the management of equivocal breast lesions. Cancer Biother Radiopharm 2004;19(5):621–6.

54. Sickles EA. Practical solutions to common mammographic problems: tailoring the examination. AJR Am J Roentgenol 1988;15(1):31–9.

55. Pearson KL, Sickles EA, Frankel SD, et al. Efficacy of step-oblique mammography for confirmation and localization of densities seen on only one standard mammographic view. AJR Am J Roentgenol 2000;174(3):745–52.

56. Sickles EA. Findings at mammographic screening on only one standard projection: outcomes analysis. Radiology 1998;208(2):471–5.

57. Newstead GM, Baute PB, Toth HK. Invasive lobular and ductal carcinoma: mammographic findings and stage at diagnosis. Radiology 1992;184(3):623–7.

58. Mendelson EB. Problem-solving ultrasound. Radiol Clin North Am 2004;42(5):909–18.

59. Mehta TS. Current uses of ultrasound in the evaluation of the breast. Radiol Clin North Am 2003;41(4):841–56.

60. ACR practice guideline for the performance of a breast ultrasound examination. Available at: http://www.acr.org/SecondaryMainMenuCategories/quality_safety/guidelines/breast/us_breast.aspx. Accessed February 5, 2010.

61. Youk JH, Kim EK, Ko KH, et al. Asymmetric mammographic findings based on the fourth edition of BI-RADS: types, evaluation, and management. Radiographics 2009;29(1):e33.

62. Sickles EA. Breast masses: mammographic evaluation. Radiology 1989;173(2):297–303.

63. American College of Radiology ACR appropriateness criteria. Available at: http://www.acr.org/SecondaryMainMenuCategories/quality_safety/app_criteria/pdf/ExpertPanelonWomensImagingBreastWorkGroup/NonpalpableBreastMassesDoc2.aspx. Accessed February 5, 2010.

64. Bassett LW. Mammographic analysis of calcifications. Radiol Clin North Am 1992;30(1):93–105.

65. Burnside ES, Ochsner JE, Fowler KJ, et al. Use of microcalcification descriptors in BI-RADS 4th edition to stratify risk of malignancy. Radiology 2007;242(2):388–95.

66. Berg WA, Arnoldus CL, Teferra E, et al. Biopsy of amorphous breast calcifications: pathologic

outcome and yield at stereotactic biopsy. Radiology 2001;221(2):495–503.

67. Stomper PC, Margolin FR. Ductal carcinoma in situ: the mammographer's perspective. AJR Am J Roentgenol 1994;162(3):585–91.

68. American College of Radiology. Breast imaging reporting and data system (BI-RADS). 4th edition. Reston (VA): American College of Radiology; 2003.

69. Bazzocchi M, Zuiani C, Panizza P, et al. Contrast-enhanced breast MRI in patients with suspicious microcalcifications on mammography: results of a multicenter trial. AJR Am J Roentgenol 2006; 186(6):1723–32.

70. Cilotti A, Iacconi C, Marini C, et al. Contrast-enhanced MR imaging in patients with BI-RADS 3-5 microcalcifications. Radiol Med 2007;112(2):272–86.

71. American College of Radiology ACR appropriateness criteria—breast microcalcifications. Available at: http://www.acr.org/SecondaryMainMenuCategories/quality_safety/app_criteria/pdf/ExpertPanelonWomensImaging BreastWorkGroup/BreastMicrocalcificationsDoc1.aspx. Accessed February 5, 2010.

72. Kuhl CK, Schrading S, Bieling HB, et al. MRI for diagnosis of pure ductal carcinoma in situ: a prospective observational study. Lancet 2007; 370(9586):485–92.

73. Schouten van der Velden AP, Boetes C, Bult P, et al. Magnetic resonance imaging in size assessment of invasive breast carcinoma with an extensive intraductal component. BMC Med Imaging 2009;7(9):5.

74. Perfetto F, Fiorentino F, Urbano F, et al. Adjunctive diagnostic value of MRI in the breast radial scar. Radiol Med 2009;114(5):757–70.

75. Leung JW, Sickles EA. Developing asymmetry identified on mammography: correlation with imaging outcome and pathologic findings. AJR Am J Roentgenol 2007;188(3):667–75.

76. Sickles EA. The spectrum of breast asymmetries: imaging features, work-up, management. Radiol Clin North Am 2007;45(5):765–71.

77. Kopans DB, Swann CA, White G, et al. Asymmetric breast tissue. Radiology 1989;171(3): 639–43.

78. Sardanelli F, Melani E, Ottonello C, et al. Magnetic resonance imaging of the breast in characterizing

positive or uncertain mammographic findings. Cancer Detect Prev 1998;22(1):39–42.

79. Heywang SH, Hilbertz T, Beck R, et al. Gd-DTPA enhanced MR imaging of the breast in patients with postoperative scarring and silicon implants. J Comput Assist Tomogr 1990;14(3):348–56.

80. Kerslake RW, Fox JN, Carleton PJ, et al. Dynamic contrast-enhanced and fat suppressed magnetic resonance imaging in suspected recurrent carcinoma of the breast: preliminary experience. Br J Radiol 1994;67(804):1158–68.

81. Whitehouse GH, Moore NR. MR imaging of the breast after surgery for breast cancer. Magn Reson Imaging Clin N Am 1994;2(4):591–603.

82. Muuller RD, Barkhausen J, Sauerwein W, et al. Assessment of local recurrence after breast-conserving therapy with MRI. J Comput Assist Tomogr 1998;22(3):408–12.

83. Preda L, Villa G, Rizzo S, et al. Magnetic resonance mammography in the evaluation of recurrence at the prior lumpectomy site after conservative surgery and radiotherapy. Breast Cancer Res 2006;8(5): R53.

84. Belli P, Constantini M, Romani M, et al. Magnetic resonance imaging in breast cancer recurrence. Breast Cancer Res Treat 2002;73(3):223–35.

85. Morakkabati N, Leutner CC, Schmiedel A, et al. Breast MR imaging during or after radiation therapy. Radiology 2003;229(3):893–901.

86. Teifke A, Lehr HA, Vomweg TW, et al. Outcome analysis and rational management of enhancing lesions incidentally detected on contrast-enhanced MRI of the breast. AJR Am J Roentgenol 2003;181(3): 655–62.

87. Brown J, Smith RC, Lee CH. Incidental enhancing lesions found on MR imaging of the breast. AJR Am J Roentgenol 2001;176(5): 1249–54.

88. Boetes C, Barentsz JO, Mus RD, et al. MR characterization of suspicious breast lesions with a gadolinium-enhanced turboFLASH subtraction technique. Radiology 1994;193(3):777–81.

89. Gilles R, Guinebretiere JM, Lucidarme O, et al. Nonpalpable breast tumors: diagnosis with contrast-enhanced subtraction dynamic MR imaging. Radiology 1994;191(3):625–31.

Probably Benign Lesions Detected on Breast MR Imaging

Peter R. Eby, MD[a,b],*, Wendy B. DeMartini, MD[a,b],
Robert L. Gutierrez, MD[a,b],
Constance D. Lehman, MD, PhD[a,b]

KEYWORDS

- Breast • MR imaging • Probably benign • Cancer

The "probably benign" Breast Imaging Reporting and Data System (BI-RADS) 3 assessment category was originally established for use in mammography. The published evidence and current practice support the use of BI-RADS 3 and short-term follow-up for specific mammographic findings that have been shown to have a chance of representing malignancy in less than 2% of cases.[1–10] Careful observation of these lesions may be preferred over biopsy to avoid the risks and costs of invasive tissue sampling. In addition, if the lesion is malignant, then the follow-up interval should be short enough that there is no change in prognosis. Therefore, current evidence supports short-interval mammographic follow-up as a valid alternative to tissue sampling when adhering to strict criteria.

In 2003 the BI-RADS atlas was revised. BI-RADS introduced the first edition lexicon for breast magnetic resonance (MR) imaging that, like its mammographic predecessor, promotes the standardization of lesion descriptors and assessment categories to facilitate reporting, communication, and research.[11] This lexicon is based on the results of the International Working Group on Breast MR imaging and the American College of Radiology Breast MR imaging Lexicon Committee.[11–14] An MR imaging BI-RADS 3 assessment category was included in this first edition to allow radiologists the option of following, rather than biopsying, some lesions noted on MR imaging. Although this approach was well established for mammographic lesions, the strict criteria for what safely constitutes BI-RADS 3 lesions had not been established for breast MR imaging. The provided definition appropriately reflected the lack of published literature pertaining to this MR imaging assessment:

A finding placed in this category is highly unlikely for malignancy and should have a very high probability of being benign. It is not expected to change over the follow-up interval, but the radiologist would prefer to establish its stability. Data are becoming available that shed light on the efficacy of short-interval follow-up. At the present time, most approaches are intuitive. These will likely undergo future modifications as more data accrue as to the validity of an approach, the interval required, and the type of findings that should be followed.

Although the lexicon represents an attempt to use similar concepts for each breast imaging modality, there are significant differences that should be considered. For example, the cost of a follow-up MR imaging is much greater than the cost of a follow-up mammogram. The average

[a] Department of Radiology, University of Washington School of Medicine, 1959 NE Pacific, Seattle, WA 98195, USA
[b] Seattle Cancer Care Alliance, 825 Eastlake Avenue East, G3-200, Seattle, WA 98109-1023, USA
* Correspondence author. Seattle Cancer Care Alliance, 825 Eastlake Avenue East, G3-200, Seattle, WA 98109-1023.
E-mail address: preby@u.washington.edu

Magn Reson Imaging Clin N Am 18 (2010) 309–321
doi:10.1016/j.mric.2010.02.006

risk of a patient undergoing screening mammography differs from a patient that has a breast MR imaging.

This article discusses the issues that are specific to MR imaging and that affect the utility of an MR imaging probably benign assessment. This aspect is especially important, as the last few years have witnessed a significant increase in the number of breast MR examinations performed nationwide as well as concerns over the indications for and outcomes of its use. The authors address these questions through a review of the data on the MR imaging BI-RADS 3 category that have emerged since the first edition of the MR imaging lexicon was published. Given the combination of the high cost of breast MR imaging and MR image–guided biopsy, it is critical that clinicians strive to determine the proper selection criteria and follow-up interval of MR imaging BI-RADS 3 lesions, to prevent unnecessary biopsies and minimize unwarranted follow-up imaging.

INCIDENCE OF MR IMAGING BI-RADS 3

Prior published reports suggest that there is significant variation in the use of the probably benign assessment, which has been applied to 14% to 34% of patients and 6.6% to 25% of examinations in prior studies.[15–22] At the upper end of this spectrum it is worth noting that as many as 1 out of every 3 patients undergoing breast MR imaging may be recommended to return for a follow-up examination. Such a strategy is unlikely to be sustainable in consideration of the cost of the examinations in dollars, time, and potential for additional false-positive findings.

Four retrospective studies tracked and reported the incidence of BI-RADS 3 even when BI-RADS 4 or 5 assessments were provided for additional lesions in that patient (Table 1).[17–19,21] These methods tracked all BI-RADS 3 lesions, even those that might not have been clinically relevant, for example, in a patient with known cancer who is planning mastectomy. The patient populations have been mixed, which may explain the wide range of BI-RADS 3 use in these studies, ranging from 14% to 24%.[17–19,21]

There have been many well-designed prospective investigations of the performance of breast MR imaging for screening high-risk patients.[15,16,20,22–31] A few of them have published data on the use and cancer yield of lesions assessed as probably benign (Table 2).[15,16,20,22] The incidence of probably benign lesions in these trials ranges from 6.6% to 25% of examinations. It should be noted that the methods for assigning and reporting BI-RADS assessments, which are then used to calculate use, vary. For example, Kriege and colleagues[20] only reported a case as probably benign if BI-RADS 3 was the most suspicious assessment given for any lesion in the examination. This method results in a lower reported rate of overall use of BI-RADS 3 compared with other retrospective trials, such as that by Eby and colleagues,[21] which reported all lesions assessed as BI-RADS 3 regardless of whether that was the highest order assessment for the patient's examination or not.

Table 1
Peer-reviewed studies designed to specifically evaluate the features and cancer yield of lesions assessed as probably benign with MR imaging

Study	Probably Benign Examinations	Probably Benign Patients	Compliance with First Short-Interval Follow-Up	Frequency of Tissue Sampling[a]	Cancer Yield[b]
Liberman et al, 2003[17]	NR	89/367 (24%)	70/89 (79%)	20/89 (22%)	9/89 (10%)
Sadowski & Kelcz, 2005[18]	NR	79/473 (17%)	68/79 (86%)	5/79 (6.3%)	4/79 (5.1%)
Eby et al, 2009[c,21]	260/2569 (10%)	236/1735 (14%)	150/236 (64%)	18/236 (7.6%)	2/236 (0.8%)
Total	260/2569 (10%)	404/2575 (15.7%)	288/404 (71.3%)	43/404 (10.6%)	15/404 (3.7%)

Abbreviation: NR, not reported.
   [a] Calculated as the number with tissue sampling divided by the number of patients.
   [b] Calculated as the number of malignancies divided by the number of patients.
   [c] Includes all 809 examinations from Eby PR, Demartini WB, Peacock S, et al. Cancer yield of probably benign breast MR examinations. J Magn Reson Imaging 2007;26(4):950–5.

Table 2
Peer-reviewed studies of screening breast MR imaging for high-risk patients that include secondary data on probably benign breast MR imaging assessments, biopsy results, and cancer yield

Study	Probably Benign Examinations	Probably Benign Patients	Frequency of Tissue Sampling[b]	Cancer Yield[c]
Kuhl et al, 2000[a],[16]	45/363 (12%)	42/198 (21%)	2/42 (4.8%)	1/42 (2.4%)
Kriege et al, 2004[a],[20]	275/4169 (6.6%)	NR/1909	12/275 (4.4%)	3/275 (1.1%)
Hartman et al, 2004[22]	19/75 (25%)	14/41 (34%)	0/14 (0%)	0/14 (0%)
Kuhl et al, 2005[d],[15]	167/1452 (11.5%)	NR/529	NR	NR

Abbreviation: NR, not reported.
[a] Examinations were only included if BI-RADS 3 was the most severe assessment.
[b] Calculated as the number with tissue sampling divided by the number of patients, except for the Kriege study where it is divided by the number of probably benign examinations.
[c] Calculated as the number of malignancies divided by the number of patients, except for the Kriege study where it is divided by the number of probably benign examinations.
[d] Includes Data from Kuhl CK, Schmutzler RK, Leutner CC, et al. Breast MR imaging screening in 192 women proved or suspected to be carriers of a breast cancer susceptibility gene: preliminary results. Radiology 2000;215(1):267–9.

For comparison, the incidence of probably benign assessments for patients undergoing mammography has been reported to range from 1.2% to 14%.[32–34] Although strict recommendations for target rate of BI-RADS 3 use in mammography are not published, it has been suggested that it should be "considerably less than 5%."[35] Kerlikowske and colleagues[36] reported that 5.2% of first and 1.7% of subsequent screening examinations included recommendation for short-interval follow-up in a multicenter study by the Breast Cancer Surveillance Consortium. If possible, one should strive to reach this low level of MR imaging BI-RADS 3 use for reasons that are described later in this article.

CANCER YIELD OF BI-RADS 3

A mix of 7 retrospective and prospective articles have included data on the MR imaging BI-RADS 3 assessment category, with a resulting wide range of cancer yields (0%–10%).[16–22] Four of these were designed, albeit retrospectively, to specifically investigate the MR imaging BI-RADS 3 assessment (see Table 1).[17–19,21] The other 3 articles include data regarding the cancer yield of MR imaging BI-RADS 3 in prospective high-risk screening MR imaging trials (see Table 2).[16,20,22]

Cancer Yield in Retrospective Studies

The cancer yield of MR imaging lesions assessed as probably benign ranges from 0.8% to 10%, and averages 3.7% in retrospective studies that specifically address the follow-up of BI-RADS 3 findings (see Table 1).[17–19,21]These results paint a mixed picture of the utility of the MR imaging BI-RADS 3 assessment. The lowest cancer yield (0.8%, 2/236) was published by Eby and colleagues.[21] This study included patients who underwent MR imaging for any reason, although the majority of examinations were performed to screen women at high risk or evaluate the extent of disease following a new diagnosis of cancer. The results suggest that the use of a BI-RADS 3 assessment is a safe alternative to biopsy. However, the very low rate of malignancy suggests that the probably benign assessment may have been used for some lesions more appropriately assessed as benign. Such a strategy, while cautious, may result in overuse of expensive medical resources and unnecessary anxiety for patients.

Liberman and colleagues,[17] on the other hand, documented the highest cancer yield of 10% (9/89) among studies of probably benign MR imaging findings. All included lesions were initially assessed as probably benign in a population of high-risk and asymptomatic patients who underwent MR imaging for screening. The risk of malignancy in the cohort of lesions that were assessed as BI-RADS 3 was higher than acceptable for probably benign mammographic findings (<2%). The study identified lesion types that would be more appropriately placed into the BI-RADS 4 category. For example, although the sample size was small, a cancer yield of 25% (1/4) was identified in lesions described as ductal nonmass-like enhancement (NMLE) and initially assessed as probably benign. The investigators subsequently recommended that ductal enhancing lesions be biopsied rather than followed.

Sadowski and Kelcz[18] reported a cancer yield of 5.1% (4/79) among probably benign lesions in a population of patients who underwent MR imaging to further evaluate a mammographic finding that was initially assessed BI-RADS 0 and "unresolved" by diagnostic mammography and/ or ultrasound.

It is important to acknowledge that each of these retrospective studies had different inclusion criteria for patient populations: screening MR imaging only (Liberman and colleagues), screening and diagnostic MR imaging (Eby and colleagues), and BI-RADS 0 mammographic and sonographic workups.[17–19,21] Because of this variability, it is not surprising that the results have also varied from an acceptable probably benign cancer yield of less than 2% to as high as 10%.

Cancer Yield in Prospective High-Risk Screening Trials

Four prospective high-risk screening trials have published data on the cancer yield in patients who received a BI-RADS 3 as the highest order assessment on screening breast MR imaging (see **Table 2**).[15,16,20,22] The yields range from 1.1% to 2.4% in large multicenter studies. However, evaluation of the probably benign assessment was not the primary purpose of these investigations. As stated earlier, the methods in some cases underreported the incidence of BI-RADS 3 lesions and, therefore, may have underreported the cancer yield as well. However, because these are prospective trials in populations of screening patients, the low cancer yield suggests that the use of the BI-RADS 3 category may be appropriate in certain clinical scenarios.

Cancer Yield and Practice Patterns

As stated, the available data arise from heterogeneous studies with undefined criteria for probably benign imaging characteristics. It is, therefore, important to place the subsequent cancer yield of such lesions into the context of the practice patterns of the interpreting radiologists. Data that result in a high use of BI-RADS 3 and a low cancer yield may reflect an over-cautious pattern of recommending follow-up for many benign lesions. In essence, this results in a BI-RADS 3 category that is comprised of benign findings and very few cancers. Alternatively, data that result in a high cancer yield can occur when some suspicious lesions are allowed to be followed—shifting

lesions that may deserve BI-RADS 4 assessments into the BI-RADS 3 category.

The primary mechanism for assessing individual or group practice patterns is an audit. Methods for performing an audit are described in the BI-RADS atlas.[11] An audit can help determine, for example, if biopsies are being recommended appropriately. Although the performance benchmarks from an audit are fairly robust for mammography, additional information will be needed to establish similar targets for MR imaging. Regular audits will be a requirement for accreditation of breast MR imaging programs by the American College of Radiology (ACR).[37]

Risks and Benefits of Short-Term Follow-Up

The mammographic BI-RADS 3 category was implemented when repeating a relatively fast and inexpensive mammogram could obviate the need for a more costly trip to the operating room for surgical excisional biopsy. Considering the need for preoperative and postoperative appointments, risk of general anesthesia, possible undesirable cosmetic outcomes, and morbidity of the procedure, the potential benefit for 98% of patients with benign lesions was large.

The development of percutaneous biopsy methods decreased the gap between follow-up imaging and tissue sampling. These techniques allow radiologists to acquire tissue samples without a visit to a surgeon or an intraoperative procedure. Risks of undesirable cosmetic outcomes are reduced along with morbidity. Compared with an operation, percutaneous tissue sampling is faster and less expensive. In 1997, Brenner and Sickles[38] estimated the cost savings of periodic mammographic follow-up versus percutaneous biopsy to be $1040. A similar study of the cost savings of follow-up breast MR imaging has not been published.

At a minimum, patients that participate in an annual high-risk screening MR imaging program and receive a BI-RADS 3 assessment may undergo a single extra breast MR imaging at 6 months in lieu of MR-guided tissue sampling. These patients may thus benefit by having follow-up MR imaging that is less expensive and invasive than a tissue sampling procedure. However, this must be balanced against the risks. The patient population undergoing MR imaging has a higher baseline level of risk for malignancy than the general population undergoing screening mammography. The high-risk group may also be younger, have higher levels of anxiety, and have more aggressive tumors. The latter is particularly critical to the safety of short-term follow-up because the stated goal is to allow imaging surveillance of a lesion without a change in prognosis. Additional research is needed to determine if a balance that is acceptable can be achieved.

LESION FEATURES

Data are not yet available that allow clinicians to definitively describe lesions that belong in the BI-RADS 3 category. The available data come from studies with variable design and criteria for what constitutes a probably benign MR imaging lesion. Despite these challenges, these preliminary studies provide thoughtful insight into the issues. As the data mature, one can begin to extrapolate some general principles about the use of probably benign assessment and initial guidance for specific lesion criteria that comprise it. In addition, the data are also helping us to suggest which lesions may be more appropriate for the BI-RADS 2 or BI-RADS 4 categories, thereby minimizing the use of short-term follow-up MR imaging.

The authors' previously published data comprise the largest study to date on the characteristics of probably benign lesions.[21] Of the 362 lesions, 168 (48%) were foci, which are lesions that, by definition, are smaller than 5 mm.[11] Of 168 foci, only one malignancy was identified (0.6%).[21] This focus contained washout kinetics during delayed phase enhancement. Additional data from that study suggest which lesions may be more appropriately placed into the BI-RADS 2 category. The authors found that the 69 foci designated BI-RADS 3 that demonstrated 100%

persistent kinetics on delayed phase enhancement were all benign.[21] This finding suggests that all persistent foci may be placed into a BI-RADS 2 category. These 69 foci were identified in 54 patients on 55 examinations. If these 69 foci had been called benign on the baseline examination, then the percentage of women recommended for short-term follow-up in this study would have decreased from 14% (236/1735) to 10% (182/1735) without missing a cancer. In addition, the probably benign cancer yield would still be less than 2% (2/182, 1.1%).[21]

Prior research by Liberman and colleagues indicates that the risk of malignancy in suspicious lesions smaller than 5 mm is less than 3%.[39] The investigators concluded that "biopsy is generally not warranted for MR imaging-detected lesions less than 5 mm." This corollary suggests that short-term follow-up may be adequate for any lesion smaller than 5 mm. However, kinetic information was not incorporated into their analysis. The authors' findings, with a larger sample of probably benign foci, support the conclusion of Liberman and colleagues and build on that prior work by adding kinetic data to the equation. The data that are currently available indicate that kinetic features can help guide decisions about the appropriate BI-RADS assessments for some lesions.

UTILIZATION PATTERNS OF BI-RADS 3

In the authors' experience, the use of the probably benign assessment has decreased slightly over

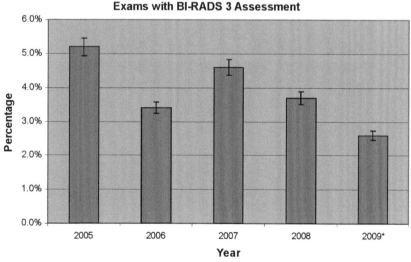

Exams with BI-RADS 3 Assessment

Fig. 1. The percentage of BI-RADS 3 examinations has decreased slightly during the last 5 years of performing breast MR imaging, and now averages approximately 3% of all breast MR imagings interpreted at the authors' institution.

time (**Fig. 1**). Anecdotal discussion with other investigators suggests a similar pattern. Several possible explanations can be considered.

For mammography, the use of the BI-RADS 3 assessments is predicated on the lack of prior films that can establish stability or growth to respectively downgrade (benign) or upgrade (suspicious) probably benign findings. Callbacks and probably benign assessments are more common among patients without comparisons. Most breast MR imaging programs have evolved and grown in recent years from a population of patients undergoing their first examination to a more mature cohort, with prior studies that can be used to establish stability or change. Warner and colleagues[29] reported a decrease in the percentage of patients with a BI-RADS 3 assessment: 7.6% of study patients were placed into this category in the first round of screening, compared with 2.9% in the second, and 2.4% in the third round. While it is clear that comparison studies are valuable for guiding BI-RADS assessments and recommendations, the MR imaging lexicon does not specifically describe the role of prior examinations when a probably benign assessment is being considered.

As with any imaging study, the most significant task for the radiologist is to ascertain the difference between what is normal and abnormal; this holds especially true for breast imaging whereby there is wide variability in the patterns of density, distribution, and enhancement of breast parenchyma from patient to patient. **Fig. 2**, for example, demonstrates findings of bilateral scattered and similar appearing foci, a pattern that was frequently assessed as probably benign in the early years of the authors' breast MR imaging program. After years of observing this pattern and the follow-up examinations that demonstrated stability or resolution in many cases, the authors now consider this to be typical of bilateral benign background parenchymal enhancement. The authors now routinely assess such cases as BI-RADS 1 (negative) with marked background parenchymal enhancement rather than assigning them BI-RADS 3 with short-term follow-up recommended.

In general, in the authors' practice one refrains from using the BI-RADS 3 assessment for

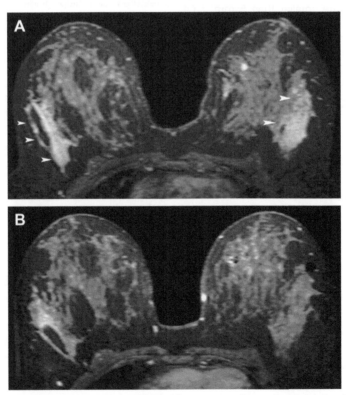

Fig. 2. High-risk screening MR imaging in this 47-year-old was assessed as probably benign for bilateral posterior lateral NMLE (*arrowheads* in *A*, axial T1 fat-suppressed postcontrast sequence). At the time of 5 month follow-up MR imaging the bilateral enhancement had significantly decreased (*B*) and was called benign. This image is an example of findings now known as background parenchymal enhancement (BPE).

examinations that are performed to evaluate the extent of disease in patients with a new diagnosis of cancer. The primary reason for this decision relates to patient care. Unresolved questions regarding the extent of ipsilateral disease or contralateral disease for a patient who is about to begin treatment can create uncertainty at best or delayed diagnosis at worst. Secondarily, if a patient receives chemotherapy or hormonal therapy, or stops taking estrogen replacement, and the lesion disappears at follow-up imaging, then it may be impossible to determine if the finding constituted benign background enhancement or treated malignancy.

Recommendations for Use of Probably Benign Assessment

The authors' approach for determining if BI-RADS 3 is an appropriate assessment begins with an evaluation of the background parenchymal enhancement (BPE). Experience has shown that there are patterns of bilateral and symmetric enhancement that represent benign BPE and do not need short-interval follow-up. For example, bilateral symmetric posterolateral regional NMLE is a typical pattern of moderate BPE (see **Fig. 2**). Multiple bilateral and diffusely distributed foci are also a common pattern that represents benign BPE (**Figs. 3** and **4**). However, there are cases, such as contralateral mastectomy or radiation therapy, in which symmetry cannot be confirmed (**Fig. 5**). When the foci are similar in size and kinetics, short-term follow-up is not necessary. However, kinetics may be especially useful to identify a single focus that is different from the rest and may contain some washout enhancement (**Fig. 6**). Similarly, an examination may contain a single focus with some washout enhancement (**Fig. 7**). It is reasonable to place these foci into the BI-RADS 3 category and follow them in 6 months if there is no prior MR imaging to establish stability (benign) or growth (suspicious).

Lesions that are distinct from the BPE should be carefully evaluated to determine the most appropriate assessment. The first step is to assess the

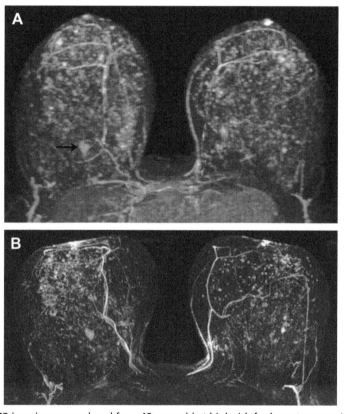

Fig. 3. A screening MR imaging was ordered for a 48-year-old at high risk for breast cancer. Axial subtraction MIP shows diffuse bilateral foci (*A*) that were designated probably benign. A known fibroadenoma was present as an oval mass in the posterior right breast (*arrow*). Follow-up MR imaging at 14 months revealed stable findings that were called benign (*B*). The diffuse bilateral foci in this case illustrate the appearance of marked BPE now known as negative.

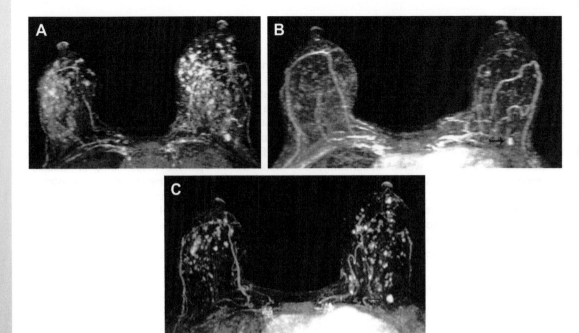

Fig. 4. A 46-year-old perimenopausal (status post hysterectomy but not oophorectomy) woman had a stereotactic biopsy for a 2-mm cluster of heterogeneous calcifications in the left breast at 9 o'clock that was diagnosed as DCIS. MR imaging to evaluate the extent of disease did not show an abnormality corresponding to the DCIS. Although the authors do not typically use BI-RADS 3 in patients with a new diagnosis of cancer, bilateral diffuse foci (*A*, axial subtraction MIP) were described as probably benign. Left lumpectomy was performed 2 weeks later. Follow-up at 7 months shows resolution of the foci on both sides (*B*). However, a mass was then seen in the posterior left breast and identified retrospectively on the initial study (*arrow*). This mass was called probably benign due to 7 months of stability. Subsequent 6-month follow-up MR imaging show continued stability of the mass and return of the bilateral foci (*C*) that were all called benign. The patient was cancer free after 3 years of additional follow-up.

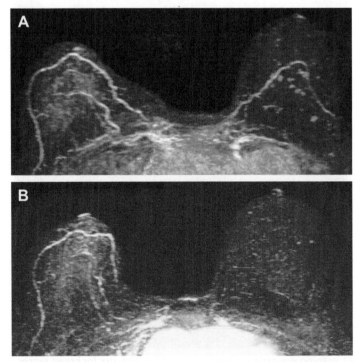

Fig. 5. MR imaging was performed for screening in a 50-year-old woman due to her history of prior right lumpectomy and radiation therapy. The axial subtraction (T1-weighted immediate postcontrast minus T1-weighted precontrast) MIP shows unilateral diffuse left scattered foci (*A*) that were called probably benign, and which had resolved at 10-month follow-up examination (*B*). (*A*) is an example of findings now considered to be mild BPE that is unilateral because of prior therapy.

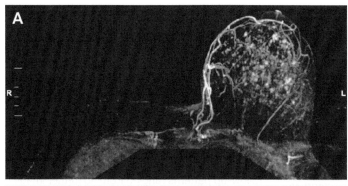

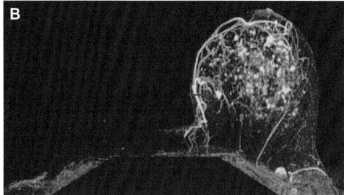

Fig. 6. High-risk screening MR imaging performed for a patient who had undergone right mastectomy demonstrates diffuse foci in the left breast on axial subtraction MIP (*A*). Although the foci are similar in size and diffuse, which suggests benignity, the lack of a contralateral breast prevents assessment of bilateral symmetry. Computer-aided evaluation (CAE) can be helpful in this scenario to determine if the kinetics of all the foci are homogeneous. CAE shows that a single upper inner focus (*red*) contains washout. This focus was assessed as probably benign. Enlargement of the focus to a mass on follow-up examination (*B*) prompted MR-guided biopsy that revealed invasive ductal carcinoma. The prognosis for the patient was unchanged.

morphology, size, stability, and distribution of the lesion(s). For example, some masses may be determined, based on reniform shape, smooth margins and fatty hilum, to be benign lymph nodes. It is common for normal lymph nodes to display delayed washout kinetics, so it is the morphologic characteristics that are critical to establishing benignity. On the other hand, some lesions have morphologies that should be considered suspicious and biopsy recommended. For example, NMLE that is linear, ductal, or segmental and masses that have an irregular shape or spiculated margins should be assessed as BI-RADS 4 and recommended for biopsy. After the clearly benign and suspicious lesions have been categorized, those that remain may be carefully considered for possible short-term follow-up.

Unilateral singular lesions without suspicious morphologic features and limited data to evaluate MR imaging stability can be appropriate for

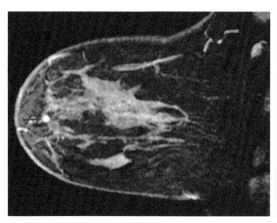

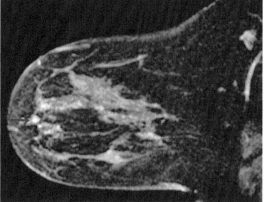

Fig. 7. MR imaging in a 49-year-old was remarkable for a single, probably benign 4-mm focus (*arrow, A*) on sagittal T1 fat-suppressed postcontrast sequence that was smaller at 7-month follow-up MR imaging (*arrow, B*) and considered benign.

BI-RADS 3 assessment. Examples of such lesions include round or oval masses with smooth margins, and focal or regional homogeneous NMLE (**Figs. 4 and 8**). Kinetic information may help determine if biopsy is indicated or if follow-up is a safe alternative. Targeted ultrasound can then be considered, at the discretion of the interpreting radiologist, to gather additional information about the lesion. In some cases, suspicious sonographic features may lead to a recommendation for biopsy. Alternatively, targeted ultrasound for round or oval masses with smooth margins and washout enhancement may reveal a classically benign intramammary lymph node with a thin, smooth cortex and an echogenic fatty hilum that can obviate the need for biopsy. If this type of MR imaging finding is not seen on ultrasound, then a BI-RADS 3 assessment is appropriate. In addition, if the lesion is seen on ultrasound and has sonographic probably benign features such as a round or oval shape, smooth margin, and parallel orientation, ultrasound can be used to follow the lesion in a more comfortable and less costly manner.

TIMING OF SHORT-INTERVAL FOLLOW-UP

When should the patient return for follow-up of probably benign breast MR imaging findings? For how long and at what frequency should they be followed? In the absence of published guidelines, such decisions are based largely on the preference of the individual radiologist. For mammography, the ACR BI-RADS atlas recommends that short-interval follow-up consist of a unilateral examination at 6 months followed by bilateral examinations at 12 and 24 months, acknowledging that some radiologists may even choose to follow to 36 months.[11] Multiple studies have shown this follow-up strategy to be safe and effective for mammography, but its applicability to MR imaging–detected lesions is unknown.[1–10] However, in the absence of published guidelines, radiologists are left with few options but to apply this strategy to breast MR imaging in some form or another.

Prior studies have reported initial short-interval follow-up times ranging between 3 and 6 months.[16–22] These preliminary reports suggest that an initial 6-month follow-up examination is often all that is needed to confirm variability or resolution of findings suspected to be related to benign BPE. There are 3 possible scenarios radiologists encounter when evaluating lesions at follow-up imaging, regardless of modality:

1. Interval decrease in size or complete resolution of the finding

2. Increase in size or otherwise suspicious change in morphology
3. No significant interval change in size or morphology.

Management of scenarios 1 and 2 is straightforward: diminishing size or resolution is highly suggestive of a benign process and the lesion can therefore be downgraded, whereas any increase in size or otherwise suspicious change in morphology should prompt biopsy. For scenario 3, the published studies report wide variability in follow-up patterns ranging from no further imaging to follow-up every 6 months for 2 years.[16–22] In addition, most of these investigators reported timing these follow-up examinations to coincide with the second week of the menstrual cycle to minimize hormonal influence on background enhancement. In the authors' practice, patients scheduled for routine screening or follow-up examinations are asked to present during days 7 to 10 of their menstrual cycle.

FOLLOW-UP COMPLIANCE

Compliance with recommended follow-up imaging can be challenging. Prior reports describe compliance with short-interval follow-up mammography ranging from 69% to 89%.[2–6] A breast MR imaging costs more and requires more time from the patient as well as placement of a peripheral intravenous catheter. In addition, some insurance companies continue to deny coverage for breast MR imaging more than once a year, even in high-risk patients. Despite these additional barriers, studies that have included data regarding compliance have shown a range of 62% to 86% of patients undergoing the recommended MR imaging follow-up, similar to the reports for mammographic compliance.[17–19,21]

SUMMARY

Use of breast MR imaging is on the increase, and its performance will continue to depend on the accuracy of a diverse group of radiologists and their ability to recommend short-interval follow-up appropriately. The data for MR imaging are not yet as robust as those for mammography. However, at this time it is reasonable to consider limiting the use of MR imaging BI-RADS 3 assessments to examinations done for screening and in situations where there are few or no prior comparisons. Bilateral symmetric findings are typical of background enhancement (BI-RADS 2) and do not need short-term follow-up. Lesions with suspicious morphologic features are more appropriately recommended for biopsy (BI-RADS 4),

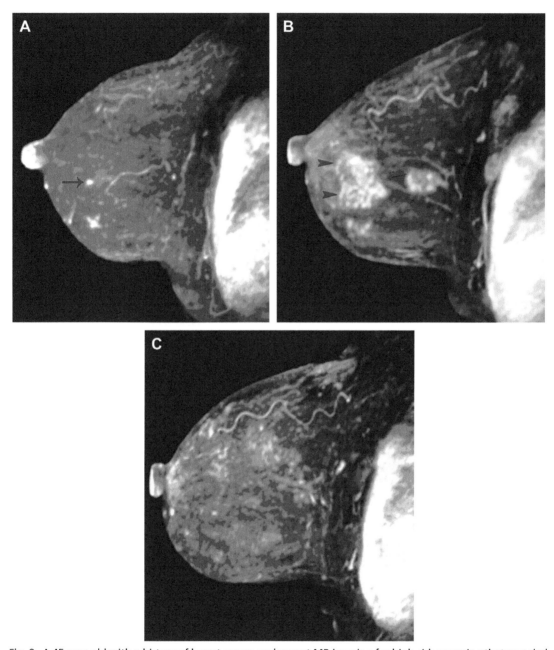

Fig. 8. A 45-year-old with a history of breast cancer underwent MR imaging for high-risk screening that revealed a single focus of enhancement in the contralateral breast, assessed as probably benign (*A*, sagittal subtraction MIP). Six-month follow-up MR imaging showed resolution of the focus. However, new regional NMLE (*B*) was described and assessed as BI-RADS 0 with a recommendation for targeted ultrasound. The ultrasound was normal at the site of NMLE, and a final assessment of probably benign was given, with a recommendation for short-term follow-up MR imaging. Eight months later, the NMLE and focus had resolved and the examination was assessed as negative (*C*). There was no evidence of malignancy after 2 more years of follow-up.

regardless of kinetic findings. Singular or asymmetric small lesions that demonstrate benign morphology but mixed kinetics, including some washout, may be considered probably benign and followed with MR imaging, with or without antecedent targeted ultrasound. Additional research is needed to determine if there are distinct morphologic and/or kinetic characteristics that can be defined as appropriate to warrant the MR imaging BI-RADS 3 assessment with an acceptable cancer yield and preservation of favorable prognosis.

REFERENCES

1. Brenner RJ. Follow-up as an alternative to biopsy for probably benign mammographically detected abnormalities. Curr Opin Radiol 1991;3(4):588–92.
2. Vizcaino I, Gadea L, Andreo L, et al. Short-term follow-up results in 795 nonpalpable probably benign lesions detected at screening mammography. Radiology 2001;219(2):475–83.
3. Varas X, Leborgne JH, Leborgne F, et al. Revisiting the mammographic follow-up of BI-RADS category 3 lesions. AJR Am J Roentgenol 2002;179(3):691–5.
4. Varas X, Leborgne F, Leborgne JH. Nonpalpable, probably benign lesions: role of follow-up mammography. Radiology 1992;184(2):409–14.
5. Sickles EA. Periodic mammographic follow-up of probably benign lesions: results in 3,184 consecutive cases. Radiology 1991;179(2):463–8.
6. Helvie MA, Pennes DR, Rebner M, et al. Mammographic follow-up of low-suspicion lesions: compliance rate and diagnostic yield. Radiology 1991; 178(1):155–8.
7. Brenner RJ, Sickles EA. Acceptability of periodic follow-up as an alternative to biopsy for mammographically detected lesions interpreted as probably benign. Radiology 1989;171(3):645–6.
8. Hall FM. Follow-up as an alternative to biopsy for mammographically detected lesions interpreted as probably benign. Radiology 1989;173(1):284–5.
9. Monticciolo DL, Caplan LS. The American College of Radiology's BI-RADS 3 classification in a nationwide screening program: current assessment and comparison with earlier use. Breast J 2004;10(2):106–10.
10. Rosen EL, Baker JA, Soo MS. Malignant lesions initially subjected to short-term mammographic follow-up. Radiology 2002;223(1):221–8.
11. D'Orsi CJ, Bassett LW, Berg WA, et al. Breast imaging reporting and data system: ACR BI-RADS. 4th edition. Reston (VA): American College of Radiology; 2003.
12. Ikeda DM, Baker DR, Daniel BL. Magnetic resonance imaging of breast cancer: clinical indications and breast MRI reporting system. J Magn Reson Imaging 2000;12(6):975–83.
13. Ikeda DM, Hylton NM, Kinkel K, et al. Development, standardization, and testing of a lexicon for reporting contrast-enhanced breast magnetic resonance imaging studies. J Magn Reson Imaging 2001; 13(6):889–95.
14. Ikeda DM. Progress report from the American College of Radiology breast MR imaging lexicon committee. Magn Reson Imaging Clin N Am 2001; 9(2):295–302, vi.
15. Kuhl CK, Schrading S, Leutner CC, et al. Mammography, breast ultrasound, and magnetic resonance imaging for surveillance of women at high familial risk for breast cancer. J Clin Oncol 2005;23(33):8469–76.
16. Kuhl CK, Schmutzler RK, Leutner CC, et al. Breast MR imaging screening in 192 women proved or suspected to be carriers of a breast cancer susceptibility gene: preliminary results. Radiology 2000; 215(1):267–79.
17. Liberman L, Morris EA, Benton CL, et al. Probably benign lesions at breast magnetic resonance imaging: preliminary experience in high-risk women. Cancer 2003;98(2):377–88.
18. Sadowski EA, Kelcz F. Frequency of malignancy in lesions classified as probably benign after dynamic contrast-enhanced breast MRI examination. J Magn Reson Imaging 2005;21(5):556–64.
19. Eby PR, Demartini WB, Peacock S, et al. Cancer yield of probably benign breast MR examinations. J Magn Reson Imaging 2007;26(4):950–5.
20. Kriege M, Brekelmans CT, Boetes C, et al. Efficacy of MRI and mammography for breast-cancer screening in women with a familial or genetic predisposition. N Engl J Med 2004;351(5):427–37.
21. Eby PR, DeMartini WB, Gutierrez RL, et al. Characteristics of probably benign breast MRI lesions. AJR Am J Roentgenol 2009;193(3):861–7.
22. Hartman AR, Daniel BL, Kurian AW, et al. Breast magnetic resonance image screening and ductal lavage in women at high genetic risk for breast carcinoma. Cancer 2004;100(3):479–89.
23. Hagen AI, Kvistad KA, Maehle L, et al. Sensitivity of MRI versus conventional screening in the diagnosis of BRCA-associated breast cancer in a national prospective series. Breast 2007;16(4):367–74.
24. Kriege M, Brekelmans CT, Boetes C, et al. Differences between first and subsequent rounds of the MRISC breast cancer screening program for women with a familial or genetic predisposition. Cancer 2006;106(11):2318–26.
25. Lehman CD, Isaacs C, Schnall MD, et al. Cancer yield of mammography, MR, and US in high-risk women: prospective multi-institution breast cancer screening study. Radiology 2007;244(2):381–8.
26. Leach MO, Boggis CR, Dixon AK, et al. Screening with magnetic resonance imaging and mammography of a UK population at high familial risk of breast cancer: a prospective multicentre cohort study (MARIBS). Lancet 2005;365(9473):1769–78.
27. Lehman CD, Blume JD, Weatherall P, et al. Screening women at high risk for breast cancer with mammography and magnetic resonance imaging. Cancer 2005;103(9):1898–905.
28. Sardanelli F, Podo F, D'Agnolo G, et al. Multicenter comparative multimodality surveillance of women at genetic-familial high risk for breast cancer (HIBCRIT study): interim results. Radiology 2007;242(3):698–715.

29. Warner E, Plewes DB, Hill KA, et al. Surveillance of BRCA1 and BRCA2 mutation carriers with magnetic resonance imaging, ultrasound, mammography, and clinical breast examination. JAMA 2004;292(11): 1317–25.

30. Tilanus-Linthorst MM, Obdeijn IM, Bartels KC, et al. First experiences in screening women at high risk for breast cancer with MR imaging. Breast Cancer Res Treat 2000;63(1):53–60.

31. Podo F, Sardanelli F, Canese R, et al. The Italian multi-centre project on evaluation of MRI and other imaging modalities in early detection of breast cancer in subjects at high genetic risk. J Exp Clin Cancer Res 2002;21(3 Suppl):115–24.

32. Caplan LS, Blackman D, Nadel M, et al. Coding mammograms using the classification "probably benign finding—short interval follow-up suggested". AJR Am J Roentgenol 1999;172(2):339–42.

33. Geller BM, Ichikawa LE, Buist DS, et al. Improving the concordance of mammography assessment and management recommendations. Radiology 2006;241(1):67–75.

34. Yasmeen S, Romano PS, Pettinger M, et al. Frequency and predictive value of a mammographic recommendation for short-interval follow-up. J Natl Cancer Inst 2003;95(6):429–36.

35. Leung JW, Sickles EA. The probably benign assessment. Radiol Clin North Am 2007;45(5): 773–89, vi.

36. Kerlikowske K, Smith-Bindman R, Abraham LA, et al. Breast cancer yield for screening mammographic examinations with recommendation for short-interval follow-up. Radiology 2005;234(3):684–92.

37. American College of Radiology Accreditation. Available at: http://www.acr.org/accreditation.aspx. Accessed December 20, 2009.

38. Brenner RJ, Sickles EA. Surveillance mammography and stereotactic core breast biopsy for probably benign lesions: a cost comparison analysis. Acad Radiol 1997;4(6):419–25.

39. Liberman L, Mason G, Morris EA, et al. Does size matter? Positive predictive value of MRI-detected breast lesions as a function of lesion size. AJR Am J Roentgenol 2006;186(2):426–30.

MR Intervention: Indications, Technique, Correlation and Histologic

Liane E. Philpotts, MD

KEYWORDS

- Breast • Breast MR imaging • Breast biopsy
- Breast interventions • Breast histology

The use of magnetic resonance (MR) imaging of the breast has increased dramatically in the last few years. Breast MR imaging offers a unique imaging technique for which many defined indications proven to benefit certain subsets of patients exist.[1–8] MR imaging provides information not available through other breast imaging modalities routinely used at present. The unique qualities of breast MR imaging, including lack of ionizing radiation or limitation by breast density, make it particularly beneficial to young and high-risk patients. Although breast MR imaging was initially hindered by the limited availability of coils, protocols, and particularly breast biopsy devices, standardized imaging and specialized equipment necessary to perform high-quality MR imaging of the breast is now readily available.

Given the unique properties of this modality, familiarity with breast MR imaging is necessary for all radiologists interpreting breast imaging. It is encouraged that those performing breast MR imaging also be capable of performing biopsies, or at least have a close association with a facility that does. Familiarity with the indications and technique of breast MR imaging biopsies is recommended for all, regardless of whether they actively perform biopsies. Optimal management of patients requires a good understanding of these

processes. In this article the indications for breast MR interventional procedures along with the techniques used are described. In addition, the histologic process encountered and recommended strategies for patient management are discussed.

INDICATIONS FOR INTERVENTIONAL MR

MR interventional procedures include both wire localization and needle biopsy. Historically, wire localization procedures were the first to be employed, as MR-compatible needle/wire sets became available.[9–11] When vacuum-assisted biopsy devices were later developed for use in magnets, this procedure quickly replaced the majority of wire localizations.[12–17] As with lesions found by palpation or other breast imaging modalities, suspicious lesions identified by MR are preferentially sampled percutaneously rather than surgically. With routine use of postbiopsy markers, sampled lesions requiring subsequent excision can easily be localized either mammographically or sonographically, thus reducing the need and indications for MR-guided wire localization. Therefore, the indications for core biopsy in general are discussed first.

Studies have shown that MR imaging has a high sensitivity for the detection of invasive carcinoma

Disclosures:
Department of Diagnostic Radiology, Yale University School of Medicine, 333 Cedar Street, PO Box 208042, New Haven, CT 06520-8042, USA
E-mail address: liane.philpotts@yale.edu

Magn Reson Imaging Clin N Am 18 (2010) 323–332
doi:10.1016/j.mric.2010.02.013
1064-9689/10/$ – see front matter © 2010 Elsevier Inc. All rights reserved.

of the breast.[6,18–25] With the higher resolution scanning now achieved with dedicated breast coils along with advances in interpretation criteria, ductal carcinoma in situ (DCIS) is being detected more frequently.[22] Lesions detected on MR imaging include enhancing masses and non-mass-like enhancement. Both can indicate malignancy and, depending on the morphology and kinetics of individual lesions along with the clinical scenario, may require biopsy. Detection of malignant disease in another quadrant to an ipsilateral cancer or in the contralateral breast can have a profound effect on surgical management (**Fig. 1**). Some MR-detected lesions will prove to be detectable by mammography or sonography, particularly what has been termed "second-look" ultrasound (US), but many will not.[26,27] For those suspicious MR-detected lesions not identified on mammography or sonography, MR-guided biopsy is indicated.

Correlation with Other Imaging Studies

Correlation with other imaging studies is the first step in management of MR-detected lesions that are suspicious enough to require biopsy. Recent mammograms should be reviewed to assess for a mammographic correlate. Sometimes, a small enhancing mass on MR can be easily determined to represent a stable mass such as a fibroadenoma or an intramammary lymph node seen on mammography. If no mammograms are available for correlation, diagnostic mammography should be performed, with particular attention to the area(s) of interest. The majority of additional MR-detected lesions, however, will usually prove not to be identified on mammography.

Focused US is probably more useful than mammography in the detection of MR-detected lesions. If a sonographic correlate is found, then biopsy is facilitated. US-guided percutaneous biopsy can be performed quicker, easier, at lower cost, and with more patient comfort than MR-guided biopsy. Second-look US has been shown to detect approximately one-quarter to one-third of MR lesions.[26,27] Detection of mass lesions is higher than that of nonmass lesions, which is not surprising given that mass lesions are more likely to represent invasive disease and nonmass lesions in situ disease. DCIS is, of course, more difficult to detect with US. Of note, the malignancy rate has been found to be higher if a US correlate is found.[26,27] However, lesions without a US correlate still have a substantial rate of malignancy such that biopsy is still necessary.

Correlation of MR-detected findings with other imaging modalities can be challenging because of the differences in patient positioning during mammography, US, and MR. Mammography is performed with the patient upright and the breast in firm compression, US with the patient supine and the breast tissues uncompressed and flattened dependently against the chest wall, and MR with the patient prone and the breasts hanging pendulously. Correlating a lesion seen on one modality with another can be challenging. It is common among interpreters of breast imaging studies to describe the distance of a lesion from the nipple. For other than the smallest breasts, this distance may change substantially among the different imaging studies because of the markedly different imaging positions. Localization of a lesion within the anterior, mid, or posterior thirds of the breast is usually adequate. Otherwise,

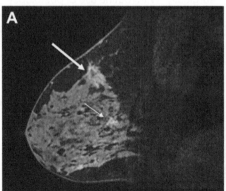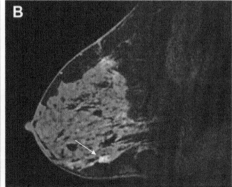

Fig. 1. (*A, B*) A 58-year old woman was recently diagnosed with ductal carcinoma in situ (DCIS) in the superior right breast (*large arrow*). Postcontrast fat-saturated T1-weighted images show 2 additional sites of linear nonmass-like enhancement elsewhere in the breast, in the central posterior and inferior areas (*small arrows*). MR-guided biopsy of both these areas also revealed DCIS.

conforming to strict nipple-lesion distances may result in markedly inaccurate areas of the evaluated breast. In particular, when performing US for MR lesions, a generous range of tissue area around the site of the measurement from the nipple is recommended as these 2 study methods have the greatest degree of differences in breast position. Use of landmarks such as cysts or other benign masses may help increase detection of MR lesions. Assessment of the glandular tissue and fat planes can also be helpful.

Confidence that a US-detected lesion correlates with the MR lesion of interest is always somewhat problematic. The differences in breast position as outlined above constitute a main reason. Detection of the smaller masses and nonmass-like enhancement by US will require sampling of more subtle sonographic lesions. Confidence that the "correct" area has been sampled will sometimes be uncertain. Studies have shown that higher rates of falsely benign findings occur with such biopsies, indicating that the MR-detected lesion was not correctly sampled. A study by Meissnitzer and colleagues[26] showed that 10 of 80 lesions that underwent US biopsy with what was considered a benign, concordant result on follow-up imaging was found not to correlate with the MR finding. On subsequent biopsy, 5 of 9 lesions were shown to be malignant. This result underscores the difficulty in correlating the 2 imaging studies. If there is a reasonable degree of uncertainty in the sonographic findings, biopsy under MR guidance may be a better option. If US biopsy is performed, then careful review of the

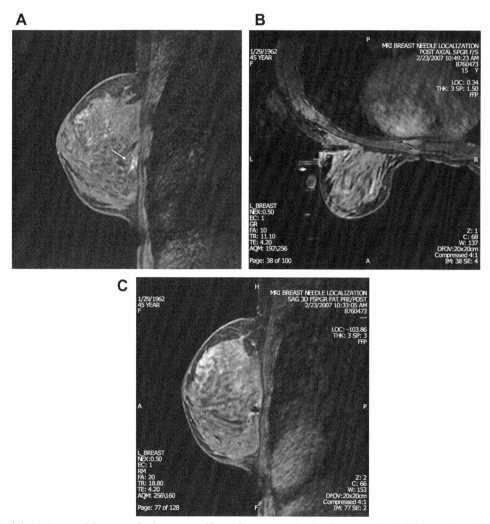

Fig. 2. (A) A 45-year-old woman had nonmass-like enhancement in the far posterior left breast (arrow). (B, C) Axial and sagittal images after needle localization and wire insertion for surgery show the close proximity of the wire to the chest wall.

histologic findings to assess for concordance is required and follow-up MR is also necessary.

Attempts at improving correlation of MR and US imaging are underway, with modification of coil design along with development of software, aiming at a greater degree of accuracy in finding lesions and confidence in assessing concordance. This upgrade should greatly improve the chance of finding lesions, increase the confidence in targeting the correct lesion, and reduce the need for follow-up MR examinations.

Core Biopsy

As stated earlier, core biopsy is the primary procedure performed under MR guidance. Wire localizations, however, may be necessary under certain circumstances. In a patient with ipsilateral newly diagnosed cancer, bracketing of areas of MR enhancement suspicious for extent of disease around the index cancer may be appropriate through MR-guided preoperative wire localization. For example, this would include areas in the same vicinity as the primary cancer not sufficiently separate to require preoperative core biopsy if management would not have been changed. Whereas technical considerations are discussed below, limitations for prone MR vacuum-assisted biopsy are similar to prone stereotactic procedures and include lesions that are far posterior or in the axillary tail as well as lesions near the nipple (**Fig. 2**). For such lesions, wire localization may be technically possible whereas vacuum-assisted biopsy would be difficult or impossible. Also, wire location rather than the larger gauge vacuum-assisted biopsy may be preferred for some superficial lesions or lesions adjacent to implants.

MR-GUIDED BIOPSY TECHNIQUE

Although it may seem intimidating to some at first, MR-guided biopsies are actually easily learned and performed. Other than the obvious differences in imaging used, the technique of patient positioning and lesion sampling with vacuum-assisted devices is markedly similar to stereotactic biopsy. Thus most radiologists performing breast biopsies will be familiar and become quickly comfortable with the technical aspects of the procedure. Lesion detection and targeting can be the most challenging part of the procedure.

Imaging and Report Review

Good quality prebiopsy MR imaging and interpretation is necessary. If imaging quality is different, particularly when performing biopsies from outside facilities, repeat MR imaging prior to

biopsy may be indicated. However, given the cost of these imaging studies along with the additional time involved to repeat the study, sometimes scheduling the patient for biopsy is more appropriate than repeating a diagnostic MR examination which, if still suspicious, would require the patient to return yet again.

Review of the preprocedure imaging and reports is necessary before starting the procedure. For cases performed at another facility, importing the study into a PACS (picture archiveing and communications system) is advised such that images are readily available for reference during the procedure. Importing the prior study into PACS permits linking of various images in various planes, particularly sagittal and axial, which is necessary for confidence in targeting during biopsy. Such a viewpoint is not always possible when viewing images directly from a disc.

Review of the prior studies is also necessary to ensure sampling of the correct lesion. Ideally, such studies should include annotated images and/or image slice numbers detailed in the report to avoid uncertainty for the performing radiologist at the time of the procedure. Also, review of the prior images allows planning when biopsy of more than one site is necessary. Whereas sampling of more than one site in the same breast is relatively easy, bilateral biopsy requires sequential sampling. Although this process is relatively quick with the coils and imaging protocols available at present, targeting and sampling of the most suspicious lesion or breast first is recommended, particularly if lesions have washout kinetics. Having a clear plan before starting the procedure can allow the technologist to image in the shortest amount of time.

Canceling or Aborting the Procedure

It is well understood that many lesions for which MR biopsy is recommended are ultimately not reproduced, thus resulting in clinicians aborting or canceling the procedure.[28] This situation occurs because there is considerable overlap in the MR appearance of normal breast glandular enhancement and other benign findings with malignant processes. Often such subtle findings, particularly nonmass-like enhancement, may represent "hormonal" breast glandular tissue and thus may not be reproduced at the time of biopsy. Other factors may include the amount of compression used, which may be slightly greater during biopsy than routine breast MR imaging, given that the fenestrated grid immobilizes the breast. Too much compression can inhibit intravascular contrast, thus decreasing lesion conspicuity. In a study by Hefler and colleagues,[28] repeat imaging was performed in 29 patients in whom MR biopsy had been canceled due to lack of enhancement. Although most of these (25/29) did not enhance on follow-up, 4 of 29 did persist and 3 of these (75%) proved to be malignant. For reasons like this, the grid should be placed firmly enough against the breast to restrict breast movement, but without being too firm to be uncomfortable for the patient or limit blood flow. If a previously noted lesion is not seen during biopsy, slight release of compression and repeat imaging should be performed before canceling the procedure. Re-injection of additional contrast if a period of time has elapsed could be considered if doing sequential breast biopsies. The efficacy of this technique, however, has not been proven in the literature. It is possible that malignant lesions could not be evident on reinjection, being obscured due to background enhancement.

T1 Imaging

After positioning the patient as comfortably as possible in the breast coil with the breast immobilized, nipple straight, and no skin folds present, T1-weighted fat-saturated sequences in the sagittal projection are generally performed. If isotropic imaging is available, software can permit ease of viewing information in multiple planes on the workstation. A precontrast sequence is recommended to check for good imaging parameters, such as fat saturation, as well as the appropriate field of view. Also, precontrast images will prove useful if subtraction images are required to detect subtle enhancing areas.

Targeting the Lesion

After the area of interest is identified, targeting the lesion simply depends on identifying the correct opening within the grid and deciding into which hole in the needle guide the probe will be inserted. Most MR procedures are approached from the lateral, or less commonly the medial direction. If a cranial approach is available, similar steps can be taken with imaging in the axial projection. If targeting is done manually on the console or workstation, scrolling through the images in the sagittal plane with a cursor placed over the lesion to the skin/grid will provide the depth information. The distance from the skin to lesion can be determined on the monitor as the difference of the slice numbers and the thickness of each slice. For example, if slice thickness is 3 mm and there are 10 images from skin to lesion, then the depth is 30 mm, or 3 cm.

For core biopsy, noting the X and Y coordinates (established as the designated hole in the needle guide) and the Z depth (determined as skin to lesion distance) is all that is necessary to initiate the biopsy. The extra depth to account for the thickness of the needle guide block (2 cm) is already added into the depth markings on the introducer sheath. In other words, the 0 position actually starts at 2 cm from the tip of the sheath, rather than the distal end.

Incision and Insertion for Vacuum-Assisted Core Biopsy

After local anesthetic is delivered both as a skin wheal and to deeper tissues along the projected needle track, a small slit in the skin is made with a scalpel. The trocar is then placed through the sheath and both are inserted together through the needle guide to the predetermined depth in the breast. Use of a slight rotation motion of the trocar facilitates penetration of the tissues with the least amount of displacement. Once inserted, the trocar is then withdrawn from the sheath and replaced with a plastic obturator for MR imaging. If using a ceramic probe (Mammotome; Ethicon Endosurgery, Cincinnati, OH, USA), which allows imaging of the actual sampling probe rather than an obturator, this will be inserted beyond the Z=0 position such that the lesion sits within the middle of the sampling trough. MR imaging is then performed to document accurate needle position in all directions. As vacuum-assisted biopsy is directional, small offsets of the lesion in the X and Y directions can be accommodated by preferential sampling in the desired direction. If the distal end of the obturator is not at the desired depth, it can be corrected by either withdrawing or advancing the sheath with the trocar reinserted.

Sampling

Sampling is quickly and easily performed with vacuum-assisted techniques. In general, circumferential sampling is performed although, as mentioned earlier, directional sampling can be performed if the lesion predominantly resides in a particular direction. Most vacuum-assisted devices used for MR are either 9- or 10-gauge. Six to 12 core samples generally are felt to be adequate for diagnostic purposes.

Repeat MR imaging is again performed to assess for completeness of sampling. Documenting adequate sampling on MR biopsy can be challenging. Visualization of small enhancing lesions can be very difficult because of the combination of local anesthetic, hemorrhage, saline, and air all present at the biopsy site (Fig. 3). If the

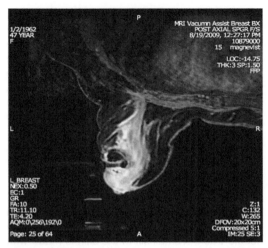

1/2/1962
47 YEAR
F

P

MRI Vacumn Assist Breast BX
POST AXIAL SPGR F/S
8/19/2009, 12:27:17 PM
10879000
15   magnevist

LOC:-14.75
THK:3 SP:1.50
FFP

L   R

L BREAST
NEX:0.50
EC:1
GR
FA:10
TR:11.10
TE:4.20
AQM:0\256\192\0
Page: 25 of 64   A

Z:1
C:132
W:265
DFOV:20x20cm
Compressed 5:1
IM:25 SE:3

Fig. 3. Postbiopsy axial T1-weighted fat-saturated image shows a large hematoma in the left breast. With air, anesthetic agent, saline, and blood occurring at the site during biopsy, determination of adequate lesion sampling can often be difficult.

enhancing lesion is felt to be inadequately sampled, the probe can be reinserted and additional samples can be obtained.

After sampling is complete, the biopsy cavity is irrigated (if using saline) and aspirated before probe removal. A biopsy marker is then deployed at the site. A final set of images is obtained to document accurate marker deployment. The metallic artifact generated by the marker clip can be difficult to differentiate from air and other biopsy site changes on fat-saturated images. Nonfat-saturated T1-weighted images may permit better visualization of the metallic clip, so this may be preferred as the last sequence.

MR-Guided Needle Localization Core Biopsy

MR-guided needle localizations are performed slightly differently than vacuum-assisted core biopsies. An MR-compatible 20-gauge hookneedle is used (Cook, Bloomington, IN, USA). This needle has centimeter markings on its length; however, unlike the sheath used for core biopsies, the thickness of the needle guide is not accounted for. Therefore, after determining lesion depth, as described above, an extra 2 cm has to be added to the depth. In addition, as with all needle localization performed with a Kopans needle, the lesion should ultimately reside within the thick portion of the wire and not the tip; therefore, an additional increment of 5 to 10 mm depth must also be added.

It is important to keep in mind that, unlike mammographically-guided wire localizations, the wire is deployed through the needle in the orthogonal projection to how it was inserted, the needle is inserted, and wire deployed all in one direction, with the breast in compression throughout. Therefore, depending on the compressibility of the breast and corresponding amount of accordion effect, the distance beyond the lesion to which the needle should be inserted varies. In general, in a fatty compressible breast the accordion effect is greater, therefore a distance of 5 mm may be adequate. In dense, less compressible tissues, a distance of 1 cm is reasonable. After documentation of accurate needle position and wire exchange, the compression of the breast may be released slightly before the last imaging series such that a better assessment of the final wire position can be made. Of course, when the patient is removed from the magnet and resumes the upright position, the wire may migrate from its position during imaging.

The wires used for MR-guided localizations are somewhat more fragile than their counterparts used in mammography or sonography, and breakage or fragmentation has been reported.[9] It is prudent to inform the surgeons of this fact, such that extra care may be taken in the operating room to avoid accidental breakage or fracture of the wire.

Software for MR-Guided Procedures

Software systems providing computer-aided detection for MR are available and commonly used in breast MR interpretation. These systems also provide targeting and tools for MR-guided procedures that greatly facilitate the biopsy process. These tools include visual guides as to precise needle insertion points and depth determination, and visual representation of the needle position in relation to the lesion (**Fig. 4**). Such programs even include warnings when there is not adequate breast thickness for appropriate needle position or trough placement. Even if such programs are routinely used, knowledge of the manual steps involved is advised to facilitate trouble-shooting or permit successful biopsy if the system is not functioning for any reason.

Superficial Lesions

Lesions that are very superficial or within the anterior breast near the nipple can be challenging for vacuum-assisted biopsy, as the entire trough must be placed within the breast to permit adequate vacuum suction and avoid sampling of

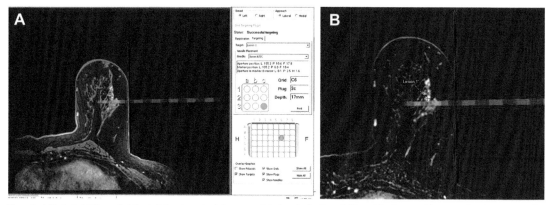

Fig. 4. (*A*) Axial T1-weighted fat-saturated image obtained during MR-guided core biopsy of a lesion in the lateral aspect of the left breast using interventional software (Aegis; Sentinelle, Toronto, Canada). Such programs aid in determination of lesion location and depth to facilitate accurate probe placement. (*B*) Close up image shows the projected position of the sampling trough (in *green*) in relation to the location of the lesion to be sampled. Pathology showed benign findings.

the skin. Techniques to accomplish such biopsies include use of the Petite Probe (Suros ATEC, Hologic, MA, USA) or techniques that permit partial closure of the sampling trough. The Petite Probe has a 12-mm sampling trough, rather than the usual 20 mm, and also has a blunt tip to prevent puncture of superficial tissues on the distal side of the breast when performing a biopsy on a thin breast. Partial trough sampling involves blocking the more superficial portion of the trough, such that the sampling area is within the breast tissue and the skin is not sucked into the trough when the vacuum is applied. Both result in smaller core samples but permit procedures to be completed that otherwise would not be possible.

For lesions that are so superficial that insertion of a wire may be impractical, a simple skin marker can be placed directly over the lesion before surgery. Rather than the metallic BB that is used mammographically or sonographically, an MR-compatible device such as a vitamin E capsule can be affixed to the skin overlying the lesion. Imaging with contrast is first performed, the area identified, and the capsule placed over the expected area. Repeat imaging can document proximity of the marker (**Fig. 5**). Adjustments in the placement of the marker can be made as necessary with repeat imaging. When accurate placement is achieved, a mark on the skin right under the capsule can be made with a surgical marking pen and the capsule taped to the skin. The pen mark is recommended in case the capsule is displaced before the patient arrives in the operating room. Such a technique may be necessary for very superficial lesions, or for those lying near implants where puncture of the implant is a concern.

HISTOLOGY CORRELATION

MR-guided biopsies, particularly core biopsies, differ from breast biopsies of other modalities in that there is less immediate confirmation that the lesion has been adequately sampled. Lesion conspicuity is dependent on enhancement in

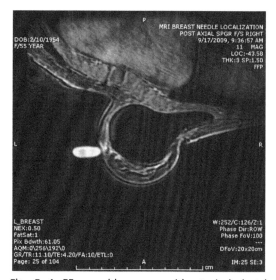

Fig. 5. A 55-year-old woman with atypical ductal hyperplasia in the left breast underwent bilateral MR imaging before surgery. Silicone implants were present. A 1-cm area of nonmass-like enhancement was noted in the lower inner quadrant of the contralateral right breast. Targeted US showed no abnormality. Given the small size of the breast, medial location, and proximity to the implant, localization of the area for surgical excision was achieved with a vitamin E capsule placed directly on the adjacent skin surface. Successful surgical excision revealed DCIS.

vivo. There is no method of imaging the core samples that confirm adequate sampling, such as is possible with specimen radiography of stereotactic core biopsy specimens. Furthermore, real-time visualization of the probe within the area of interest such as during US-guided biopsies is not possible with MR-guided procedures. Imaging of the obturator provides only indirect documentation of the area of the breast where sampling will occur. Tissue displacement may occur when the probe replaces the obturator and could result in sampling of adjacent tissues unbeknownst to the performing radiologist. With MR-guided wire localizations and surgical removal, there is also uncertainty in target removal. Although specimen radiography, including sliced specimen radiography, has been attempted by some, it is accepted that adequate documentation of lesion removal is not possible by imaging means.[29] Therefore, there is far less degree of confidence of accurate and adequate sampling of lesions in MR procedures than with those done with other modalities. For those reasons, careful assessment of histologic results and determination of concordance is of critical importance in MR-guided procedures.

If malignancy is diagnosed, surgical or therapeutic management can then be determined. Despite careful targeting and meticulous technique, upgrades of DCIS to invasive disease on MR-guided core biopsy will inevitably occur.[13,17,30–32] This rate has been reported to be 17% and, as with other imaging modalities, can be problematic if node sampling has to be performed as an additional surgical procedure.

Benign Diagnosis Considerations

More problematic is the management of cases of high-risk findings and some of the benign diagnoses. If the pathologic assessment yields benign histology, review of the original MR imaging and biopsy imaging is advised to reassess the level of suspicion and adequacy of sampling. Reports such as "benign adipose tissue" should be viewed with suspicion for the possibility of a missed lesion. Benign parenchymal tissue is a known false-positive cause of enhancement, and may be considered concordant depending on the initial imaging findings and degree of suspicion.

A study by Li and colleagues[33] showed that follow-up of 177 lesions considered benign and concordant at MR-guided core biopsy revealed 17 that required a repeat biopsy. Of these, 4 (24%) were found to be malignant; 2 were invasive disease, and 2 were DCIS. Only 2 lesions were rebiopsied because of interval growth or change on MR imaging at 6 and 12 months. The

remaining 2 were rebiopsied because of increasingly suspicious mammographic and sonographic findings and concern for a missed lesion during MR biopsy. The investigators concluded that repeat imaging earlier than 6 months is probably not justified. Studies like this underscore the need for accurate technique and follow-up of all MR biopsies along with correlation with other imaging studies.

For cases that are felt to be discordant or possibly missed, repeat biopsy or surgical excision is recommended as soon as can be reasonably tolerated by the patient. Although assessing concordance is important in all image-guided biopsies, it is particularly important for MR-guided biopsies as the confidence in targeting is never as great. Rebiopsy of cases considered discordant on MR biopsy has shown malignancy rates of 13% to 44%.[17,34–36]

Certain high-risk lesions are causes of false-positive findings on MR and include papilloma, lobular intraepithelial hyperplasia, radial scar, and atypical hyperplasia. Although the management of some of these high-risk lesions may be controversial, that of atypical ductal hyperplasia (ADH) is generally agreed to be surgical excision. Given the uncertainties in targeting and sampling during the procedure outlined above along with the lack of documentation of specimen adequacy, sampling error during MR biopsy is probably more common than with either stereotactic or US guidance. The pathologic differentiation of ADH from DCIS can be a quantifiable one. Atypical cellular changes measuring more than 2 mm or more than 2 ducts can be reported as DCIS whereas lesser amounts of disease may be called ADH. For this reason, adequate sampling can be crucial in making the correct diagnosis.

ADH has been reported in 3% to 9% of MR biopsies.[12,13,31,32,36–39] The upgrade rate of atypical ductal hyperplasia in MR core biopsies in these studies has been found to range from 25% to 100%, greater than that found in other biopsy modalities. This result is probably partly caused by the sampling error mentioned above in addition to the higher risk status of patients undergoing MR imaging and, possibly, the more extensive nature of disease often being targeted. Liberman and colleagues[39] found no factors that were able to predict which patients or lesions were more likely to be upgraded. Therefore, surgical excision of lesions containing atypical hyperplasias is strongly recommended.

The management of other high-risk causes of false positives such as papillomas, lobular intraepithelial hyperplasia, and radial scars is more controversial. Liberman and colleagues[12] found one upgrade to DCIS in a patient with papilloma diagnosed on 9-gauge vacuum-assisted MR biopsy that may have been an incidental finding. Mahoney[36] also found 1 upgrade out of 3 papillary lesions found on 10-gauge vacuum-assisted MR biopsy as well as 1 lobular carcinoma in situ upgraded to invasive ductal carcinoma. These high-risk histologic findings may account for the imaging findings or may be incidental. Excision of such high-risk lesions should probably be considered until there is more information in the published literature. In certain cases, if patients are not undergoing surgery for other concurrent disease and instead will be undergoing close imaging follow-up, surveillance may be adequate. More data on the management of such lesions found on MR biopsy is needed.

In summary, comfort with MR-guided biopsies is a necessity for the breast imager, as MR imaging of the breast is playing an ever-increasing role in management of patients. Correct use of MR-guided vacuum-assisted core needle biopsies and wire localizations, as well as comfort with the technical aspects, are essential. These techniques have marked similarities to other imaging-guided biopsies and can be easily mastered. Careful histologic correlation and follow-up of patients is particularly important in this population of patients.

REFERENCES

1. Lee SG, Orel SG, Woo IJ, et al. MR imaging screening of the contralateral breast in patients with newly diagnosed breast cancer: preliminary results. Radiology 2003;226:773–8.
2. Liberman L, Morris EA, Kim CM, et al. MR imaging findings in the contralateral breast of women with recently diagnosed breast cancer. AJR Am J Roentgenol 2003;180:333–41.
3. Tillman GF, Orel SG, Schnall MD, et al. Effect of breast magnetic resonance imaging on the clinical management of women with early-stage breast carcinoma. J Clin Oncol 2002;20:3413–23.
4. Bedrosian I, Mick R, Orel SG, et al. Changes in the surgical management of patients with breast carcinoma based on preoperative magnetic resonance imaging. Cancer 2003;98:468–73.
5. Lee JM, Orel SG, Czerniecki BJ, et al. MRI before reexcision surgery in patients with breast cancer. AJR Am J Roentgenol 2004;182:473–80.
6. Kuhl C. The current status of breast MR imaging. Part I. Choice of technique, image interpretation, diagnostic accuracy, and transfer to clinical practice. Radiology 2007;244:356.
7. Kuhl CK, Schmutzler RK, Leutner CC, et al. Breast MR imaging screening in 192 women proved or suspected to be carriers of a breast cancer susceptibility gene: preliminary results. Radiology 2000;215:267.
8. Lee CH, Smith RC, Levine JA, et al. Clinical usefulness of MR imaging of the breast in the evaluation of the problematic mammogram. AJR Am J Roentgenol 1999;173:1323.
9. Morris EA, Liberman L, Dershaw DD, et al. Preoperative MR imaging-guided needle localization of breast lesions. [see comment]. AJR Am J Roentgenol 2002;178:1211–20.
10. Liberman L, Morris EA, Lee MJ, et al. Breast lesions detected on MR imaging: features and positive predictive value. AJR Am J Roentgenol 2002;179:171–8.
11. Bedrosian I, Schlencker J, Spitz FR, et al. Magnetic resonance imaging-guided biopsy of mammographically and clinically occult breast lesions. Ann Surg Oncol 2002;9:457–61.
12. Liberman L, Bracero N, Morris E, et al. MRI-guided 9-gauge vacuum-assisted breast biopsy: Initial clinical experience. AJR Am J Roentgenol 2005;185:183–93.
13. Lehman CD, Deperi ER, Peacock S, et al. Clinical experience with MRI-guided vacuum-assisted breast biopsy. AJR Am J Roentgenol 2005;184:1782–7.
14. Ghate SV, Rosen EL, Soo MS, et al. MRI-guided vacuum-assisted breast biopsy with a handheld portable biopsy system. AJR Am J Roentgenol 2006;186:1733–6.
15. Perlet C, Schneider P, Amaya B, et al. MR-guided vacuum biopsy of 206 contrast-enhancing breast lesions. Fortschr Geb Rontgenstr Nuklearmed. Rofo 2002;174:88–95.
16. Perlet C, Heinig A, Prat X, et al. Multicenter study for the evaluation of a dedicated biopsy device for MR-guided vacuum biopsy of the breast. Eur Radiol 2002;12:1463–70.
17. Orel SG, Rosen M, Mies C, et al. MR imaging-guided 9-gauge vacuum-assisted core-needle breast biopsy: initial experience. Radiology 2006;238:54–61.
18. Mainiero MB, Philpotts LE, Lee CH, et al. Stereotaxic core needle biopsy of breast microcalcifications: correlation of target accuracy and diagnosis with lesion size. Radiology 1996;198:665–9.
19. Morris EA, Liberman L, Ballon DJ, et al. MRI of occult breast carcinoma in a high-risk population. AJR Am J Roentgenol 2003;181:619–26.
20. Weinstein SP, Orel SG, Heller R, et al. MR imaging of the breast in patients with invasive lobular carcinoma. AJR Am J Roentgenol 2001;176:399–406.
21. Morris E, Liberman L, Breast MRI. Diagnosis and intervention. New York: Springer; 2005. 280–6.
22. Kuhl CK. Science to practice: why do purely intraductal cancers enhance on breast MR images? Radiology 2009;253:281.

23. Kuhl CK. MRI for diagnosis of pure ductal carcinoma in situ: a prospective observational study. Lancet 2007;370:485.

24. Orel SG, Mendonca MH, Reynolds C, et al. MR imaging of ductal carcinoma in situ. Radiology 1997;202:413–20.

25. Liberman L, Morris EA, Dershaw DD, et al. Ductal enhancement on MR imaging of the breast. AJR Am J Roentgenol 2003;181:519–25.

26. Meissnitzer M, Dershaw DD, Lee C, et al. Targeted ultrasound of the breast in women with abnormal MRI findings for whom biopsy has been recommended. AJR Am J Roentgenol 2009;193:1025.

27. LaTrenta LR, Menell JH, Morris EA, et al. Breast lesions detected with MR imaging: Utility and histopathologic importance of identification with US. Radiology 2003;227:856–61.

28. Hefler L, Casselman J, Amaya B, et al. Follow-up of breast lesions detected by MRI not biopsied due to absent enhancement of contrast medium. Eur Radiol 2003;13:344.

29. Erguvan-Dogan B, Whitman GJ, Nguyen VA, et al. Specimen radiography in confirmation of MRI-guided needle localization and surgical excision of breast lesions. AJR Am J Roentgenol 2006;187:339–44.

30. Lee J, Kaplan J, Murray M, et al. Underestimation of DCIS at MRI-guided vacuum-assisted breast biopsy. AJR Am J Roentgenol 2007;189:468.

31. Perretta T, Pistolese CA, Bolacchi F, et al. MR imaging-guided 10-gauge vacuum-assisted breast biopsy: histological characterisation [serial online]. Radiol Med 2008;113:830.

32. Liberman L, Morris E, Dershaw DD, et al. Fast MRI-guided vacuum-assisted breast biopsy: Initial experience. AJR Am J Roentgenol 2003;181:1283.

33. Li J, Dershaw DD, Lee C, et al. MRI follow-up after concordant, histologically benign diagnosis of breast lesions sampled by MRI-guided biopsy. AJR Am J Roentgenol 2009;193:850.

34. Han B, Schnall MD, Orel SG, et al. Outcome of MRI-guided breast biopsy. AJR Am J Roentgenol 2008;191:1798–804.

35. Lee J, Kaplan J, Murray M, et al. Imaging histologic discordance at MRI-guided 9-gauge vacuum-assisted breast biopsy. AJR Am J Roentgenol 2007;189:852.

36. Mahoney MC. Initial clinical experience with a new MRI vacuum-assisted breast biopsy device [serial online]. J Magn Reson Imaging 2008;28:900.

37. Liberman L, Cohen MA, Dershaw DD, et al. Atypical ductal hyperplasia diagnosed at stereotaxic core biopsy of breast lesions: an indication for surgical biopsy. AJR Am J Roentgenol 1995;164:1111–3.

38. Perlet C, Heywang-Kobrunner S, Heinig A, et al. Magnetic resonance-guided, vacuum-assisted breast biopsy: results from a European multicenter study of 538 lesions. Cancer 2006;106:982.

39. Liberman L, Holland AE, Marian D, et al. Underestimation of atypical ductal hyperplasia at MRI-guided 9-gauge vacuum-assisted breast. AJR Am J Roentgenol 2007;188:684–90.

Index

Note: Page numbers of article titles are in **boldface** type.

doi:10.1016/S1064-9689(10)00024-3
1064-9689/10/$ – see front matter © 2010 Elsevier Inc. All rights reserved.

mri.theclinics.com

Moving?

Make sure your subscription moves with you!

To notify us of your new address, find your **Clinics Account Number** (located on your mailing label above your name), and contact customer service at:

Email: journalscustomerservice-usa@elsevier.com

800-654-2452 (subscribers in the U.S. & Canada)
314-447-8871 (subscribers outside of the U.S. & Canada)

Fax number: 314-447-8029

Elsevier Health Sciences Division
Subscription Customer Service
3251 Riverport Lane
Maryland Heights, MO 63043

*To ensure uninterrupted delivery of your subscription, please notify us at least 4 weeks in advance of move.

Printed and bound by CPI Group (UK) Ltd, Croydon, CR0 4YY

03/10/2024

01040361-0018